For Eileen

Paddy Doyle was born in Wexford in 1951. In 1974 he married and now lives in Dublin with his wife Eileen and their three children, Shane, Niall and Ronan. In 1983 he received the first Christy Brown Memorial Prize for literature. Shortly afterwards he resigned from his job in CIE and today conducts seminars and awareness projects for medical students in Trinity College, Dublin. He is cur-

THE GOD SQUAD

Paddy Doyle

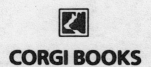

CORGI BOOKS

THE GOD SQUAD
A CORGI BOOK : 0 552 13582 8

Originally published in Ireland by The Raven Arts Press

PRINTING HISTORY
Raven Arts Press edition published 1988
Corgi edition published 1989
Corgi edition reprinted 1989
Corgi edition reprinted 1990
Corgi edition reprinted 1991
Corgi edition reprinted 1993
Corgi edition reprinted 1994
Corgi edition reprinted 1995

This book is set in 10/11 pt Mallard by Busby Typesetting, Exeter.

Corgi Books are published by Transworld Publishers Ltd,
61– 63 Uxbridge Road, London W5 5SA,
in Australia by Transworld Publishers (Australia) Pty Ltd,
15– 25 Helles Avenue, Moorebank, NSW 2170,
and in New Zealand by Transworld Publishers (NZ) Ltd,
3 William Pickering Drive, Albany, Auckland.

Printed and bound in Great Britain by
Cox & Wyman Ltd, Reading, Berkshire

PROLOGUE

For years I had believed my uncle to be dead. Attempts at correspondence, spanning over twenty years and including an invitation to my wedding in 1974, had failed to bring any response. So that Sunday in 1983 as I drove with my family from Dublin my feelings were of trepidation. The phone call telling me he was still alive and in hospital in Wexford had come about because of the media exposure surrounding my being awarded the first Christy Brown Award for Literature.

How was he going to react to me – or I to him? I was aware of going to see a man who was ill, but even more aware that he was the sole living relative I had – apart from my younger sister. He surely would give me the information I needed about my parents and my past.

On arrival at the hospital, crowds were lining the grounds for the removal of the remains of a local dignitary of the church. I left my wife and children in the car and moved through them, overhearing their comments about my appearance on The Late Late Show the previous night.

I was nervous and waited outside the ward before asking a senior nurse to tell him I had arrived, explaining to her who I was and the number of years that had elapsed since he and I had last met.

As soon as I entered the ward we recognized each other and he began to cry. He was in some pain following the removal of his appendix and obviously distressed at seeing me. After awkwardly discussing his health, I asked him about my parents. At first he ignored my questions about them and would only reply repeatedly 'You'll be alright when I'm gone'. Finally I forced him to tell me that my mother had died of 'the disease' but he just wept when asked about my father,

7

avoiding the question in every way he could. Eventually he revealed where my mother was buried but still consistently refused to say anything about my father. When I asked about photographs he said there were none.

Back in Dublin the suspicion of a conspiracy of silence which I had long held was reinforced and I was convinced that whatever happened to my parents had been deliberately concealed from me by the silence of a whole society and time. I knew so little that I even began to wonder if the man I called 'uncle' could in fact be my father. I discussed what had happened with a doctor friend and we decided that there had to be a way of getting to the truth. I was a man with no past. There must be someone who knew why I was sent to an Industrial School and somebody who could explain the origins or cause of my disability. Previous attempts at such ventures had failed. What past I did have amounted to a birth and baptismal certificate. Enquiries about medical records had yielded no results. I had no reason to believe that things would be any different this time.

Yet gradually the truth began to filter through as the thirty year conspiracy of silence slowly cracked. Unexpectedly I learned of the deaths of both parents in a letter from someone who did know of my past. Though the information was scant it was filling great gaps. I began to delve further and with the help and support of my wife, I intensified my search.

I discovered that on the morning of August 15th, 1955, I was taken to the District Court in County Wexford, where I was found to be in possession of a guardian who did not exercise proper guardianship. Two days after my appearance an Order of Detention in a Certified Industrial School was drawn up and brought to the house I was staying in by a Garda for legal execution. The form was signed by the Justice of the Court. I was four years and three months old at the time.

In early June of that year my mother had died from cancer of the breast and six weeks later my father committed suicide by hanging himself from an alder tree at the back of a barn on a farm where he worked as a labourer. I was taken into court by a woman who was later described as 'a sort of an aunt'.

Earlier at the inquest into my father's death, my mother's brother who had lived with us had given a statement which I have in my possession. Part of it reads:

'I left the house at 8.15 a.m. this morning 15/7/1955. When I was leaving Patrick Doyle was in bed. On my return to the house this evening at 9.15 p.m. Patrick Doyle was not in the house. I looked around the back of the house and later went to the haggard where I found him with a rope around his neck hanging from an alder tree on the fence. I felt one of his hands and it was cold. His feet were about two feet off the ground.

I didn't cut down the body. I sent word to the village with a little girl that was passing for someone to come down to me. Someone arrived in about 15 minutes. A priest from the nearby parish cut down the body. Since the deceased man's wife died about six weeks ago he has been worrying about her ever since. He was a labourer by occupation and about 52 years of age.'

A doctor had told the inquest that he had been called to the farm by the Gardai and after an examination had estimated that the time of death had been some twelve hours earlier. It appears that I witnessed the suicide and may have been found wandering on the farm in great distress.

It had taken me thirty years to discover the truth about the deaths of both my parents even though a death such as my father's was likely to have made the local, if not the national newspapers, of the time. With that in mind I searched through old copies of *The Wexford People* in the National Library. There in the July 1955 edition I read the details of my father's suicide, and the other events surrounding it. While searching through these papers I tried to find a death notice for my mother, but did not succeed. Reading a journalist's report of the event made me realize that this was not a secret, unheard of event, but a public domain issue.

I began to pressurise my uncle for photographs, certain there must be some and that he could tell me where to look. A letter arrived at my home, containing a short note and two photographs: one of myself with a group of children on my First Communion day, the other of two women and a child in a buggy. The child was me, and the woman standing behind was my mother. Until then I had no idea what my mother looked like. Though she had obviously been a part of my early life, I had no memory of her. At 35 years of age I was seeing my mother for the first time. I didn't cry, nor was I jolted in any way. Despite my best efforts I have as yet been unable to get a photograph of my father. I still have no idea of what he looked like, my only memories of him are those that haunted me as a child. A faceless man hanging dead. A fierce determination set in to get any information I could, which eventually resulted in my obtaining the original Order of Detention, rust marks from a paper clip etched on it, statements of witnesses given at the coroner's court and other papers pertaining to his death.

There were many times during the course of writing this book, that I questioned what I was doing, often frightened by the chill running through my body as I wrote. The support I received from people, particularly Eileen, my wife, was limitless. The impact of having to absorb one shock after another was at times very painful for her and she cried enough for both of us.

Many people familiar with the effects of institutional care, particularly Industrial Schools, will say that I have gone too easy on them. Lives have been ruined by the tyrannical rule and lack of love in such places. People have been scarred for life. Others will wonder why I bothered to delve into the past at all.

This book spans just six years of my life. There was almost consistent trauma, ranging from the death of both my parents, to the isolation of hospital wards and brain surgery. Such surgery was not just traumatic, but debilitating also. One procedure could not be completed because of the breakdown of the apparatus, prompting me to wonder why it was not attempted again when the apparatus was repaired.

It is important to point out that interspersed with this trauma were moments of great love and affection. From the gentle kiss of a young nurse to the soft hand of a caring nun. It may well be the case that these were the moments which preserved my sanity and gave me something to live for.

This book is not an attempt to point the finger, to blame, or even to criticise any individual or group of people. Neither is it intended to make a judgement on what happened to me. It is about a society's abdication of responsibility to a child. The fact that I was that child, and that the book is about my life is largely irrelevant. The probability is that there were, and still are, thousands of 'mes'.

Paddy Doyle,
Dublin,
Sept. 1988.

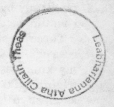

CHAPTER ONE

I lay flat on my back on the narrow cast iron bed in the dormitory of St Michael's Industrial School in Cappoquin. The thin horse-hair mattress was barely adequate to separate my thin body from its taut criss-cross wire springs. My eyes were fixed on the ceiling, the paint flaking just above the bed. From a room below the sound of children singing seeped through the floor-boards.

In the distance a train hooted, heralding its imminent arrival at the station just beyond the high granite walls of the school. I turned towards the tall sashed window a few feet from my bed. Through watery eyes I noticed the sun was shining, though the dormitory was cold and dark. The train hooted again, louder as it drew nearer the station, panting and hissing through the stillness of the day.

It had been three weeks since my uncle had driven me here in the black Morris Minor owned by his employer. In his pocket he carried the order of detention from the District Court in Wexford sentencing me to seven years in custody. The charge against me was of being found having a guardian who did not exercise proper guardianship. I was then four years and three months old. I remember being terrified of the nuns from the moment I entered the Industrial School and clinging to my uncle, pleading with him to take me home. A tall, thin evil looking nun had come towards me and forced my hand away from his before gripping my jumper at the neck to ensure that I could not grab hold of him again. I'd screamed and kicked in an attempt to free myself, but the more I struggled, the tighter her hold became. She told my uncle that I would settle down just as soon as he left. I can remember trying to get free of her and follow my uncle. But the nun held me firmly by the ear lobe and warned me to stop, otherwise I would receive a 'good flaking'.

Three weeks had taught me the meaning of that phrase. I rose cautiously from my bed, rubbed my eyes and cheeks with my knuckles and went towards the window. I stood back, frightened that I might be seen from the yard below. I moved as close to it as I felt it was safe to do.

The granite wall glistened in the sunlight like a million jewels. I pressed my face against the window and watched the approaching train. The sun shone onto its black rounded front like a spotlight. The shiny, black funnel belched out a mixture of smoke and steam that hung above the tender in a large plume of grey and white, and when the colours merged to black and soared into the sky the cloud cast a dark shadow across the grey concrete of the school yard. Behind the glossy tender, the wagons laden with sugar beet rattled along, zig-zagging awkwardly in contrast to the graceful, steady movement of the engine. A screeching of the wheels on the tracks and a loud prolonged hissing brought the engine to a halt. I noticed the sparks made by the wheels as they skidded along, igniting in the dark shadow of the underframe. A final banging of the wagons as each one buffetted into the one ahead of it, then silence. Total silence. Two men in blackened boiler suits jumped cautiously from the tender and stood briefly in the hot sunshine as both rubbed their foreheads with a sleeve. Before leaving the train each in turn slapped the great tender on its belly as a farmer would a cow, or a jockey a horse, a sign of affection, the beast had done her job well.

I counted the wagons as the tender took water from the great red-oxide tank overhead. There were fifteen, and a guard's van at the rear. Each one filled with sugar beet, mud baked by the combination of hot sun and drying breeze. The stillness of the moment was broken by a sudden rush of feet into the yard below the dormitory window. I backed away from the window though I still looked out as the other children ran about the yard screaming their excitement. Some of them tried to climb the wall to get a better view but their efforts were brought to an abrupt halt by the swish of a cane from one of the nuns patrolling the yard like a black shadow. One boy who

14

was midway up the wall fell to the ground writhing in pain having felt the full force of Mother Paul's cane across his calf muscles. He lay curled up, on the ground screaming and gripping his leg tightly. The other boys stood still, frozen in terror.

I watched. I knew the pain of the bamboo and the horror of being beaten until it was no longer possible to stand it. As blow after blow landed, I trembled, fully convinced that I would receive similar punishment when Mother Paul came to the dormitory. I went back to bed and pulled the covers over my head in an attempt to escape the piercing, painful screams. Finally the screaming stopped. I lay waiting for the footsteps.

'Well Master Doyle . . . are you finished now or would you prefer to spend more time here on your own?'

Startled by the sound of Mother Paul's voice, I turned down the bedcovers. Her tall black clad figure stood beside my bed, her wrinkled hand carrying the cane that she kept partially hidden up the long loose sleeve of her habit. She stared coldly down at me, her icy-blue eyes seeming magnified through the thick lenses of her rimless spectacles. Her long pointed nose threatened to drip its watery contents onto my bed but was halted by the swift use of her check-coloured handkerchief. Her wicked-looking face was gripped tightly in the habit of the Sisters of Mercy. The black habit was pulled tight at the waist by a leather belt.

'Get up out of that bed then this instant,' she roared, 'and I don't want to hear another word from you about a man hanging from a tree. It's not good for the other children and, besides, people don't do that sort of thing.'

'But there was . . .'

The nun's mouth tensed visibly. 'That is enough, I warn you. Get dressed and get down to the assembly hall immediately.'

'Yes Mother,' I said.

She left as I started to dress. Once I had my boots laced up I walked slowly through the dormitory stopping as I reached the door that led to the room where Mother Paul and Mother Michael slept. Gripped by curiosity my eyes fixed on the large oak door with a big iron key protruding from its lock. On the tips of my boots I approached, gripped the key and turned it, trying to ensure it would make no sound. It clicked, the noise sounding much louder than it really was in the emptiness of the large room. I cupped the knob in my hands and turned it slowly before gently pushing the door open. I walked into the carpeted room, its whiteness glaring when compared to the drabness of the dormitory. Walls and ceiling were painted in a gloss white and the only thing hanging on the wall was a large wooden crucifix. On a press beside the white quilted beds was a statue of the Virgin Mary, a golden rosary beads entwined in her hands. I looked at the statue. Its pale blue eyes appeared to be watching my every move. I moved uneasily back out of the room closing the door gently before locking it and walking down the wooden stairs to the assembly hall.

The hall was a big room with bare floorboards and large sashed windows that rattled whenever there was even the slightest breeze.The walls were wood-panelled and painted black to about three feet above floor level. The remainder was painted dark grey. The only furniture was two chairs which were used by the nun who was in charge of the children or by another nun who played the piano, thumping out chords and shouting at us to sing. In a sudden movement she would stop playing and jump to her feet usually knocking her chair over as she did. Her finger wagged and in a voice that rose in pitch with each word she would say, 'There is a crow in amongst you and when I find out who it is he is going to have sore ears.'

'What kept you?' Mother Paul snapped. I hesitated before answering, 'I couldn't get my boots tied, there was a knot in the laces Mother.'

'I sincerely hope that is the truth,' she leered.

'Yes Mother.'

'Get over here and learn this song before Miss Sharpe comes back from her holidays, she will expect you all to know it.'

As I approached the piano she suddenly slapped me in the face.

'Where were you?'

I looked at her, surprised by the question and the sharpness in her voice.

'I asked you a question and when I ask someone a question I expect to get an answer. Is that clear?'

'Yes Mother.'

'Now tell everyone where you were and why you were late.'

'I was in the dormitory.'

She slapped me viciously across the face again. Then at the top of her voice Mother Paul shouted 'I was in the dormitory . . . What?'

'Mother,' I responded, my voice trembling. 'I was in the dormitory Mother.'

'Louder' she demanded.

'I was in the dormitory Mother, then.'

'Why? Tell everyone why you were sent to the dormitory,' she demanded.

'For making up stories Mother,' I said.

She hit me again.

'For telling lies, that's why. Is that the reason?'

'Yes Mother.'

'What were the lies you were telling? I want everyone to hear.'

I could barely speak, my voice shook and tears welled in my eyes. My bottom lip quivered and I began to cry.

'Speak up child' she demanded.

'I said I saw a man hanging from a tree.'

I stood there shaking.

'This little pup is a liar,' Mother Paul said to the other frightened children as she held me by my ear. 'And everyone here knows what happens to people who tell lies.' There was silence.

'What happens to children who tells lies?' she asked.

'They go to hell,' they all answered. The nun smiled.

'Not only that,' she continued, 'but they burn in its flames for ever and ever. That is what is going to happen to this little liar. He is going to burn forever in hell if he doesn't stop. Always remember to tell the truth.'

She pulled me over to the piano and struck the chords of

a song I knew well, one which the nuns began to teach me shortly after I entered the school.

'Stop whinging immediately and sing,' Mother Paul ordered.

As I did my voice trembled. I stood straight, with my hands crossed in front of me as I had been taught to do whenever I was asked to sing for visitors. My voice was a pleasant boy-soprano type which the nuns appeared to take great pleasure demonstrating for visitors to the school.

> 'A Mother's Love is a blessing,
> No matter where you roam,
> Keep her while she's living
> You'll miss her when she's gone,
> Love her as in childhood,
> Though feeble old and grey,
> For you'll never miss a Mother's Love
> till she's buried beneath the clay.'

Mother Paul waved her hand and the rest of the children joined in the remaining verses.

When we had finished singing Mother Paul reminded us that as we had no parents it fell to the nuns to give us the guidance and grace that would make us into fine young men. Nuns were married to God she said as she raised her right hand to show a thin silver ring. Nuns did not have children in the way mothers had. 'Each of you was sent to St Michael's by God and you will be trained in the manner He would like. Mark my words, you will all one day be proud to have been a part of this school.'

Two years after being admitted to St Michael's I had become familiar with its routine. The official report on me for that year says; 'A bright little lad. Made his first Holy Communion when barely over 6 years.' For the year 1958 the same report remarks; 'A very bright little boy, quiet and intelligent. Able to serve Mass in the Parish Church. Promoted in school.' I found it easier to mix with the other children as each day passed and I joined in whatever games I could.

One day, as I heard the beet train pulling into the station I climbed the wall to get a better look at it and to see if I could get either the driver or the fireman to throw some sugar beet over. I shouted, and a lump of beet sailed over the wall landing in the school yard. There was a rush to get it but I decided that as I was the one who had asked for it I should have it, and furthermore I would decide who I was going to share it with. Because the mud was so dry it was easy to remove from the beet. My efforts at breaking it up for distribution among my friends proved more difficult than I had expected. I put it on the ground and banged the heel of my boot down hard on it hoping it would break but it didn't. A jagged edge of the wall proved more useful. Soon lumps of beet were being scattered around the ground. Hungry grasping hands picked up the pieces and if they were small enough they were stuffed into waiting mouths. Those who did get some of it moved to a secluded part of the yard to suck and chew large bits of the creamy-coloured beet.

The group of which I was a part broke up. Mother Paul was coming towards me. The sun cast her long shadow on the ground as I dropped the beet I was eating. In one hand she had her cane and under the other arm she was carrying the school dog, a Jack Russell, called Toby. The dog barked and I froze, pressing my back hard against the wall. The dog barked again. I was terrified. I hated dogs. I wanted to run but I couldn't move. The long cane of Mother Paul pressed into my shoulder pinning me where I stood.

'Will you look at him,' she leered as the other children gathered around.

'This pup who is so brave when it comes to stealing from the train is afraid of his life of a tiny dog.'

She pointed to the dog, and as I attempted to run he growled. Mother Paul jeered. She told me that just as I had been created by God so had the dog, then she stroked his head gently and moved closer to me. I screamed with fright, causing the dog to growl and almost leap from her arms.

'Nice Toby,' Mother Paul said. 'Do you like this dog?' she asked.

'No Mother.'

She hit me across the legs with her cane and I shrieked

with pain. She hit me again. And seeing my fear she grinned. There was an evil look on her face.

'Say you like little Toby,' she ordered.

I paused for a minute, my fear gradually turning to rage. Mother Paul looked at me through slit eyes and purple thin lips. She hit out again. I ran towards her and kicked her as hard as I could across the shin. The crack of my boot echoed around the now silent yard. She grimaced and dropped the dog. It ran for cover as I ran across the yard. Before I could make my way into the assembly hall I was grabbed and held by another nun until Mother Paul arrived limping and red-faced. She held me by the ear and, as I tried to kick her again and again, she twisted it until I was almost motionless. She lashed out at me with her cane hitting me across the back of the knees. I fell to the ground, screaming and writhing in agony.

'Get up off that ground you filthy, dirty little pup,' she yelled. 'You will get what any little brat would get for kicking a holy nun. Mark my words, you will be sorry.' She ordered the rest of the children inside, shouting at them that the punishment I was going to get would ensure that none of them would do what I had done; kick a woman chosen by God to do his work.

In the assembly hall she looked around for somewhere to vent her anger. She ordered a group of children to bring her a table which was in one corner of the room. When it was placed to her satisfaction she addressed the rest of the boys while holding me firmly by my ear.

'This child,' she poked her cane into my ribs before continuing, 'is possessed by an evil demon.' She paused to allow the magnitude of what she had said to sink deep into the minds of the other children.

'He has the devil inside him and it is my duty to him and to God in Heaven to get it out. He must be punished and severely so. He must ask God for forgiveness for the terrible sin he has committed.' She ordered me to strip. I stood motionless. Mother Paul slammed her cane onto the table in front of her.

'Strip child,' she shouted.

20

I began to take off my clothes. First my heavy grey jumper, then the grey shirt.

'Come on, come on, I haven't all day. Get those trousers, boots and socks off immediately.'

I stood there shivering, a combination of cold and fear. My ribs protruded through my skin as though I was under-nourished. My skin was white except for red patches where I had been hit or jabbed by the cane.

'Get onto that table,' she demanded.

I lay on it naked, allowing my arms to hang over its side until I was told to bring them onto the table and down either side of my body. She gazed at me, a perverse grin on her face.

'Roll over on to your face and let this be a lesson to you.'

Her long cane whistled through the air and in the moment before it made contact every muscle in my body tensed and I became rigid. I squirmed and the first vicious blow stung, but I did not cry out.

'Never, never, as long as you live must you assault a holy nun in that manner.'

A second, third and fourth painful lash of the bamboo, and I could feel my skin burning. For some reason I cannot understand I refused to cry out. The number of times I was struck increased until it was impossible to count, just as it was difficult to separate one blow from the next. I remained silent, until the pain became unbearable and I finally screamed. I was being struck everywhere from the back of my neck down to my heels.

'Now,' she said, 'the devil is coming out of him.' The ferocity and frequency of the blows lessened until eventually I rolled off the table and onto the floor. Mother Paul looked pleased.

'That is how to get the devil out of someone like him. Only Satan himself would make a child behave the way he did. It will be a long time before he'll kick a nun again. Stand up and get your clothes on immediately,' she yelled before warning the other boys that they would receive the same treatment if they didn't keep quiet. I dressed in the silence, the coarse bulls wool trousers hurting my legs as I pulled them on. When I was clothed she pulled me to her by my ear and told the other children that I was being put into the coal shed for the

21

remainder of the day. She led me away, holding my ear tightly between her thumb and forefinger.

She fumbled through the pockets of her black habit for a key to fit the padlocked door. Impatiently, she undid the lock and threw the door open.

'Get in and stay there. Pray. Say an Act of Contrition so that God may forgive you.'

She slammed the door. In the darkness I could hear the bolt being slid across and the lock applied. I stood and listened to her footsteps fading.

In any other circumstances I would have been terrified of the darkness. Now it came as a blessing, a place of refuge from the terror of my persecutor. I sat on the dusty blackened floor and wept. The pain of the punishment was unbearable. My flesh stung, and though I could not see, I was certain my skin had blistered. I hated that nun, and I said it. I wished her damned in hell to burn forever.

The only light that entered the coal shed was from under the door and through a cracked slate in the roof. I moved under this slit of light and stared at it, straining my eyes, until they became tired. Within minutes I was in a deep sleep. The darkness, the cold or the dampness didn't matter to me. Peace mattered.

A noise woke me. The rattle of keys mingled with the distinct sound of the long Rosary Beads worn by the nuns. The light through the roof had gone grey and I guessed that it was evening. The chill evening air crept under the door making me feel cold. The bolt slapped back and the door was flung open. What little light there was hurt my eyes and I had difficulty in focusing on the black clad figure standing with arms outstretched, framed by the rotting wood of the doorway. Her voice was sharp and icy as she ordered me to get out of the shed and go straight to the dormitory without supper. I moved as quickly as I could across the yard, through the assembly hall and up the stairs.

It was quiet, all the other boys were in their beds and the lights had been turned off. Heavy black roller blinds covered the windows ensuring that no light penetrated the vast room containing sixty beds. Twelve in each row, head to foot. A big statue of the Sacred Heart stood imposingly in one corner, the red light at his feet casting an eerie shadow onto the ceiling. I began to undress. I removed my heavy black boots and placed them carefully beneath the bed, taking care not to bang them off the chamber pot. I folded the rest of my clothes and left them at the foot of my bed.

Because of the soreness of my body and hunger, I had great difficulty in getting to sleep, constantly moving in an attempt to find a comfortable position. Just as I was about to fall asleep I heard Mother Paul's voice beside my bed asking if I had said my night prayers. When I replied that I had not, she immediately ordered me out of bed to kneel on the bare floor with my hands joined. I was not allowed to lean against the bed for support. My flimsy, striped night-shirt was a poor barrier against the cold. I said the prayer I had been taught since the day I arrived in St Michael's;

> 'Now I lay me down to sleep,
> I pray the Lord, my soul to keep,
> If I should die before I wake,
> I pray the Lord, my soul to take.
> God bless the nuns who are so good to me.'

I blessed myself and got back into bed.

It was the practice each night in St Michael's Industrial School for a nun to walk around the dormitory at eleven o'clock, ringing a large brass bell. The purpose was to awaken the boys and get them out of bed to sit on white enamelled chamber pots. We hunched on the floorboards urging our bladders or bowels to act so that we could return to bed. Many children used to fall asleep, others neglected to position their penises properly, and urinated over the rim, sending a stream of water along the floor. I liked to create a well between my legs by pressing my thighs tightly together thus allowing the urine to gather. It was a warm pleasurable feeling. Any child who wet the floor or whose nightshirt became damp received a clatter on the face from the patrolling nun as she checked those of us who had finished and held our pots for her to examine the contents. Often boys cried, as they pushed and strained to 'do' something.

One night the boy in the bed next to mine screamed, and each time he did he was slapped on the bare backside by one of the two nuns attending to him. I turned my head slowly. A ball of blood hung from his anus like a half-inflated scarlet balloon. He screamed as the nuns took it in turn to attempt to push it back up inside his body. Once he had been taken care of he was told he would be punished for what he had done. It was 'only a prolapsed bowel,' Mother Paul said, as she returned to her own room. I was so terrified by the experience that the unfamiliar words stuck in my mind.

CHAPTER TWO

The children in St Michael's were divided into two groups, those between six and ten and children under six years of age. I was just over six and so I was regarded as one of the 'big boys'. As such, I was given charge of a younger child. My 'charge' was a small curly-headed blonde boy I knew only as Eugene. The day he was put into my 'care' Mother Paul told me that I must take good care of him, see that he went to the toilet when he wanted to and ensure that he was kept clean, especially before and after meals. Eugene latched onto me and annoyed me by following me constantly but if I said anything to him he would start crying. I did everything I could to stop him and he was cute enough to know that I wouldn't want any of the nuns to hear him cry. One day while we were all out in the yard I left Eugene alone to play with a group of boys of my own age. I liked to play priests and altar boys and I treated the game as though it were an actual religious ceremony. I always regarded it as good training for the day I would become a priest. Halfway through the game Eugene's voice rang in my ears. So did Mother Paul's. I ran to where the child stood. A circle of children had gathered around him. I broke through and saw Eugene standing in a mound of his own excrement and urine. Tears ran in torrents from his pale blue eyes. He was dirty from the tops of his legs to the heels of his boots. Mother Paul screamed at me to clean him up, but before doing that I was to clean the yard. I stood looking at the child, my hand tightly pressed across my mouth to prevent myself from vomiting. My stomach heaving, I ran off to get a bucket of sawdust and a shovel. When I returned Eugene was still standing like a statue, yelling. I dug the shovel into the galvanised bucket of sawdust and scattered it at his feet. Then holding my breath, I told him to move, and when he was out of the way I scooped up the excrement and dumped it into the bucket. Then I took the child by the hand and brought him to the toilet. I had to take off his boots and socks, his jumper and shirt and finally his trousers. As he stood naked with much of his body covered in his own excrement, I vomited onto the cement floor. He became hysterical and to stop him being overheard I slapped my hand across his mouth and begged him not to scream. I cleaned him with some old papers that had been left in the toilet for that purpose. I held my nose with the fingers of one hand and rubbed off as much excrement as I could with the dry newspaper.

'Why are you holding your nose?' Eugene asked me.

'Because I don't like the smell,' I answered, gripping my nose tightly with the thumb and forefinger of my right hand.

'Why?' he asked.

'Because it stinks, that's why.'

He laughed at the emphasis on the word 'stinks'.

I went to the tap that hung from the wall to get some water to clean him. I turned its brass handle, and as I did it swayed on its length of lead piping.

I soaked an old newspaper in the freezing water and rubbed the child's body with it. His pale skin erupted in goose-pimples and his teeth chattered uncontrollably. He cried from the cold but there was nothing I could do. When I was finished, I warned him not to tell anyone that I had been sick. He said he wouldn't, but just to stress the point as best I could, I told him that if he opened his mouth I would kill him. Once he had committed himself not to tell anyone, I further warned him that if he told now, he would be lying and that lies would ensure instant death. Then when he was dead he would go to hell. He looked straight into my eyes and then asked me if the devil really had horns.

'He has,' I said positively, 'and he might come and stick them in you if you tell anyone that I was sick.' By the look on Eugene's face as I spoke, I knew he would not say a word about what happened in the toilet. He watched me as I swirled his dirty clothes around in a bucket of cold water to rinse them. When they were clean I threw the dirty water down the drain, wrung out the clothes and shook them to remove the wrinkles. As soon as he was dressed in clean clothes he ran out of the toilet, content.

The toilets in St Michael's were stark and cold. The rough cement floor matched the even rougher cement walls. Ventilation was by means of an eighteen inch diameter hole in the wall with thick circular iron bars across it. We urinated against a cement wall which was flushed down every now and then via a piece of pipe with holes at intervals of about an inch. Sometimes I was given the task of washing down these stinking toilets. I had to use a hand held deck-scrub and a bucket of water into which some Jeyes Fluid had been added. The waste closet was a large wooden bench with three holes cut out of it.

We sat, three at a time, with maybe another six waiting to take our places when we were finished. No partition separated one boy from the next. When one finished he shouted to the rest to 'have a look and see if you can see it floating down'. Whoever was sitting on the last hole was shouted off it so that we could all watch as the brown lumps of waste floated away. If two lumps happened to be racing towards the outlet at the same time it was certain there would be an argument as to who won. There were arguments about winners; 'He couldn't have done anything. Look, his face isn't even red and he didn't grunt either. Everyone grunts when they're going to the toilet.'

I walked back to the assembly hall with Eugene by the hand. Mother Michael had relieved Mother Paul and she had gathered the children around the gramaphone. A record turned on its deck and the voice of John McCormack filled the hall. 'Machusla, Machusla, your sweet voice is calling, calling me softly . . .'

'Where were you?' Mother Michael demanded to know. 'I was in the toilet . . . cleaning my charge,' I answered.

'I hope he is properly cleaned and that his clothes are washed?' She took Eugene from me and sent him to the front of the group of children with the instruction that he listen to the music, then she told me to take a message across to the convent.

'Give it to Mother Ita,' she said, handing me a small parcel, 'and come straight back. Her bell is three rings,' she said, before remarking that I should know it anyway. I did know. Groups of us often played games guessing what different nuns 'bells' were. Before leaving the assembly hall I had to remove my heavy black boots and put on a pair of white-soled canvas shoes.

Even though it was a part of the same building, the area of St Michael's where the nuns resided was totally different to that where we lived. The corridor leading to the convent smelled of wax from the polished floor and from the candles that burned in their holders at the feet of the statues that stood stoically against the dark wood panelled walls. My light shoes squeaked as I walked along the parquet floor. I tried to lighten my step by walking on my toes, fearful of breaking the silence. I stopped and looked out of one of the windows at the well-kept gardens, a large circular flower-bed covered with a variety of flowers swayed gently in the breeze. From the centre of this magnificent display rose a large grey painted cross and high in the air a crucified Christ, the dead custodian of St Michael's and of the world. I gazed at this pathetic figure, his head hanging to one side crowned with thorns, his face spattered with blood, painted in bright red on sunken cheeks. His emaciated body was held to the cross by three nails that were inadequate to support the weight as it leaned slightly forward. Birds flew above the statue landing on the crown of thorns or on the outstretched arms, carelessly chattering as they did so. A robin landed and I remembered the story told so often by the nuns of how this tiny creature came to have a red breast; he was trying to pluck the thorns from the head of Christ at the time of his Crucifixion.

The corridor became narrow and much darker. A flickering light was given off from a candle burning at the feet of a large statue of the Virgin Mary. I looked around for a bell but could see none. A round brass gong hung from a silver chain and to one side there was a stick with a padded leather-bound head. I picked it up and banged the gong once, twice, then a third and final time.

I had hardly replaced the stick when a nun rushed towards me. She placed her hands on the gong to stop its sound reverberating through the convent.

'I have this message for Mother Ita,' I said, handing over the package which I had been given.

'I am Mother Ita,' she replied, her breath quickening and her voice beginning to rise.

'Who told you to ring the gong, you stupid child?'

'Mother Michael said that your bell was three.'

'It is, it is, but my God child do you not know the difference yet between a bell and a gong?'

I remained silent. She grabbed me by the arm, led me across the corridor to where an ornate piece of rope hung through a small hole in the ceiling, and held the tasselled end of the rope close to my face.

'This, you stupid child . . . is a bell!'

'Yes Mother,' I answered.

'That over there,' she said turning, 'is a gong.'

Then she pointed to a small printed sign on the wall and asked me to read it.

'Bell' I said.

'Yes, B.E.L.L.' and with the back of her hand she slapped me across the face. 'That gong is an ornament and it is not meant to be rung, you have disturbed Jesus in the Tabernacle. The very least you could do is go to the chapel and say that you are sorry.'

The chapel was small and dimly lit by a stained-glass window depicting a cross. On either side of this there were two other smaller windows on which the black roller blinds were pulled down. The flame from the ever-burning sanctuary lamp which hung from the ceiling on its triangular chain hardly moved in the still air. The big statues made the chapel look smaller than it actually was. St Michael the Archangel, triumphant, his foot firmly placed on the back of a serpent. A snake, once the most beautiful saint in Heaven banished to eternal damnation for the sin of pride. Lucifer, serpent, symbol of evil, the devil. Out of the corner of my eye I could see the nun was watching me, and to give the impression that I was praying I bowed my head and moved my lips, certain that she would be impressed. After some minutes I found that I was actually praying.

'Lord, if it be your holy will, please don't let me get into trouble.' I was always taught that it would be wrong to ask God for anything without first prefacing the request with the words 'if it be your holy will'. Mother Ita got up from where she was kneeling but I remained in prayer just to reassure her that I was serious about what I was doing. As we left the chapel I noticed she had calmed a great deal. She ran her fingers through my hair and asked me if I was one of the new altar boys.

'Yes Mother,' I replied.

'What age are you?' she inquired.

'Six and a little bit' I replied confidentially.

'Well,' she said, 'didn't Jesus himself make the odd mistake, I'm sure He'll see His way to forgiving you.'

'You can tell Mother Michael that there is no message.'

I walked quickly, and on my way back to the assembly hall stopped again to look out at the figure nailed to the Cross, with a sparrow now perched on one of the outstretched arms, resting.

Twice each week we went for long walks along the country roads outside St Michael's. Before leaving we were instructed on the need to be clean, and how to behave when we were out. To salute a priest, if we met one, by raising one hand to our forehead and bringing it down sharply to our side, just as a soldier would in the army. The walk we took happened to be the same one as the priests took to say their offices from thick, black, leather-bound missals, with page-edges gilted in gold.

Lined up two-abreast, we were inspected by Mother Paul and Mother Michael. Trailing boot-laces had to be tied properly. Hair, not properly combed was fixed with the black combs each of the nuns carried. I hated having my hair done by them, their strokes were heavy and the teeth hurt my scalp. When I tried to shift away from either of the nuns they gripped my chin tightly so that I could not move. Snotty noses were wiped with checkered handkerchiefs to mutterings of 'dirty little pup'. I tried to find a place mid-way down the line for these walks to avoid being constantly under the eye of the leading nun, or the one at the end of the procession. This allowed a certain amount of freedom to chat with some of the other boys, and at the same time for a degree of alertness in case either of the nuns checked the line during the walk.

The large grey wooden gates swung open and enthusiastically we filed out. Talking was strictly forbidden unless we were told that it was alright. The walk was always the same, about a mile and a half out along the road and if the weather was fine we would stop in one of the many fields in the area for twenty minutes or half an hour. During this time we were allowed to break into groups and chat to each other. If the weather was not to the liking of the nuns we turned around and went back to Saint Michael's. I loved the freedom of the open fields. I picked buttercups and held them under other boys' chins to see if they were brave or cowardly. A bright yellow reflection from the skin was a sure sign of bravery, less bright the mark of a coward.

On those rare occasions when they were so engrossed in conversation that they took little notice of us, we used to sneak across the field near to a derelict house. It was a bungalow, with the path which at one time had led to its door now covered with grass and weeds. All of its windows were broken and the frames hung precariously outward. The roof was in poor condition. The slates from the apex had slid down and broken through the rusty iron guttering. Some of the others and I used to gather stones and when we got the chance we'd throw them at the roof where they landed with a sharp clack. I would turn quickly towards the nuns, watching them as they tried to discover what the noise was. I believed that the house was haunted and a banshee lived in it. Every time a stone struck the roof I ran, terrified that the banshee would appear.

Just like the other boys I was sure there was a huge hole in the floor of the house, and that any children caught would be thrown into it. Every time I got anywhere near this house I was filled with feelings of terror and a peculiar sense of delight. The fun ended with the call to 'line up'. Two by two we marched back to St Michael's and confinement.

There were days when the strict regime of the school was less in evidence. First Communion day was one. On 29th of May 1957, a few months after my sixth birthday, the day before I made my first communion, I was marched to the bathroom with eight other boys. Before any of us were stripped for a bath we had to have our heads treated for lice, whether we had any or not. The lotion used was like urine to look at and had a very strong smell. It stung as it trickled down my forehead and into my eyes. I clenched them shut as I groped for something to wipe them with. Once my hair had been soaked in this foul-smelling liquid I was stripped and ordered into the bath. The heavy hand of a nun rubbed the rough flannel over my body, nudging me to lift my arms so that she could wash beneath them. Then I had to stand up, the water reaching just half-way up my shins. Naked, cold and embarrassed I let the rest of my body be scrubbed. Mother Paul said it was important that I be 'spick and span' before Jesus entered my body.

In the bathroom there were two cast-iron baths stained from the constant dripping of water and chipped-off enamel from use over many years. It was a big room with black and red quarry tiles on the floor and dark green painted walls. There was no heating. Every second Saturday as many as sixty children waited their turn to be washed. Everyone stripped at the same time. As one child got out of the bath so another stepped into the ever clouding dirty water. Each child had to dry himself and it was not unusual to have three or four boys waiting for the same towel, their bodies shivering as the carbolic stained water ran down their bodies onto the cold floor.

I was nervous from the moment I entered the confession box to make my first confession, afraid that I would say something wrong.

'Yes?' a gruff voice said.

I took a deep breath and began; 'Bless me Father for I have sinned. This is my first confession Father. Father I told lies, Father I was disobedient, for these and all the sins of my life I humbly ask pardon of God.'

I was not actually aware of having told lies or of having

been disobedient but these were the words I had been taught in the weeks leading up to my confession. Then on the day, I recited them like a poem I had learned at school. The priest began his absolution prayer while I said an Act of Contrition. His mumbling distracted me and I lost my way halfway into the prayer I had rehearsed so often. He didn't notice, and if he did, he didn't seem to care.

On the morning of my First Communion I was not allowed to eat or drink anything. Mother Paul came into the dormitory, her arms laden with clothes. Jumpers, shirts, dicky-bows and ties as well as trousers and jackets. She tried various outfits on me before deciding that a coarse grey wool suit would look best. Instead of the usual heavy boots I was given a pair of shiny black shoes and knee length white socks to wear. She put her two fingers into a jar of Brylcream and rubbed it into my hair before parting it at one side and then warning me not to touch it. From that moment on I was to prepare for Jesus by praying and asking him to make me worthy to receive him. Before leaving for the Church I was reminded that He only stayed in my soul for fifteen minutes. It was important, during those minutes that I prayed for anything I wanted. The importance of praying for those who looked after me was stressed. Then there were those who had died and gone to God, those that were in Purgatory. I had to pray for the souls who had gone to Limbo, babies who died before they were baptized, and who would never see God. She impressed on me the importance of praying for those who had gone to Hell because they had not led good lives. Protestants too needed prayer so that they would believe in the Blessed Virgin.

On no account was I to touch the Sacred Host with my teeth. Great care was to be exercised to ensure that the host did not fall out of my mouth and even if it did I was never to touch it with my hands. Only the priest could do that. If it became stuck on the roof of my mouth it was permissible for me to gently peel it away using my tongue.

Having gone to the altar-rails and taken the white host into my mouth I returned solemnly to my seat where I bowed my head and closed my eyes. My prayers were a sort of a test for Jesus. I never did pray for the nuns. Nor did I pray for the souls of those who had died in a state of sin and, as for Protestants, I never mentioned them. I was very specific about what I wanted. I asked Him to bring me an apple and an orange and sixpence. I had seen apples and oranges but never tasted either. Despite the fervour of my prayer, the fruits never materialized and I only got half the money I asked for.

Later in the day, Miss Sharpe, our singing teacher, brought us out for a walk through the town. It was a hot sunny day and the local people who were standing at their hall doors stared at us. Groups of local children laughed and jeered, mocking our clothes. Some of the older people gave us money. I got a thrupenny bit and, if I could manage to hide it, I was going to buy three ice-pops. Miss Sharpe went into a shop and bought a bag of sweets while we waited outside gaping through the window. We walked until we came to a field where she suggested we go in and sit down. She sat on the grass for a while and then moved to where there was a big grey boulder. She sat up on it and called us to gather round her so that she could share out the sweets. Before doing that she asked had any of us got any money, I admitted that I had and she took it from me saying that it was part payment for the sweets. We were not allowed to have money. She gave us two sweets each and said that she would raffle the remainder before we went home. Just as St Michael's was home for us so it was for her. We gathered daisies and made them into a long chain, looping one through the pinched-out stem of the other. I pulled some grass from the field and tossed it into the air, explaining to one of the other boys that this was how farmers tested to see which way the wind was blowing.

I lay on the grass propped up with my hand under my chin and my elbow dug firmly into the ground. My eyes shifted in the direction of Miss Sharpe. I noticed her sandaled feet and as I looked up along her leg I could see where her stocking-top was gathered and held by a suspender. Her bare thigh was pure white in contrast with the tan colour of the stocking and the pale yellow colour of her knickers which were elasticated firmly higher up her leg. I wanted to tell one of the other boys but I decided against, just in case he told on me. I watched for as long as I thought it was safe to, enjoying the sensations that rippled through my body. Something inside suggested that the pleasure I was getting from watching this lady was sinful, but that didn't matter. The feeling of pleasure outweighed everything.

Eventually I got up and went over to a part of the field where some of the boys had gathered. Our supervisor did not seem to mind. In a hole in a stone wall we could hear the buzzing of what we presumed to be a hive of bees or wasps, nobody knew the difference. I couldn't resist the temptation to poke a long piece of stick into the hole. As I probed around the buzzing intensified and, too late, one of the boys warned me that they would emerge and sting the life out of us.

The insects streamed from the hole and we all ran, pursued by them. Agitated wasps bent on revenge stung most of us, and as they did we screamed. My own face and legs were sore and I found it difficult to run as Miss Sharpe ushered us from the field, her headscarf tied tightly about her face.

Curious villagers watched as we were walked back down the town, each of us holding a different part of our bodies.

'What happened the poor children?' an old lady asked.

'Wasps,' Miss Sharpe replied acidly, 'they got stung.'

'Ah sure God help them.'

'Indeed,' Miss Sharpe said, 'God help them.'

One by one, stung and weeping we walked through the gates of St Michael's. Hearing us, Mother Paul rushed out and demanded to know what all the commotion was about? Miss Sharpe told her what happened.

'Well now,' the nun intoned, 'we all know that wasps and bees don't sting for nothing, and we all know, don't we, that some little devil has to disturb them? Is anyone going to own up?' she said as she swung her pointed finger round the group of us. No one spoke. She waited, then reminded us that it was not long since Jesus came to visit us.

'It's as well to be aware,' she continued, 'that He knows.' She ordered us to the dispensary saying that whatever pain or suffering we were enduring was entirely of our own making. We would have to put up with it until she was ready to attend to us.

The dispensary was a small room where any cuts or grazes

were dressed, usually with iodine and a big lump of cotton wool held in position with a piece of sticking plaster. It was a dark room, with many presses, all of which had glass doors. On the shelves inside, bottles of different colours and shape were carefully labelled and fitted with cork stoppers. Cotton wool was wrapped in purple paper, its whiteness contrasting sharply with the colour of its wrapper. The air smelled heavily of disinfectant.

As we sat and waited on the wooden benches I warned the others not to say a word. The doors were flung open and Mother Paul rushed in to attend to us. As she dabbed iodine onto the various stings she said she hoped that there was no one telling lies. Nobody was. Nobody was saying anything. I felt a great sense of relief as I left the room, my stings had been anointed and I was not found out. As I walked down the short passage which would bring me to the school yard Mother Paul shouted after me to tell the other boys that they were to take off their communion clothes, fold them, and leave them ready for her to collect. I was glad to get out of the coarse wool suit as the rough hems on the trousers had scorched my legs, and the jacket felt heavy across my shoulders. Communion day was over.

CHAPTER THREE

Much of the time in St Michael's was given to training us to be altar boys and to serve Mass in the local parish church. I often spent three or four hours a day learning the Latin responses. A small fat nun gave out the responses in a monotonous voice and made me repeat them. Another hour was set aside for the practice of the ritualistic movements necessary on the altar during Mass. I learned the foreign words without the least understanding of what they meant. I knelt, stood, bowed, joined my hands while the nun played the role of priest. I learned to move the large missal and brass stand from one side of the altar to the other at the right moment and at the right speed. Reverence for the blessed sacrament was everything. I was constantly reminded of the need to keep my hands clean and my hair combed. My hands would not just be carrying cruets of wine or a chalice full of white hosts. The wine would become the blood of Christ and the hosts his body. When I was not moving sacred items I had to kneel absolutely still, with my hands joined and my eyes fixed on the crucified Christ just over the tabernacle. Being an altar boy gave me a sense of importance. I loved it, loved the stillness of early morning in the town. The sun shone low in the eastern sky, slanting its way across dark slated roofs and onto the narrow streets of Cappoquin. As I started my walk the streets were silent except for the sound of my hob-nailed boots click-clacking on the pavement. The neat rows of houses looked as though nobody lived in them, their curtains still drawn. As I neared the church, which was about ten minutes walk from the Industrial School, people opened their hall doors to check the weather or to sweep the dust from the pavement in front of their houses. Some greeted me,

37

others didn't say anything and I often felt that they were trying to avoid me. I used to hear people refer to me as 'one of the children from the orphanage', which was the phrase locals used to soften the brutal reality of the industrial school in their midst.

The church was on a hill overlooking the town. It was surrounded by black railings that always had the appearance of being newly painted. Moist, glistening cobwebs had formed between the rails during the night and I loved to cup my hand and scoop them off, trying not to damage them as I did. I examined the cobwebs closely to see what had been trapped there. There were small flies and midges, dead or dying. Breakfast for a hungry spider was ruined many a time due to my clumsy efforts at replacing the web between the rails from which I had taken it. My attempts at delicacy could not match those of the original spinner of the beautiful silken webs.

The sacristy was at the back of the church and the first thing I had to do on entering it was bless myself and then remove my heavy boots and replace them with soft plimsoll runners. My soutane and surplice were in a cupboard, ironed and starched, ready for me to wear. If there was time before or between Masses the sacristan would allow the altar boys out into the church yard for a game of handball, always stressing the importance of keeping clean and tidy. Playing with a ball in a snow white surplice was difficult, there was always the risk of getting it dirty from a hopping ball or a fall. If that happened an angry sacristan would forbid the serving of Mass. Since that was a risk I was not prepared to take I very seldom played handball.

The priest robed for mass, constantly praying as he put on each vestment. The amice, the alb, the cincture, the stole, and the chasuble, each with its own significance and its own prayer. If he wanted assistance it was always given to him. Some priests preferred to robe without help.

I stood at the sacristy door looking into the darkened church slowly filling with morning worshippers. They genuflected in the centre of the church and then men and women went to their respective sides of the centre aisle. The women wore head scarves. The men took off their hats or caps as they entered the church. The sacristan put on some lights, the brown bakelite switches clicking loudly in the silence, then he struck a match and lit the white taper wick fitted to the top of a smooth dark brown wooden pole. Slowly and solemnly I walked out of the sacristy and ascended the red carpeted steps to light the three candles on either side of the altar. The congregation moved and even though I had my back to them, I could feel their eyes on me.

In the sacristy the priest waited for the altar boys to lead him onto the altar. His hands were joined tightly and his index fingers pressed hard against his well-shaven chin. His eyes were lowered and his head bowed. Priests, once vested, seldom spoke, and when they did it was usually to say that something was wrong.

The congregation rose to its feet as every light was switched on, the brightest ones being over the altar. If it was an 'Ordinary Mass' there would be only two altar boys serving, and as I was normally on the right hand side of the priest, I would be more involved in the ritual than the other boy. I had to move the missal, ring the bells at the offertory and communion, sound the gong at the consecration and hold the platen under the chins of the people receiving communion. It was a role I thoroughly enjoyed. I always felt as though I was on a stage performing for an audience. I knew that there would be a nun from the school there, they always attended the Masses being served by any of 'their children'.

One morning, when Mass was over, I disrobed, taking great care about how I hung my soutane and surplice. Walking down the town I noticed Mother Paul ahead of me and deliberately slowed my pace so as not to catch up with her. Some people were polishing the brass fittings on their front doors, and as the day threatened to be hot and sunny, they covered their 'scumbled' or painted halldoors in colourful canvas sheets with holes for the bell, knocker and doorknob to protrude. I heard men and women comment on how the sun caused the paint to blister.

As I neared St Michael's, I noticed Mother Paul standing, beckoning me to hurry. I was gripped with fear as I quickened my step. Thoughts of what I could have done wrong now ran through my mind. Once I had caught up with her, she told me to walk in front of her.

'You were very good on the altar this morning. I am going to suggest to the sacristan that you be allowed to do more altar boy duties in future. You can be a very good child when you want to be.'

I walked ahead, smiling to myself. It was the first time she had ever praised me for anything. I was just six and a half when I began serving Mass. The ease with which I mastered Latin was a topic of conversation among nuns and priests. Altar boys were highly regarded in the community. I was proud of myself and delighted in being referred to as the 'little altar boy'.

I was thin and often jeered at by other children. Those from the town were the worst offenders referring to me as 'a skinny little orphan'. The jeering hurt and I was often close to tears. That would have suited my tormentors but I was not prepared to give in to them.

Sunday was my favourite day for serving. Flowers adorned the altar in brass vases and many more candles burned than for weekday masses. The crowd was bigger and the organ droned constantly in the background. The sound of the choir singing filled the church and added to the pomp of the occasion. Instead of the usual black and white, the altar boys wore bright red soutanes and well-starched pure white surplices. The priests vestments were also more colourful than usual. A white chasuble with a golden cross embroidered on the back and the scripted letters I.H.S. in the centre.

Before Mass, the priest spent a great deal of time going through the big red missal from which he would read. The chosen sections were marked, each with a different coloured ribbon. A final check through it and he nodded to the sacristan indicating that the book could be placed on the heavy brass stand and brought to the altar. He carried it and as he placed it on the right hand side of the altar he checked that all candles had been lit. On this religious stage everything had to be correct.

Once I reached the altar there was tension and drama.

There was the fear of forgetting a line, a response, the thought that a wine cruet might slip from my hand. My heart raced as I rang the bell to warn the congregation of the approaching consecration, that part of the Mass when white host and red wine became the body and blood of Jesus Christ. Transubstantiation. The silence was palpable. I struck the brass domed gong firmly; Bong. Heads down. Bong. The white host held aloft as the bowed heads looked up momentarily, in adoration. Bong, eyes and heads lowered again. Now the priest prayed over the chalice of wine. Bong, he genuflected, Bong, each head rose and gave praise to the gold cup containing the blood of Jesus Christ. A final bong and the solemnity and tension of the Consecration gave way to a restless shifting of bodies, clearing of throats, and the distinctive sound of people blowing their noses.

Before the distribution of Communion two altar boys draped stiffly-starched cloths over the marble top of the altar rails. The bell sounded, indicating to people that it was time to approach the altar rails. Men and women left their seats on the different sides of the church and took their places on either side of the centre gate leading onto the altar. Men on the right, women on the left. I often carried the gold paten which I held under the chins of those receiving Communion, in case the host fell. As I walked carefully backwards with the priest, I couldn't help noticing the various ways people offered their tongues to receive the host. The men seemed to be in a hurry and opened their mouths rapidly, unleashing their tongues on the white host like a lizard whipping up its prey. Their tongues were dirty, yellow tobacco-stained and rough in appearance. Women were much less hurried and more reverent in their approach. There was a sensuality about the way they parted their lips and put out their tongues. They usually left the altar rails slowly, walking on the toes of their shoes, so as not to break the silence with their stiletto heels. The men were heavy footed.

Hands joined, heads bowed, the entire congregation spent the next fifteen minutes in silent prayer, each undoubtedly requesting a different favour from the Visitor now within their bodies.

Every week-day after serving mass I had to call into the local post office to collect any letters or parcels there might be for the Industrial School. It was a quaint old building serving the townspeople as a newsagents, a hardware store and a confectioners. The exterior was painted dark green with the words 'Oifig an Phoist' beautifully written in gold lettering over the entrance. There was a gold harp at the beginning and end of the hand-painted sign. The window display consisted of some faded cigarette packets, magazines and newspapers, discoloured by the sun. The entrance was through a double sided door, one side of which was always open. When the breadman came it was necessary to open both sides, or when the sacks of mail were very bulky. I had to wait as the postman and the shop owner sorted through the letters, stacking them according to the particular area of the town they were going to. Each batch was then put into sacks with the letters P&T imprinted on them in heavy black printing ink. The local postman became a particular friend to me. He was a small, chubby, man, always smiling, chatting, or singing. Whenever he saw me he'd say, 'How's me man this morning then,' before remarking to the other people in the shop that one day I would be the best postman the town had ever seen. When he asked me if I was going to be a postman when I grew up, I said I wasn't. I was going to be a priest.

'A priest, begob,' he replied, 'Well I suppose you could do worse.'

He used to take me by the hand and bring me over to the counter where the cakes were, eclairs with chocolate, tarts with jam seeping through their crusty sides, fairy cakes and currant buns.

'What'll ye have?' he would ask.

After spending some time scanning the wooden trays I would normally settle for a currant cake covered in sugar. The postman paid for it and I'd sit down to eat it while he packed the bag that I was to carry. He told me not to leave a trace of it as he didn't want 'them nuns' coming up the road after him.

'I've nothing against nuns, son, I love them really, at a distance.' He roared laughing.

I always felt uneasy sitting there eating cakes and I used to stuff them into my mouth as quickly as I could, afraid that some of the local people might mention to the nuns that they had seen me. There was no doubt in my mind as to what the consequences of that would be. The postman insisted that I carry the post like a 'real Postman'. 'Over yer shoulder, that way it won't feel so heavy.' I did as he instructed and when I was ready to leave he'd clap his hands together before saying 'Right now begob, you're away with it.'

Instead of going back into the school I would have to go to the convent door and hand in the bag containing letters and parcels. It was a big oak door, with very ornate and well-maintained brass fittings. The bellpush was set into a circular brass disc with the words 'press' etched into its white convex shaped button. I pressed it and waited. I heard the lock being opened and prepared to hand over the bag. The nun that took the post from me never spoke to me nor I to her. She closed the door and I walked the few yards further on to the grey gates leading into the yard of St Michael's. As I crossed the yard I could hear the sound of mugs and plates being collected through the large open windows. After a few minutes silence the collective voices of the other children chanted grace after meals.

After delivering the post one Friday morning, I knocked on the kitchen door. A fat, small, wrinkled faced nun opened it and glowered at me. I told her I had been answering mass and that I had missed breakfast. My excuse was a good one. I would get my porridge, my dripping-covered bread and a mug of cocoa.

'Wait,' she snapped as she let the door slam. I stood, looking around the large grey dining room, for the first time noticing how big it really was. Everyone was gone, the tables were cleared. In the distance I could hear the other children playing. The kitchen door swung open and a tin plate of porridge was pushed into my hands.

'Leave it at one of the tables and come back for cocoa and bread.'

I did as instructed. The porridge was cold and very lumpy, the bread greasy and the cocoa had a skin on its surface. As

43

I ate, the sweating nun emerged from the kitchen carrying a brown bottle, from which she poured a thick dark liquid. She tossed a tablespoon of syrup of figs into my mouth.

'Lick that spoon clean and swallow,' she demanded. I hated the stuff and made no secret of that. I used to hold it in my mouth hoping the nun would go away so that I could spit it out. She stayed, watching, until my mouth was empty. Everyone got a spoonful of syrup of figs once a week. As I was washing my mug and plate she asked me to take a message up the town for her. She didn't wait for an answer, just rushed back into the kitchen and emerged a few moments later carrying a canework basket, with a live chicken inside.

'You know where the other convent is?' she asked.

'Yes,' I hesitated before adding 'Mother'. My eyes were riveted on the basket. She held it up for me to take from her and when I didn't take it immediately she left it on the floor. The top was held closed with two leather straps and buckles. The chicken poked its head out through a grille on one side. Then it began to flutter about, frightened. I lifted the basket, holding the grille section towards my legs, thus allowing the chicken to take a peck at me. I jumped, and quickly turned it the other way round.

'Give that message to Mother Immaculate,' she said.

I walked out of the dining hall, through the assembly hall into the yard where I was immediately surrounded by inquisitive children.

'What's in the basket? Where are you going?' Some laughed at the difficulty I was having in holding the basket steady. It was heavy and I had to stop repeatedly in order to change it from one hand to the other.

The street near the school was quiet, and the houses on each side of it basked in the sun. At one of the houses two old men leaned over their half door, both smoking pipes and wearing hats. They took it in turns to spit out onto the street or greet people going by. I had often heard the older boys talk about these men. They were brothers, known as the two Toms. Tom Dee and Tom Tee. I had heard more than once that they had a big hole in the floor just inside the door of their house and that one of their 'Tricks' was to try and lure children in, so they would fall into it. Once dead, the children were fed to the greyhounds they kept in the backyard. I believed the story and shivered as I walked by, even though I was on the opposite side of the street. Out of the corner of my eye I watched, just in case one of them chased me.

An inquisitive dog sniffed at the basket. As he barked the bird became frightened and fluttered furiously. I was still terrified of dogs.

'Go away,' I said.

My heartbeat quickened and my breath became uneven and hurried. I became very frightened. The barking dog attracted more dogs and as they followed me I began to run. They ran too, snapping at the chicken. I held the basket high in the air and screamed. Some of the dogs jumped, bared their teeth and growled viciously again. People rushed to their front doors, some said that none of the dogs would bite, others told me to stop running. One man tried to stop me by saying that it was the chicken they were after. Nothing they said eased my fear. I continued running.

Ahead of me I could see the green gate leading into the convent. When I reached it I grabbed the latch and quickly pushed the gate open. I kicked out at the dogs to get them away from me before banging the gate shut. I stood with my back to the wooden gate listening to the barking animals. I was perspiring heavily and as I looked at the basket now lying on the gravel path I began to cry uncontrollably, sobbing hysterically, fighting for each breath.

I badly needed to go to the toilet. I undid the braces holding the buttons at the back of my trousers. In this hunched position, I defecated on the gravel. There was never toilet paper supplied in the school, but out there in the open I instinctively wanted to wipe my backside and looked around for something I could use, there was nothing. I pulled my trousers back on and stuffed my shirt inside them before using my foot to shift some stones into a pile to cover the stool. Just as I was finishing off the gravel mound I heard footsteps coming towards me from around a bend on the walkway to the convent.

I grabbed the basket and took a quick glance at the pile of

stones, pressed lightly on it with my foot, picked up the basket, and was just about to move off when a tall nun asked me what I was doing.

'It's a message for Mother Immaculate.' I answered nervously.

'I am Mother Immaculate,' she said and reached out to take the basket. It was then she noticed the pile of stones.

'What is this?' she said, pointing. I told her about being chased by the dogs, that I was tired, and had sat down to play with the stones. Then she asked me to leave the basket down, before walking towards the heaped stones.

She kicked them. I watched as her shoe became embedded in the mixture of gravel and excrement. Her anger at me was obvious from the expression on her face.

'You filthy dirty little pup,' she said, 'you will be severely punished for this.'

I tried to speak but she wouldn't allow me to. I wanted to explain how frightened I had been, and how I couldn't help doing what I had done, but she wouldn't listen. I offered an apology but she ignored me.

She rushed over to a patch of grass and dragged her shoe back and forth through it trying to clean it. 'You will pay for this, you dirty brat. As sure as there is a God in Heaven, you'll pay for this.' The idea of running did occur to me but I realized that such a move would make my situation worse. Mother Immaculate strode forward and grabbed me by the ear-lobe.

'If I had a dog's lead I'd put it around your neck,' she said, 'because it's only dogs that do what you have done.'

The basket remained on the ground as she opened the gate, and began walking me back down the town while holding me by the ear.

Inside St Michael's I was pushed towards the part of the yard where Mother Paul was sitting.

'What has the pup done now, Mother Immaculate?' she inquired.

The two nuns discussed what had happened and I could see Mother Paul become more and more annoyed. They both looked down at Mother Immaculate's shoe and then at me. Mother Paul grabbed me as the other nun left.

'Why didn't you go to the toilet before you left?' she asked.

'Because I didn't want to Mother,' I answered.

'But you should have gone,' she yelled, as she hit me across the face, 'instead of behaving like a wild animal.'

I remained silent. I saw the cane slide down from under her sleeve and it swished across my legs.

'That hurts,' I shouted.

'It will hurt a lot more I promise before I'm finished with you. You're no better than a dog.' She hit me with the cane again before ordering me to go to the dormitory and wait for her. As I walked away from her she shouted, 'You should be ashamed of yourself, an altar boy. You're a disgrace. And you better start walking properly or you'll get more of this cane than you bargained for.' Nothing had ever been said to me before about my manner of walking. I bowed my head and watched my feet. I could see nothing wrong, yet somehow I had become conscious of every step I was taking, and was aware that unless I changed the way I walked, Mother Paul would be even more severe in her punishment of me.

As I slowly made my way up the long wooden stairs to the dormitory I was followed by another boy.

'Mother Paul said you're not to lie on your bed, or sit on it. You're to stand beside it until she has time to deal with you.'

The dormitory was cold and dark even though the sun was shining. I stood by my bed as I had been told, too frightened to do anything else. From the dining room, I could smell food and hear the sounds of the other boys having dinner. I was hungry. When dinner was finished I could hear them playing 'tig'. I knew that others would be playing priests and altar boys. I wondered who was acting as priest, since it was usually me who played that role.

I began to cry remembering the last time I had been beaten, the stinging of the cane and the nun's taunting as she delighted in my terror. Without warning the image returned of a man's body trembling violently as it hung from a short length of rope tied to an alder tree. It became so real that I was certain I could touch it. I shifted uneasily from one foot to the other, trying desperately to block out the vision. I trembled violently and then screamed, a high-pitched, piercing cry that echoed through the stillness of the dormitory down to the assembly hall. As I yelled at the image to 'get away,' Mother Paul grabbed me tightly by the shoulders and slapped me across the face.

'What in the name of God,' she shouted, 'is the matter with you?'

'I saw the man hanging.'

'What man?' she asked.

'I don't know Mother, just a man.'

She hit me again. 'This nonsense will have to stop, it's distressing the other children. What you are seeing is just in your imagination. People don't hang themselves. You're here for us to look after because your parents are dead. You'll see them again when you die, provided you get to heaven and that is where they are.'

I remained silent. She told me to get undressed and prepare to take the punishment I deserved. I trembled, taking my clothes off, from both the cold and the knowledge of what I knew I was going to have to endure. Mother Paul walked towards the dormitory door, took a large key from the pocket of her habit and locked it. I hadn't finished undressing by the time she returned to my bedside. She became agitated and shouted at me to hurry.

'The sooner we get this over,' she said, 'the sooner I can be getting on with my work.'

Once undressed, I lay on my side. Mother Paul told me to lie face down. I noticed a tremor in her voice, a nervous excitement.

'I'm only going to give you a light spanking,' she said, 'as long as you promise not to tell anyone I let you off with the punishment you should be getting.'

I didn't answer her. I tensed my body and waited for the cane to strike, but it didn't. Her hand slapped me gently on the bare backside, then with the other hand she rubbed the area she had just hit. I was nervous, desperately anxious, and unsure. I could hear her breath, deep and rushing through her nostrils. She ran her fingers down the centre of my back and out towards my shoulder-blades. Then she eased them along the full length of my body in long, gentle, sweeping movements.

'Lie over on your back,' she said.

I turned slowly and looked into her flushed face. She held my limp penis in her hand and drew back the foreskin. It hurt slightly but I was too frightened to say anything.

'You must make sure that you do this every time you are washing yourself, it's very important to keep that part of your body clean.' She moved the skin backwards and forwards until I had an erection. A sensation I had never experienced swept through my body causing me to squirm and writhe involuntarily. When it had passed I sobbed uncontrollably, frightened at what had happened.

She explained that what I had experienced sometimes happened to boys and men when they are washing their 'private parts' and added that it was not a sin.

'Sometimes boys and men play with themselves for pleasure. Not only is that a sin, it is a mortal sin which can only be forgiven by a Bishop in confession. It is up to him to decide whether to give absolution or not. If he doesn't, then that black stain will remain on your soul forever. If that happened you certainly would never see your Father or Mother again with God in Heaven. Now get dressed, and remember, nobody is to be told I let you off so lightly.' She unlocked the dormitory door and watched as I dressed.

Downstairs, in the assembly hall, I could hear the other children playing, and when I had my clothes on I walked towards the door leading to the stairs. As I passed her, Mother Paul hit me across the back of the head with the full force of her hand and, losing my footing, I fell down the stairs. I tried to break my fall as I tumbled but could not. I landed on my back in the Hall. She rushed down the stairs after me shouting, 'you filthy dirty pup.'

I got to my feet and ran.

'Stop, stop,' she screamed, 'before I have to deal with you again.' Her tenderness in the dormitory had evaporated and was now replaced by a rage I had not seen in her before. When she eventually caught me she hit me across the face and I ran away from her. She shouted at some of the other boys to catch me. One grabbed my jumper and held it until she took over.

'How many times am I going to have to ask you to stop dragging that foot after you?' She struck me again, this time on the right side of my face.

'If you don't stop dragging it then as sure as God is in Heaven, I'll ensure that you don't serve Mass again.'

The idea of not being allowed to serve Mass hurt more than the physical punishment. Walking away, I looked down at my feet and wondered what I was doing wrong.

Mother Paul brushed past me and indicated with her finger that I was to follow. She walked towards the boiler room, opened the doors and pushed me inside. I tripped and fell. She didn't wait to see if I was alright. The doors closed and I heard her putting a brush across the two handles so that I could not open them. I remained on the floor crying for a few minutes before realizing the torture was finished.

The boiler room was dark except for a weary yellow flame trying to ignite the coals which had been stacked in the grate of the black range. Through the iron bars of the door I watched the flame leaping and bobbing. Slowly the coals lit and the room warmed, I was content in the heat and happy to remain where I was for a long time. I thought of hell as I watched the coals redden and once again I wished Mother Paul would go straight there and burn.

As the heat of the fire intensified, so did the noise. An eerie howl as the hot air was drawn up the chimney. I found a piece of old newspaper on the floor and began to tear it into little pieces which I tossed into the fire. It burned quickly, before its blackened remains rose on the hot air currents and disappeared.

The peace of the boiler room was broken by the sound of the brush being removed from the door. Mother Paul pushed the doors open, allowing the colder air of the outside to sweep through the room and chill the warmth I had been so comfortable in.

She told me to go to the dining room and have my supper. When I was finished, the boots belonging to the other boys had to be polished and shone. One of the other boys would help me.

I took my place at the table, waiting for the big jug of cocoa to come around to fill my tin mug. The bread was coated in lard that stuck to the roof of my mouth as I ate it, allowing the weak, watery cocoa to take the greasy feeling from my mouth.

Like every meal, it was taken in silence. After supper as I walked out of the dining room, Mother Paul grabbed me by the arm and asked me if there was something wrong with my boots.

I told her they were a bit tight and that they were hurting my toes. They were not hurting me at all but I felt I had to offer some excuse in order to avoid further punishment.

'Go to Mr O'Rourke in the morning and see if he can do anything about them for you,' she said.

'Yes Mother,' I replied.

When all the other boys were gone to the dormitory, John Cleary and I began the twice weekly task of polishing and shining their boots. On this occasion he did the polishing and I the shining. One by one, pair by pair, until all sixty pairs were finished. Then they had to be put into boxes on the wall, each box with its number corresponding to a tag on the back of every pair. It was a tedious and tiring process, but to relieve the boredom we chatted quietly to each other. Cleary asked why Mother Paul had called me a dirty little pup.

'Because of the big gick I did under the stones up in the other convent.'

'What gick?' he laughed.

'The one that Mother Immaculate stuck her foot in,' I said. John laughed hysterically. 'Shut up,' I said, knowing we would get into trouble if caught laughing or talking when we were supposed to be doing something. Invariably, when we were laughing, one or other of the nuns would accuse us of laughing or jeering at them, or talking about something dirty. Once we had finished and tidied away the tins of polish and brushes, we went to bed. It was late and most of the other boys were asleep. With a fleeting 'goodnight' we parted, he to one end of the big room and I to the other. At the sound of a nun approaching I took my hands from under the bedcovers and folded them prayer-like across my chest. She reminded me to include in my prayers all those who were so good to me, particularly the nuns who looked after me. Because of the fear of dying that had been instilled from my first days in the school, the prayer I said most fervently each night was; 'If I should die before I wake . . .' Mother Paul frequently reminded us that we could never tell the day, or the hour, when God would call.

Mr O'Rourke was the convent handy-man. He did everything from farming the few acres of land the nuns had, to weeding the flowerbeds at the front of the convent. I went looking for him to see if he could do anything about my boots. He was an elderly man with wrinkled pock-marked skin and an almost bald head on which he wore a cap with the peak to one side. He was a quiet, soft spoken, shy man. The first place I went to look for him was the farm. In the distance I saw him leading two horses as he steered a plough. The smell of freshly-turned earth was evident. Overhead a flock of birds swooped and dived to pick the succulent worms unearthed by the plough. I stood at the edge of the field watching man and animals move in unison. I watched birds fighting over juicy worms and waved to him but he didn't notice. He was puffing contentedly at his pipe and concentrating on the furrow he was ploughing. When he eventually noticed me he took the pipe from his mouth, held it in his hand and spat onto the ploughed clay before waving back. Once finished, the horses were freed to roam an adjoining field. He walked towards me. The crests and troughs in the field exaggerated his limp, giving his body a deformed appearance. He greeted me with an affectionate toothless smile, inquiring what the nuns wanted this time. I told him that Mother Paul had sent me to him to see if he could do anything about my boots because they were too tight.

'What I like about the ploughing is this,' he said. 'It's grand to be out there on your own with the smell of the clay. I get away from the nuns for a while and I can smoke me ould pipe without a bother. Mind now, I wouldn't say that to them, but I know you won't say a word to anyone.'

He lifted his cap and wiped his head with the back of his right arm. Both of us stood there for a while looking out over the field he had just finished working on. The birds continued to land, grab at a worm and resume their flight, pursued by a more aggressive flyer anxious to have everything his way.

'Come on so, me lad, and we'll see what we can do for ye.' He led the way through the convent orchard to a greenhouse where we both sat down on a wooden bench. He told me he knew me from serving Mass in the local church.

'What's this they call ye?'

'Pat,' I answered.

'That's a great name, Patrick. That's the man they say drove all the snakes out of Ireland. Did ye know that?'

'I did,' I answered.

He asked me to give him a look at the boots. I undid the laces as he scraped out the bowl of his pipe with a penknife. I sat there in my stockinged feet watching him cut slices from a block of tobacco and then rub it delicately between his palms before pressing it into the bowl of his pipe. He struck a match and waited a few seconds, explaining to me that a pipe should never be lit while there is still sulphur on the match – 'It gives the tobacco a horrid taste.'

Slowly he sucked on the pipe and drew the flame from the match into the bowl. I could see the tobacco redden and as he released the smoke from his mouth, the greenhouse was temporarily filled in a ghostly mist. He waved his hand to disperse the smoke and picked up one of my boots. He pulled the leather in an effort to stretch it and, with his penknife, scraped at the inside, taking away tiny slivers of leather. He did the same with the second boot, and told me to put them on to see how they felt.

'They're fine,' I said. He suggested that we walk through the orchard just to be certain, and to see if there might be anything worth eating.

It was too early in the year for fruit to be ripe but that did not prevent me biting into a pear he picked from a fan-shaped tree growing against a wall bathed in sunshine.

'D'ye see them goosegogs,' Mr O'Rourke said as we passed

a bush laden with green gooseberries, 'them's the lads that'd give ye a right pain in the belly.'

I couldn't resist the temptation to take one. It was sour and I immediately spat out the piece I had bitten off. The old man laughed as I threw away what was left.

'They're a great man for to clean out the bowels, better than any bottle ye could buy.' He laughed and I laughed too, though I didn't understand what he meant. He asked if I would be serving mass the following morning and when I told him I would he pressed a multi-sided threepenny piece into my hand saying that it was for spending on the way back from church. He warned me in a good humoured way not to let the nuns see the money. I agreed.

'I better be getting on with me work before them nuns is coming after me with the cane. Now begob that wouldn't do at all.' He laughed loudly as we went our different directions, he into the orchard and I back to the concrete yard where there was a game of football going on. A big statue of the Sacred Heart with arms outstretched looked down on the match. I gazed back at the statue and read the plaque underneath: 'Suffer little children to come unto me' with the date 1876. Then I checked my feet, trying to ensure that I was walking properly. I couldn't be certain anymore.

CHAPTER FOUR

The only respite I had from the daily grind of St Michael's was when I became ill. I was about seven when I contracted measles, and on seeing the raspberry-like rash covering my body, Mother Paul immediately ordered me out of the main dormitory and into a smaller room with twelve beds, which was reserved for any of us who became ill. The 'sick bay' was cleaner and brighter than the main dormitory. Instead of bare floor boards it had a brightly patterned linoleum. The reason for the lino became obvious as more children were ill. Many of them were so bad that they vomited repeatedly onto the floor much to the annoyance of the nuns and the dislike of the boys who were not sick and had to clean it up. Being sick had advantages; the food was better. The porridge was warmer and sweeter and somehow the bread seemed fresher. Dinner was the most improved meal of all. Instead of the usual sloppy stew, anyone who was sick was given pandy; a mixture of finely mashed potato, milk and butter, with a little salt. It was served on plastic plates instead of the usual tin ones.

I lay quietly in the small dormitory listening to the sounds from the yard as the other boys played. A bell summoned them to dinner and everything was quiet. In the stillness I heard the sound of the train making its way into the station. The dark roller blinds were pulled down as protection from bright light. Mother Paul told us that bright light would be very bad for our eyes while we had measles. As I listened to the train's puffing and panting I couldn't resist going to the window and lifting one corner of the blind.

The light hurt my eyes at first, I had grown so used to the darkness, but despite that I persisted. The familiar cloud of smoke billowed into the air to be dispersed around the yard and replaced by another. The whistle sounded and the brake was applied causing the wheels to screech. The following wagons banged roughly into each other. Within minutes everything was silent as the tender filled with water in preparation for another journey. The room I was in was so close to the station and the day so still, that I could hear the driver and his mate discussing where they would go for a drink.

On the stairs I heard the dull thud of heavy boots, I knew it wasn't a nun, because of the absence of the jangle of her long rosary beads hitting off her habit as she walked, but just as a precaution I got back into bed. John Cleary came into the room carrying a tray with a plate of pandy on it. He mimicked Mother Paul as he left it down on my bed, first puckering his mouth, then squinting his eyes and, in a squeaky high pitched voice, saying 'I want to see every bit of that eaten, not a trace is to be left on the plate. Do you understand child?' Before he left the room he asked me to breath on him so that he would get the measles too.

Gradually the sick bay filled with red faced boys; some really sick, others just with a rash. It was not usual for us to have pillows on our beds; we didn't have any in the main dormitory, and as more of us became bored just lying in bed with nothing to do, I decided on a pillow-fight. I challenged one of the boys and when he refused, stood on my bed shouting, 'coward, coward' to provoke him. He couldn't resist swinging his pillow at me and, as I stooped to pick up mine, he hit me and knocked me onto the floor. I attempted to get back into bed while he belted me to the encouragement of the other boys. Eventually I managed to get back onto the bed and was caught up in the excitement and anger of the fight. I gripped the corners of the pillow-case firmly and dug my feet into the mattress before swinging as hard as I could. He ducked and the pillow crashed into the iron framed head of the bed, its light cover bursting open and the feathers floating around the room. I was left holding an empty pillowcase.

Some of the boys laughed. I panicked and asked them to help me put them back. I pleaded that if they didn't I would get into awful trouble. Realizing I wasn't going to get help, I rushed around the room gathering fistfuls of feathers and stuffing them into the cover they had exploded from. Those I could not collect I blew along the floor until they were underneath the beds. Mother Paul arrived into the dormitory to inquire how we were. Nervously I told her that I was feeling a bit better before adding that I thought my pillow was torn.

'I tried to fix it,' I said, 'but some of the feathers fell out'. She looked at me suspiciously, but said nothing, took the pillow and walked out of the room. I wondered if she would bring a different pillow. She did not. Once better, I was immediately doing my usual jobs around St Michael's, polishing floors, looking after Eugene, and doing messages for the nuns. One evening as I was polishing the boots, not long after being sick, I developed a severe ear ache, but was afraid to say anything in case I would be accused of trying to get back into sick bay or escape doing my jobs. It was difficult to concentrate as the pain intensified. I cried as I polished the boots, occasionally rubbing my ear violently.

'What is the crying for, Pat Doyle?' Mother Paul asked.

'I have a pain in my ear Mother.'

'You are just over the measles - you couldn't have a pain.'

'But I have Mother, honest,' I pleaded.

She admonished me, suggesting that if I concentrated more on what I was doing the pain would vanish.

'Offer it up for the Holy Souls in Purgatory,' she said before leaving me to finish the boots.

In bed the pain worsened. I pulled at my ear and swayed my head from side to side in an attempt to get relief. Eventually I screamed; 'My ear, it's killing me.'

Mother Paul ran into the dormitory.

'Jesus, Mary and Joseph, child,' she exclaimed, 'what in God's name are you trying to do?'

'I can't help it,' I said.

'You'll get nothing for the pain until you stop that crying,' she insisted.

'I can't.'

'You better try a little harder.'

I managed to control my crying long enough for her to get some tablets, which she gave me from her hand.

'Drink this,' she said, handing me a tin mug containing a mixture of warm milk and porter which I found difficult to take. The taste sickened me and I was certain I would vomit.

'I think I'm going to be sick,' I said

'If you vomit, my lad, you will lie in it for the night.'

Not long after taking the tablets and the drink, I went into a deep sleep.

When I woke the next morning it was to feel Mother Paul's hand resting on my forehead. She asked about the pain and whether it was gone.

'Yes Mother,' I answered.

She took my head in her hands and tilted it to one side to look into my ears.

'Is it any wonder,' she exclaimed, 'that you have earache. Those ears are filthy, absolutely filthy!'

She took some cotton wool and a tweezers from a small box, wrapped the tip in cotton wool and probed into my ear, removing the accumulated wax. Then she gave me two more tablets. They began to dissolve on my tongue. I stuck it out to show her the difficulty I was having trying to swallow them. She rushed into her room and returned with a glass of water. I drank quickly until the taste of the tablets was gone, then I went more slowly, enjoying the cold smoothness of the glass.

'Come on,' the impatient nun said, 'hurry up.'

I gulped down the remaining mouthful of water. It was the first time in my life I had been given a glass to drink from.

A month or two later I was given the duties of senior altar boy for a High Mass. Throughout the week I was excited and careful not to bring any trouble upon myself which would jeopardize the chance I had so often thought about. At play time I got together with some other boys to practice serving. Walking with solemn slowness and carrying imaginary missals I rehearsed every move. I genuflected reverently, barely touching the concrete yard with my right knee as I gave the proper responses to the prayers being mumbled by another boy who was acting as priest.

In preparation for Benediction I pretended to swing the

thurible. My hands swayed gently, ensuring that the imaginary instrument gave off just the right amount of incense. I rang imaginary bells, not too loud: that might annoy the Bishop. I visualized him holding the gold monstrance aloft, the white host in its centre, and I swung my thurible, head bowed in the presence of God. I had always been told never to look at the host for longer than a couple of seconds as it would be irreverent to do otherwise. I sang the Tantum Ergo, softly to myself. Sunday would be for real. No pretending. Though I was nervous I was also excited.

On Sunday morning I got up early and dressed in the clothes which had been left out for me by the nuns, before washing my face and hands in cold water. I dried them with a coarse piece of white cloth which hurt my face when I rubbed it. So that I could receive communion, I had nothing to eat or drink.

I walked quickly through the town, weaving in and out between couples on their way to Mass. The men were dressed in their Sunday suits and their shoes shone in the early morning sunlight. The women too were dressed in their best clothes. Bright coloured dresses covered by darker coloured overcoats, with stiletto heels tapping sharply on the pavement. Most of them wore scarves, some had white or black mantillas held on by a single strand – the clip hidden in their permed hair.

The altar was brightly lit and almost overcrowded with brass and cut-glass vases containing a variety of flowers. Colourful carnations and leafy ferns lined each side of the steps leading up to it. The red carpet, cross shaped, and held in position by brass bars looked even redder than usual. The dome shaped brass gong stood out majestically on its white marble pedestal. The sacristan, usually clad in just a black soutane, wore a bright red one and a pure white surplice.

There were sixteen altar boys, all dressed in red and white. Just before Mass began the sacristan asked me to bring the red missal and brass stand to the altar. Positioning it carefully to the right of the tabernacle, I tidied the coloured marking-ribbons so they hung neatly down onto the white altar cloth. I returned to the sacristy and took my place at the head of one of the rows of eight boys.

The congregation stood as we walked slowly onto the altar followed by the priests and finally the Bishop. Each of the servers took his position at the bottom step as the Bishop went to the centre of the altar to begin the sacred ritual. Two priests helped as the Bishop put three measures of incense into the thurible which I held open. Once he was finished I allowed the silver lid to slip slowly into the closed position before handing it to a priest, who passed it to the Bishop. With great solemnity, the celebrant swung it gently towards each part of the altar. A blessing, or perhaps an exorcism. The con-celebrants blessed each other before returning the thurible to me. The Bishop stood before me on the highest step of the altar, as I knelt on the lowest and gently swung the thurible at him.

The organist struck a single chord and, after a momentary silence, the Bishop chanted the opening lines of a prayer before the voices of the choir filled the church with the appropriate response. He sat while one of the priests read the epistle. I watched closely waiting for the moment he would lay his hand on the altar cloth, an indication that he was nearing the end of the reading and a signal to me to ascend the steps from the side and move the missal to the Gospel side of the altar.

I lifted the missal and stand, bowed and prepared to descend the centre steps. On the second step I tripped and fell face down. I watched helplessly as the missal slid across the polished mosaic floor, its ribbons trailing like the tail of some exotic bird. The noise of the stand reverberated through the silent church. I could feel every pair of eyes on me as I got to my feet to collect the missal. Several of the priests who were con-celebrating pushed me away, discreetly whispering to me to go back and kneel in my place. There were many minutes of silence as the ribbons were replaced at the appropriate pages. I watched, disgusted that something like this should have happened. I knew the nuns from the school would be at Mass and was certain I would be in the worst possible trouble. I prayed. Eventually I was overcome by fear and fainted.

When I came to, Mother Paul and Mother Michael were

standing over me. Just as one was about to say something to me, a priest came into the sacristy. I was petrified. He stretched out his hand, placed it gently on my shoulder and asked if I was alright.

'Yes Father,' I answered.

'What happened was an accident,' he said, 'there's nothing to worry about.'

As soon as he was gone, Mother Michael said, 'You have disgraced Saint Michael's.'

'I didn't mean it,' I replied.

'Let me tell you this,' Mother Paul said sternly, 'and remember it. You will never ever again set foot inside an altar rails.'

She could not have known it at the time but her words were prophetic.

As the rest of the boys took off their vestments in the sacristy, Mother Paul left saying she would deal with me later. Some of the boys played handball after Mass and I decided to join in, but was told to 'get lost'. They jeered me for falling and then fainting. When they saw that I was almost crying they became even more vocal in their taunting. 'Orphan, orphan,' they jeered as I walked from the church-yard. As they continued to jeer I became enraged and ran back towards them, kicking and punching as many as I could. The sacristan rushed from the sacristy and pulled me off one boy I was threatening to kill. I was shaking with anger, shocked by my sudden outburst of temper. I wondered briefly if the sacristan would tell the nuns about the incident, before deciding I didn't care.

I walked through the town, hands in my pockets and head bowed, desperately aware of being watched by the entire community. Down the street Mother Paul was waiting.

'Get your hands out of your pockets and lift up your head, God knows you're bad enough. You're a disgrace to yourself, worse still, you're a disgrace to the school.'

Hard as she tried, she could not keep her voice down and it rose gradually with every word. People passing looked at her, then at me.

'If you had lifted your feet the way I have been telling you to, none of this would have happened, but you didn't. No, you made a fool of yourself and you brought digrace on all of us.' She reminded me for the second time that I would never set foot inside the rails of an altar again but this time she added, 'as long as I am alive.' She jabbed me with her sharp pointed finger and made me walk in front of her.

'Lift your head, put back your shoulders and in the name of Almighty God will you lift that foot of yours,' she said.

On Sunday afternoon visitors came to St Michael's. They were usually relations of some of the nuns or well-to-do people from the locality. Very occasionally a relation of one of the boys would turn up. When visitors did arrive we were expected to provide entertainment for them by singing or putting on a short play. I felt important being on show. I always sang the same songs; 'A Mother's Love is A Blessing' or 'Two Little Orphans', which delighted the nuns and their guests. Mother Michael, smiled while playing the piano and scowled if I didn't reach the notes as she liked me to.

Everyone clapped politely when I was finished and I bowed to them as I had been trained to do. If there was time we would put on a short play, 'Tweedledum and Tweedledee' that finished with all of us singing 'Little Mister Baggy Britches'. Some people laughed out loud while others smiled politely. When the show was finished, a trolley containing china cups, and plates stacked with cakes was brought into the hall. We remained on the stage as the visitors ate and drank. The voice of John McCormack singing 'Ave Maria' crackled through the horn of the black gramophone at the side of the stage, which Miss Sharpe wound up before lowering the heavy needle onto the record's edge. She quietly warned us not to stare at people eating, then, as she stood out of sight of nuns and visitors, she spoke about McCormack's sweet voice and the crispness of his diction. A clear voice that never missed a note or lacked breath. He opened his mouth when he sung, he took deep breaths, he didn't sing through his teeth or his nose. His voice flowed, never wavering.

It was not uncommon for Miss Sharpe to become completely carried away as she listened to her favourite singer. Whenever she was minding us she used to put his records on and it was at such times that some of us would take the opportunity to try and look up her skirt. Quiet arguments arose about the colour of her knickers. We'd dare each other to look up her skirt, taking turns, nervous of being caught.

I had been given a miraculous medal for my Communion. As Mother Paul put the silver medal with its blue string, around my neck, she reminded me of its significance. It was the symbol of purity and chastity. I used to take it off, and slide it across the floor as near to Miss Sharpe's feet as I could get it. As she stood entranced by the music I'd pick up the medal and at the same time look up her skirt. If she did notice me I was certain I would be able to explain my presence by saying that I had dropped the medal. Afterwards we'd group together and laugh at what we had seen.

There were times when she wouldn't notice the record had finished or that we were all talking. She'd become annoyed when she realized we were not in the least interested in the music and order us out into the yard, apparently unperturbed by the fact that it was raining heavily.

'It's spilling.' I'd say, pointing to the windows.

'Get out,' she'd shout, 'a drop of rain is not going to kill you.'

I ran around the wet yard, chasing leaves that had been prematurely blown down or skidding into wet and slimy clusters of them, enjoying trying to remain upright and laughing when I landed arse first on the ground.

There was one part of the yard that was always dry because a section of the building protruded out over it. Here I would squat down on my haunches and with my arms outstretched get two other boys to pull me along the concrete. In the twilight, or winter dark, the studs on the soles and heels of my boots would leave a trail of sparks in their wake. Causing sparks was one of the things I enjoyed doing most. To create them I had to run as fast as I could and kick the heel of one boot hard against the ground.

Like many of the other boys I often came in from the yard with my hair plastered flat down onto my head and my clothes soaked, but nobody seemed to care. It was not uncommon for us to sit and eat our evening meal with rain water dripping from our clothing onto the dining hall floor.

CHAPTER FIVE

In May 1958 most of the older boys in the school were told to write to a relative. Many of us had never met the people we were being asked to write to, and even if we did, couldn't remember them. The letter writing was supervised by Mother Michael, the nun responsible for our schooling, and their purpose was to ask for a two week holiday away from St Michael's. All the letters were written under her close supervision.

She told me to write to my aunt Mary. I looked at her, surprised.

'Don't look so stunned,' she said, 'you do have an aunt as well as an uncle.'

It was three years since I had arrived in the school and though I remembered my uncle, I had never heard of any aunt. Mother Michael wrote a standard letter on the blackboard which she instructed us to copy. The address was in the top right hand corner and the date underneath.

'Dear . . .' she had written, telling us that 'the blank line is for you to fill the name of the person to whom you are writing.'

'Dear Aunt Mary,' I wrote, before looking at the blackboard to copy what was written on it.

'I hope you are well as I am myself, thank Dog. I would like to come and spend a fortnight with you if you would not mind. I will be good, and do everything I am told. Mother Michael and Mother Paul send you their good wishes. I am very happy here, the Nuns are very good to me. I pray for you every night. I look forward to hearing from you soon,

I remain,

Your nephew,

Patrick.'

Mother Michael went around checking the letters. She slapped her wooden ruler down on the desk of one of the boys near me. It made a sharp crack which startled the other boys.

'Always a capital G for God,' she shouted.

She picked up my letter, and asked me to spell God.

'G.O.D.' I answered confidently. She walked to the top of the classroom with my letter in her hand.

'This is more of this fellow's clowning,' she said. 'Not only does he tell lies and bring the school into disrepute, now he has taken to making fun of God Himself.' I watched her face redden as she rushed towards my desk. Thinking she was going to hit me, I cowered. She banged her clenched fist on the desk.

'Spell God.' she demanded again.

'G.O.D.' I said.

She handed me the letter and asked me to read the first sentence. As soon as I looked at it I realized my mistake. I reached for my pen to correct it.

'Read,' she shouted.

'Dear Aunt Mary,

I hope you are well as I am myself, thank Dog.' Some of the boys laughed, but stopped suddenly when she said there was nothing to laugh about. She referred to what I had written as blasphemy, one of the most serious of all sins. Kneeling at the top of the classroom, I was forced to say an 'Act of Contrition' before being given six slaps, three on each hand. Then I collected all the letters and left them on her table.

I was startled the day Mother Paul told me my Uncle was coming to bring me for a two week holiday to my aunt's house in Wexford. I was uncertain about whether I wanted to go or not. On the one hand I was delighted to get away from the almost constant punishment, but on the other I knew I would miss the companionship of the boys. Because I knew nothing about my aunt I was nervous of having to spend a holiday with her. Life in Saint Michael's was by now familiar. I had come to accept it as normal.

It was a Sunday. Breakfast was served at eight o'clock instead of seven which allowed time to get to early mass beforehand. I waited in line with the rest of the boys to have my dish filled with porridge from a heavy stainless steel cauldron. I walked carefully to my place, carrying my bowl with my eyes fixed on its floating contents. My steps were slow and deliberate, I didn't want to spill it. Having eaten the porridge and scraped the bowl clean, I passed the dish to the boy beside who passed his on until there was a pile of dishes stacked at the end of the long table. The nun in charge of the kitchen served cocoa and bread, and when breakfast was finished, four boys were sent to the scullery to wash up. Any other day I would almost certainly have been one of the four, but as I was going on holidays I had to keep myself clean which meant that I didn't have to do any work at all.

At dinner time I was not allowed to eat with my companions. I was told to remain in the yard where I walked around wondering what my holiday was going to be like. I looked up towards the top floor of the L shaped building to the statue of the Sacred Heart. Even in the bright sunlight the building looked cold and grey. I quietly walked up the fire escape so that I could see into the dining hall. Everyone was eating. The orchard was at the other end of the yard. I had often noticed the nuns walking through it as they said their prayers. I walked to its railings and pressed my face tightly against the black bars, almost putting my head through. Amongst the trees and bushes I saw the familiar limping figure of Mr O'Rourke. He was dressd in a dark blue suit with a heavy grey stripe through it. He saw me and immediately came forward.

'Well, be the hokey, aren't you the real smasher to-day.' I told him I was going away to stay with my aunt for two weeks. He bent his wrinkled face low towards me and said, 'Sure won't it be grand for ye to have a bit of a holiday. I wouldn't mind an ould holiday away from them nuns meself.' He laughed. 'Now,' he continued, 'for a fella that's going on his holidays, ye don't look all that happy.'

Before I could answer he slipped his wrinkled hand through the railings and unfolded it.

'Go on,' he urged, 'them's a grand goosegog, not sour like they were the last time. Why aren't ye having the dinner?'

'I'm going to have it with the nuns when my uncle comes.'

The old man's face beamed, his smile revealing the only two teeth he had, both badly decayed.

'Dinner with the nuns, begob. Them's the people that knows how to feed ye, china cups and plates and the best of silver. I had me own dinner with them a couple of times and I can tell ye this, 'tis better than I'd ever get at home. Make the best of it, it's not often you'll get the chance.' I nodded. He turned his back to me and looked round the orchard, 'When I started here there was nothing only them goosegog bushes.' I could feel his pride as he looked around at the apple and pear trees. 'Them gravel paths weren't there either, now begob the nuns is using them for praying on. I wonder do they ever think of me while they're sayin' the rosary.' Before we parted, he told me that while I was away my feet would grow, and I would have to have the boots fixed again when I got back. Then he limped away through the fruit trees and out of sight. By early afternoon I was hungry and growing more anxious at the thought of going to stay with someone I didn't know. I tried to get into the pantry for a slice of bread but my nerve failed. I was afraid of being caught and each time decided it wouldn't be worth the risk. I waited in the yard for my Uncle. By three o'clock I felt weak and had cramps in my stomach, by four the pain was unbearable and I cried. Mother Paul noticed me.

'What's the crying about now?'

'I'm hungry Mother and I have pains in my stomach.'

'Don't be ridiculous,' she said. 'Offer it up for the black babies out in Africa who never get a bit to eat. Go to the kitchen and wait until your uncle comes. The last thing the poor man wants is to turn up and find you crying like a baby.'

The kitchen was hot and filled with steam. The sun shone through a window that looked out onto a yard packed with cardboard boxes laden with the withered leaves of cabbage and galvanized bins overflowing with other food debris. The cook, a small rotund figure took little notice of me beyond casting the occasional glance over the top of her glasses. I tried to ensure I was not in her way. She wore a white apron over her black habit and had her sleeves rolled up. I watched as she mixed a large bowl of flour and water, her red face perspiring continuously as she used her apron to wipe it. She scattered flour over a rectangular board and tossed a big lump of dough onto it, kneading it vigorously until it was ready for baking.

The kitchen door opened and Mother Paul signalled to me. I went towards her and we walked to a room in the convent where my uncle was waiting.

'And you thought he was never going to come?' she said, smiling at my uncle. Three years had passed since I had last seen him.

'Are you not going to greet your uncle?' she asked.

'Hello,' I said.

He stretched out his hand and took mine. His grip was loose and nervous. His face was tanned, weathered, and deeply wrinkled while his hands looked rough though his skin was soft. Every few seconds, he rubbed his almost bald head with his right hand, and as he did, I noticed it was pitted with tiny black marks.

'We'll go and have something to eat Mr Furlong,' Mother Paul said, 'You must be hungry. I know one little man who certainly is.' She walked between us along polished corridors to the dining room, opened its oak door and invited my uncle to go in. He stood aside and insisted that she go in first. She gave both of us a chair at the circular table covered in a white cloth. I noticed the delicate china cups and saucers that Mr O'Rourke had referred to. There were silver knives and forks and spoons. A small round straw basket in the centre of the table contained fruit which was stacked in a pyramid and decorated at the edges with green and black grapes.

'I'm just going to leave you for a second,' Mother Paul said. 'I want to get some of the other nuns to join us.' During the short time I was alone with my uncle neither of us spoke. Mother Paul returned with two other nuns which she introduced to him but not to me. They sat down and made polite conversation with my uncle who seemed distinctly ill at ease, never sure of what to say. Before eating the nuns said Grace. I joined in but my uncle just kept his head bowed. We had soup first, the adults taking theirs from a bowl while I was given a half-filled cup. For dinner there was bacon and cabbage with potatoes.

'Eat up Pat,' Mother Paul kept saying to me, and though I was hungry it was hard to eat. The system I had become used to was gone and I was tense and nervous without it. When the nuns spoke about the weather my uncle answered them, otherwise he said very little but listened intently as Mother Paul spoke of how I was getting on in school.

'He is a very bright child and I can say that he is a credit to us.' She did not say anything else about me and I was relieved. After dinner she asked my uncle if he would like to wash his hands while she took me to the toilet. The toilet was spotless and the air laden with the scent of disinfectant. The walls were tiled up to the ceiling and there was white tissue hanging from a chrome toilet roll holder. I undid my trousers and sat up on the boilet bowl. Mother Paul stood in front of me urging me to make sure I 'went'.

'You have a long journey ahead and you can't expect to be stopping every few miles just because you want to go to the toilet.' I sat there, my hands firmly gripping the seat. I clenched my fists and gritted my teeth as I willed my bowels to empty. After much forcing I succeeded and then stood up to re-fasten my trousers.

'Wipe yourself,' Mother Paul snapped before she realized that I had no idea of what she meant. She took a small piece of tissue from the roll and folded it in two, 'Every time you go to the toilet, you must wipe your backside. Don't forget that.' In my time in St Michael's I never used toilet paper but just pulled my trousers up when finished.

We returned to the dining room and Mother Paul's face beamed.

'I think he's ready for the journey now Mr Furlong,' she said, looking at the clock on the mantelpiece. 'I'm sure you'll want to be getting away.' My uncle thanked her and the other nuns for the dinner, before she accompanied us to a black Morris Minor waiting outside the convent. There was a man sitting in the drivers seat.

'You should have come in and had something to eat,' Mother Paul said.

'Not at all, Mother' he said. I had never heard an adult use the word 'mother' to address a nun before.

'Are you sure you won't come in and have just a cup of tea?'

'No Mother, no. Thanks very much all the same, but I won't.' I got into the back of the car and my uncle sat in the front passenger seat. The engine started and slowly the car moved away. Mother Paul waved and as I looked back at her, I saw her lips mime 'be good'.

We gradually gathered speed along the road I had so often walked. I sat silently, looking through the windows at people out for their Sunday walks. The sun was getting lower in the sky. Both the driver and my uncle pulled their peaked caps down so as to shade their eyes. The towns and villages we drove through were strangely quiet. Mothers watched from their front doors, shouting occasionally at any of the children who were in danger of getting their Sunday clothes soiled.

'How are ye doing?' my uncle asked.

'Fine,' I answered. 'What time will we get there?'

'It's about three hours journey,' he said, and the driver nodded to confirm that. My uncle spoke to him.

'We might get to stop somewhere along the way.'

'Aye,' the driver said. Then they both got into conversation about farming and horses, cows and milking, and then hurling and football.

During that journey my uncle must have remembered the last time we had travelled along the same road. He could never have forgotten my pitiful cries and my attempts to break free of the person holding on to me in the back seat. He must have remembered my kicking at the interior panels of the car, hysterical at being taken away from where I had spent the early part of my life. Looking back now, my presence must have brought back many frightening and nightmarish things to him. How he had discovered my father hanging and his own incapacity to console me as I roamed around the farm screaming, with my face marked from rubbing and my clothes dirty and wet. The young girl who happened to be passing the gate of the farmyard whom he had pleaded with to go and get help without telling what he needed it for. The guards, the doctor and the priest. The coroners court where he had to relive the sordid business over again before the coroner pronounced that Patrick Doyle had died from asphyxiation due to hanging.

The car stopped and my uncle suggested we get out for something to drink and 'maybe a bit to eat'. We went into a public house, filled with men having their Sunday evening drink. A dense pall of cigarette smoke hung in the air. The chattering of the various groups fused into one cacophonous sound. Both men ordered their drinks at the bar while I took a seat at a small wooden table. My uncle brought me down a large bottle of lemonade and a bag of potato crisps before joining his friend at the bar.

After a few drinks the two men went to the toilet and I followed them. The stench of stale urine was choking, ammonia catching my breath. I was unsure of how to use the toilets so I waited for my uncle to start. As he undid his buttons, so did I. I copied his movements as he shuffled nearer the urinal and thought it unusual that he made no effort to prevent me from seeing his penis. I watched him hold it and withdraw the foreskin. At first I had difficulty in passing any water at all and it was only when I heard the sound next to me that I relaxed enough to be able to go to the toilet. When he was finished he shook his penis vigorously before replacing it in his trousers and buttoning his flies.

I watched as the two men poured black porter from brown bottles into sparkling clean glasses. A dirty looking yellowish froth formed on top and when this reached the top of the glass they stopped pouring. They sat looking at their drinks like two priests about to offer wine up to God during Mass. My uncle nodded to me. I drank the lemonade slowly, its tingling sensation a new experience for me. He walked down from the counter and handed me a large bar of chocolate. I took it and thanked him. The two men lifted their glasses slowly, their mouths hugging the rims as they poured the porter down. They had four drinks and I finished the large bottle of Taylor Keith before we all went to the toilet and resumed our journey. By the time we reached Wexford town it was getting dark. Lights shone from houses where people had not yet drawn the curtains. The narrowness of the streets amazed me and

I told my uncle so. 'What time is it when two cars meet on the main street in Wexford?' he asked, as the driver and himself laughed.

'I don't know,' I answered.

'Tin to Tin.'

The car turned into a sleepy cul-de-sac and came to a halt outside a whitewashed, pebble dashed, semi-detached house. There were brass fittings on the red hall door with the number six above the letter box. White lace curtains hung partially open on the windows. My uncle got out of the car, opened the little iron gate and walked up the narrow concrete path to the front door. I watched as he waited for an answer to his knock. An old woman opened the door and shook his hand. They chatted for a while before he came back to the car and let me out. I didn't like the look of the woman, there was something about the entire situation that made me desperately want to be back in Saint Michael's.

In the neat parlour, she offered my uncle a cup of tea which she poured from a decorative silver teapot. She gave me a glass of milk and a plain biscuit. They chatted to one another while I looked around the room at the various statues that sat in every available space. My aunt looked at me and remarked to my uncle that I didn't have much to say. 'He's a quiet lad anyway and it'll take him a few days to settle in,' he replied.

My aunt had long grey hair which she kept tied up in a neat bun at the back of her head. I watched her fingers tremble as she lifted the cup to her thin lips. The purple veins in her hands showed through her wrinkled flesh. They were prominent and lumpy looking. Her knuckles were white and swollen. She had difficulty in pouring tea and in lifting her own cup to drink. On the finger of her left hand a shining gold wedding ring had embedded itself into her aging skin. Instead of shoes, she had pink slippers on her feet. She moved slowly as she gathered the cups and saucers to bring them to the kitchen. My uncle rose from his chair told her that he would call some day and take me to the shops. Then he wished me good luck and left. She walked to the hall door with him and waved as he drove away from the front of the house.

72

'Now,' she said as she came back into the room, 'I think it is time for bed, but before that we will say our night prayers. I'm sure you say yours every night in the School.'

'I do,' I answered. She opened the drawer of one of the cabinets and took out a black Rosary beads. She held the crucifix in her hand, looked at it and blessed herself, pressing it to her forehead, her breast and each of her shoulders. She moved a chair from under the table and used it for support as she knelt on the carpeted floor. Once I was kneeling she began the Rosary.

'In the Name of the Father, and of the Son, and of the Holy Ghost. Thou, O Lord will open my lips.' She looked crossly at me when I didn't answer.

'Do you know the Rosary at all?' she snapped.

'I know the Our Father, the Hail Mary and the Glory be to the Father,' I replied.

'And my tongue shall announce his praise,' she answered herself before starting into the Five Joyful Mysteries – The Resurrection, the Ascension and so on. Ten hail Marys for each, sandwiched between an Our Father and a Glory be to the Father. She said the first half of each prayer and I the second. At first I was nervous and my voice trembled but I became more confident as I went along.

After the Rosary she led me up the softly-carpeted stairs to the bedroom. It was spotlessly clean and sparsely furnished with just a single bed and a two drawer wooden dresser. There was a silver framed picture of the Blessed Virgin on the wall.

'You better go to the bathroom,' she said, pushing open one of the doors that led off the small landing.

'Wash yourself and be sure to go to the toilet.' When I came out she was waiting in my room. There was a man's shirt on my bed which she told me to wear to bed. I began to undress by taking off my jumper and shirt. I was just going to drop my trousers when she said; 'Wait! Put on this first.' She held the shirt over my head and told me I must be modest always. I got into bed, immediately noticing the softness of the mattress and the freshness of the sheets and pillow cover. My aunt left the door open, and the landing light on. In the next room I heard her moving about, opening and shutting presses and drawers. When I heard her door open I closed my eyes and pretended to be asleep. She stood looking into my room before turning to go to the bathroom, leaving the door open after her. I could see her long grey hair brushed straight down almost to her waist. Her back was stooped and her pale skin contrasted sharply with the dark colour of her dressing gown. When she emerged from the bathroom she was carrying a glass of water with her false teeth in it. Her appearance frightened me, particularly her sunken cheeks and I prayed that I could go back to the other boys. I slept fitfully that night, aware that the person I was staying with fitted my idea of a banshee. As I tried to sleep I had the very real feeling that I had been in the house before and that this woman had been a part of my earlier life.

Outside the rain beat against the window. I looked towards the curtains and watched them swell slightly in the breeze that pierced the gaps in the window. My aunt coughed, a feeble rattling cough. I turned around in my bed, then turned the pillow. Its coolness relaxed me and I drifted into sleep.

The morning sun shone into the room through a gap in the curtains. Birds whistled and chirped. I wanted to get up but I felt it would be the wrong thing to do. I was used to being told when to get up so I decided to stay in bed until I was called. Eventually she called my name from the bottom of the stairs. As I dressed, strange smells and sounds attracted my attention. Sizzling and a kind of spitting. It was only when I got down to the kitchen that I discovered what the smells were. My aunt's hair was neatly pinned in a bun again as she cooked breakfast. I stood beside her for a moment and watched.

'What are they?' I asked. She looked at me.

'Do you not know?' she asked.

'No.'

'Rasher, sausage and egg,' she said. 'Now go over to the table and get yourself some cornflakes.' From a box on the table I spilled some into a bowl and began to eat them.

'Why didn't you put some milk and sugar on them?' she asked as she poured some from a white jug with a blue line around the neck of it.

'I never had these before,' I said. She took little notice of what I said. I had difficulty trying to eat the fry as I had never used a knife or fork before. Everything I had eaten up to now was taken off a spoon. My aunt offered me tea which I took out of curiosity, before deciding I didn't like it. She gave me a glass of milk instead. As we walked to church she told me that every morning for twenty years, since her husband died, she had gone to Mass, no matter how bad the weather was. She didn't always go to communion because she found the long fast beforehand 'a bit much'. She was dressed in a heavy black coat and hat with a huge pin through it. She explained to people she met that I was an orphan staying with her for a fortnight's holidays. They patted my head and remarked that I was a great boy all the same.

After Mass she did her shopping, calling to the butcher's first and asking him for a 'nice piece of bacon'. He wrapped it in brown paper, tied it with string, then handed it to me. I was glad to get out of the shop. I felt sick at the sight of carcasses of cows and pigs hanging from hooks on tubular steel bars, and the blood stained aprons of the men serving behind the counter. Next we went to the greengrocers where she spent a long time talking to another woman about me. Every few seconds the women looked down and when my aunt realized I was listening, she reprimanded me. The woman asked her what my parents died from and she replied that my mother had died of a heart attack and my father the same way shortly afterwards.

This was the first time I heard how my parents died, and though it seemed to have great significance for the woman it made no impact on me.

In the newsagents my aunt was greeted by name. Without having to ask for anything, the girl behind the counter handed her a copy of the 'Wexford People' with her name written in biro in the top right hand corner. A woman who noticed me looking through the comics asked me to pick one.

My aunt interrupted saying, 'Pat doesn't mind what he gets.'

The lady pressed me again to choose a comic.

'The Eagle,' I said.

'Did he say thanks?' my aunt asked.

'Of course he did.'

There was a steep hill from the town up to my aunt's house, and she had great difficulty in walking up. Every few minutes she stopped to catch her breath. I became worried at one point because she seemed to be a long time holding onto a railing and my anxiety must have registered with her because she said,

'Don't worry, it's just that I'm not as young as I used to be.' I was carrying all the messages but I didn't mind. I would have done anything to ensure that nothing happened to her while I was there. When we got back to the cul-de-sac where she lived she told me to go and play with the rest of the children who lived on the street. I was reluctant and, pretending I didn't hear her, opened the gate leading to the house and walked quickly up the narrow concrete path. I waited for her to open the hall door.

'You go out and play,' she said again. 'I'm going in to have a rest and I'll call you when dinner is ready.'

I watched the other children. A boy on a tricycle was racing a girl on a scooter. There was a lot of noise as the boys cheered for the boy and the girls for the girl. When the race was over and they had crossed the imaginary line they began to jeer at each other, disputing who had won.

A dark haired, fresh faced girl approached me. 'Did you see the race?'

'Yes,' I said.

'Who won?' she asked.

I pointed to the girl on the scooter and the girls cheered. The boys, annoyed at my judgement, began to jeer.

'Look at the stupid clothes he has on him,' they laughed.

The girl who had spoken to me in the first instance told them to 'shut up'.

'Look at his big farmer's boots,' they jeered again.

'Shut up,' the girl pleaded again.

'He's just a cissy,' they taunted.

I was so different from them. I was dressed in a grey heavy suit which I was given in the Industrial School. It was dreary and drab-looking compared to their bright cotton colours. Many of them were in their bare feet or in leather sandals.

Eventually they agreed to let me play with them. The boy who owned the tricycle asked me if I would like a go on it but I declined. I didn't want to make a total fool of myself by demonstrating my inability to ride it. Then they wanted me to race with them but I refused even though I was a good runner and had won races in school. I often ran in heavy boots before but was not prepared to do so now in case they jeered again.

'What's your name?' the dark haired girl asked.

'Pat,' I said.

'Does everyone call you Pat?'

'Mostly.'

'My Daddy's name is Patrick but everyone calls him Pat except my Mammy. What's your Daddy's name?'

'He's dead,' I answered, and before she could ask any more questions told her that my mother was dead too and I was just on holidays with my aunt Mary for a fortnight.

'What's your name?' I asked.

'Well,' she said, 'My real name is Maria but everyone calls me Ria.'

'Where do you live?' she asked.

'In an orphanage. It's a good bit away from here, my uncle said it was about ninety miles.'

'Who minds you?'

'Nuns do.'

'I hate nuns, they're always giving out,' she said.

'Sometimes they're cross and sometimes they're alright.'

My aunt called me for dinner and I left Ria, promising to be out again later. As soon as I got into the house I asked my aunt if I could go back out when I had my dinner eaten.

'No,' she said, 'I want to bring you up to the convent to see your sister Ann.'

It was the first time in my life that anybody had ever told me I had a sister.

CHAPTER SIX

My sister was just over two years old when my mother died, aged forty two, from cancer of the breast. She was taken into an orphanage in Wexford, run by the Sisters of Mercy, where she remained until her mid-teens. She would have been five the first evening I saw her.

Having washed up after dinner my aunt brought me to the bathroom where she cleaned my face and combed my hair. She told me to sit in a chair in the parlour and wait until she was ready. I watched her check in the mirror over the mantelpiece to see if her face was alright and her hat was on properly. As she was tidying loose strands of her hair she muttered about my uncle never being around when he was needed.

'How far is it to the convent?' I asked.

She sighed wearily. 'A mile, or maybe a bit more.' It was a hot sunny day and I knew that she did not like having to walk so far. I hoped she would decide not to go.

We walked along a country road, bounded by hedgerows and broken occasionally by a half-built house or an old-fashioned bungalow. My aunt hardly spoke at all. She allowed me to walk ahead of her and as I did I wondered again what my sister was like. Would she know me or I know her? What would I say to her? I didn't even know then if she was younger or older than me.

The green bushes of the country road merged into a high granite wall. My aunt called me and brushed my suit down with the palms of her gloved hands. She took off one glove and spat gently onto her hand before pressing my hair down. She warned me to be on my best behaviour. I could hear the sounds of children playing, their screams breaking the silence of the countryside. My aunt held my hand firmly and walked through the wrought iron gates of Saint Mary's Orphanage for Girls.

As we crossed the yard everything became quiet. The girls stared at us.

'Who are you looking for Miss?' one of them asked.

'The nun,' my aunt answered.

The girl ran off and I felt embarrassed standing in the yard with so many girls watching me. I wondered if one of them was my sister. A nun in the familiar habit of the Sisters of Mercy rushed out of a single storey building to one side of the yard and came towards us. As she walked I could hear her telling the girls to get on with whatever they were doing. She shook my aunt's hand warmly and after some minutes of conversation between them, the nun told one of the girls to get Ann Doyle.

'Come to see your sister, have you?'

'Yes Mother,' I said.

As we walked towards the convent door two girls approached us. The nun indicated to one of them to go away. Then she smiled at me. 'Well, this is your sister, have you nothing to say to her?'

We stared at each other.

'Are the pair of ye just going to stand there gaping at each other or have ye lost ye're tongues?' the nun said.

She suggested to my aunt that we be left together and both of them went into the convent.

In the school yard we tried to say something to one another but it was difficult. We did not know each other and were conscious of the girls watching us. My sister was very pretty. She had fair hair which had been put in ringlets. She wore a lovely daintily patterned dress and a white cardigan that was a few sizes too big for her. We didn't speak but when someone suggested a game of chasing we both joined in. The girls yelled as I pursued them. I ran after my sister and, when I caught her, shouted: 'You're out.' She looked disappointed and was on the verge of tears. A bigger girl suggested that she should have a second chance because she was my sister, and was smaller than me. I was pleased.

The nun and my aunt came out of the convent and the game stopped immediately. She called my sister and I to her and asked if we had found anything to talk about.

'Not really Mother,' I said.

'You don't mean to tell me that you have nothing to say to your sister after all the years ye have been away from each other.'

My aunt tried to encourage me to say something but the words would not come. The years had created a great distance between us and we were being asked to bridge it in a short time. My sister's pale, freckled face reddened shyly as she smiled revealing two prominent front teeth.

'As sure as God,' the nun said, 'there's no doubt but they are brother and sister.'

'Oh without a doubt,' my aunt agreed.

A sudden shower sent the girls scurrying for cover into the sheds on either side of the yard and instinctively I followed them. The nun and my aunt dashed back into the convent. In the rush to get out of the rain I sat on a bench beside my sister and, without realizing it, we began talking to each other.

'Do you like it here?' I asked.

'Yes,' she replied, 'sometimes.'

She and some of the other girls remarked on how I addressed the nun as 'Mother'. They laughed and said they always referred to the nuns as 'Sister'.

'Do you ever get hit or sent to bed without any supper?' I asked.

'Only if you're really bold.'

'I'm always getting hit and locked in the coal shed. Once I got locked into the boiler house.'

'The big girls get slapped sometimes,' she said 'but not the little ones.'

'It doesn't matter if you are big or small in our school, you still get slapped,' I replied, before a group of bigger girls joined in our conversation.

'I got slapped once for not having the laces of my shoes tied right. I wouldn't like to tell you where they slapped me,' one girl said, laughing.

She didn't have to. I knew.

80

When the rain stopped we played chasing again and in the middle of the game the nun and my aunt Mary emerged into the bright sunlight. I walked towards them and the nun insisted that my sister come with me.

'Have the pair of ye made friends?' she asked.

'Yes Mother,' I answered.

'And will you come and see Ann again before you finish your holidays.'

My aunt said that I would. As I was about to leave St Mary's the nun suggested that I kiss my sister goodbye. I was embarrassed and very conscious of the older girls giggling. I refused to do so.

'Sure he has a girlfriend across the road from me,' my Aunt said.

'Is that what he's up to? Wait till I tell Mother Paul.' Both of them laughed but I was terrified that something would be said about my friendship with Ria.

'Now he's no good Mrs Boyle is he? He wouldn't even give his own sister a kiss.'

The old woman nodded her agreement, exchanged a few more words and then took my hand to leave. I turned and waved to my sister, happy to have met her.

That evening before saying the Rosary and going to bed I went out into the back graden of my aunt's house. Overgrown blackberry bushes stooped under the weight of fruit and the air smelled sweet. Having eaten some berries, I reached cautiously through a gooseberry bush and plucked some of its fruit, and though they were not quite ripe I ate them. The bitterness reminded me of Mr O'Rourke and the garden at St Michael's. I rolled the fruits around my mouth, enjoying their taste and the feel of their hairy texture on my tongue.

The raspberries were less difficult to get at. I picked a handful and ate them. I loved the garden, its smells and the long uncut grass rubbing against my leg where my stocking had slipped down. I lay down for a few minutes munching a blade of grass and allowing my nose to be tickled by it which made me sneeze. My aunt knocked on the kitchen window with her ring and beckoned me to come inside.

'Will you look at the state of you,' she said and took me

81

into the kitchen to clean my face, particularly around my mouth.

'You couldn't say the Rosary with a face like that,' she said.

During the night I woke with a violent pain in my stomach. I was desperate to go to the toilet, but was afraid to get out of bed in the darkness of the house. Then I remembered the chamber pot beneath the bed which my aunt told me to use if I needed to to go to the toilet during the night. I groped around until I found it, raised the shirt I was wearing and sat on the pot. My bowels emptied hurriedly and I missed the pot almost completely. The pain was intense but I could not shout for help. When it passed I stood up to try and see the extent of the mess. I could feel my feet wet from the faeces on the carpet, and when I lifted the pot up my hands were soiled from dirt on its outside. The smell in the room was almost unbearable, a sour sickening stench. I wanted to go to the bathroom to clean myself before my aunt discovered what had happened, but decided to wait until morning and try to get up before she did. I slept erratically that night, waking and looking towards the window for any sign of morning.

'Jesus, Mary and Saint Joseph,' my aunt shouted. 'What is that awful smell?'

I was startled out of the sleep I had never intended to go into by her shrill voice.

'Have you dirtied the bed?' she asked.

'Just a bit,' I said, explaining that I had wanted to use the toilet during the night but was afraid of the dark.

'I used the pot under the bed,' I said.

'You stupid child, that pot is for passing water. Get out of the bed.'

When she pulled the curtains open I realized the full extent of the mess I had made. My shirt had dried out and become caked to my skin, the carpet was hard where the faeces had dried into it.

'Oh my Jesus, the carpet, the carpet! How am I going to clean that? I should never have taken you, you dirty thing. Is it any wonder your father and mother couldn't put up with you.'

'I couldn't help it,' I said, 'it came too quick.'

'Get out of this room quick. Take that pot with you, empty it and clean yourself.'

As I carried the pot out of the bedroom, I turned and apologised, offering to clean the carpet.

'Get out of my sight,' she said.

I stood naked in the bathroom washing myself. The door opened and my aunt watched.

'Just wait until I write to Mother Paul and tell her what happened.'

I continued washing, unaware of my nakedness until she reprimanded me. 'It is a sin for a man to be naked in front of a woman, you should have a towel around you.'

My aunt didn't speak at all during breakfast except to tell me that I could not go out onto the avenue to play and that she was getting in touch with my uncle to arrange for me to be brought back to the school as soon as possible.

On Friday evening Ria came to the house to find out if I was sick. I heard her telling my aunt that her mother had asked her to call, since she had not seen me for a couple of days.

'He's going back tomorrow.'

'Tomorrow!' Ria exclaimed. 'He told me he was staying for two weeks.'

'He was but the nuns need him back in the convent to serve at High Mass.' I was afraid my aunt was going to say why I was being sent back and was relieved when she didn't.

'Can he come over to my house later on?' Ria asked.

'We'll see,' she said 'I'll have to get him cleaned up and make sure that he gets to bed before the long journey. I'll bring him over for a few minutes later on.'

'Thanks, Mrs Boyle,' the girl said, before the door closed. My aunt gave me a stern warning about how I was to behave in the O'Neills' house. I presumed it was alright for me to go and, walking towards the hall door, I opened it.

'Wait,' she said.

She put on her coat and checked again in the mirror to see if her hat was alright. Then she took my hand and led me across the road. Ria's mother and father wondered why I was going home so soon.

'Oh', she said. 'You know the nuns.'

I sat quietly in one of the soft armchairs in the front room and Ria sat on the arm of it.

'Will you write to me?' she asked.

'I will if I'm let,' I answered. 'I don't know if I would be allowed.' Mr and Mrs O'Neill gave me a glass of lemonade and some biscuits and as my aunt led me out of their house Mr O'Neill handed me a ten shilling note. My aunt suggested that she should mind it for me. It was the last I saw of it.

Back in her house we knelt to say the Rosary and as it was Friday, she said the Five Sorrowful Mysteries; The Agony in the Garden, The Scourging at the Pillar, The Crowning with Thorns, The Carrying of the Cross, and finally, The Crucifixion. When the Rosary was finished she brought me upstairs for a bath. She washed my chest and my back, my arms and legs. Then with the face cloth she rubbed hard between each of my toes. When I protested that she was hurting me she replied that she couldn't send me home dirty.

'Wash between your legs yourself,' she said handing me the flannel. As soon as I stepped out of the bath she wrapped me in a long white towel and dried me quickly. She offered me a drink of milk and a piece of bread before going to bed, and as I went upstairs she reminded me to go to the toilet.

Early next morning my uncle called to collect me. He was alone and, judging by the conversation between my aunt and himself, didn't really want to drive me back to Waterford. As they talked I got into the car and within minutes I was on my way back to St Michael's.

Before leaving Wexford town, my uncle stopped at one of the larger shops and invited me to pick anything I liked from the shelves stacked with toys and books. I told him that I would like a football.

'And what else?' he asked.

'An Annual,' I said.

'Pick whichever one you like,' he said.

I picked a cowboy one and handed it to him. He gave it to the shop assistant who put both items in a bag. On the way out of the shop he bought me a large ice-cream cone which I licked as we walked along the street. Someone bumped into me and the cornet fell onto the footpath and when I was about to retrieve it someone stood in it.

It was mid-afternoon before the car drew up outside the high grey gates of St Michael's. My uncle pushed them but they were locked. He pulled the car halfway onto the pathway and switched off the engine. We both walked to the convent door and he rang the bell. It was answered by one of the nuns who had eaten with us on the day he had called to collect me.

'Mr Furlong,' she said, surprised, 'and Pat.' She showed us into the parlour saying that she would get Mother Paul.

In the centre of the highly polished parquet floor there was a mahogany table with six chairs around it. Everything shone and smelt of wax polish. On the wall over the beautiful ornate white marble mantelpiece was a large gilt framed picture of a woman dressed in the habit of the Sisters of Mercy. Beneath the picture a brass plate had the words 'Our Foundress'.

'Are ye glad to be back?' my uncle asked, his voice barely audible.

'It's alright.'

'Next year ye can come again, you'll be bigger and maybe you'll enjoy yourself better.'

I nodded.

The door of the parlour swung open and Mother Paul came in to greet my uncle. The vindictive look on her face frightened me.

'I'm awful sorry, Mr Furlong,' she said, 'I had no idea this would happen. I was sure the child wouldn't have been any bother.' She took a letter from her pocket and told him that it was from my aunt. 'It just arrived in this morning's post. The poor woman is distracted, God help her.'

She offered my uncle tea but he declined and, when he noticed I had not got my presents, told Mother Paul that he was just slipping out to the car for a second before heading off. While he was out, Mother Paul glared at me and through clenched teeth told me that I 'was in for it'. 'You are going to be a very sorry lad before I'm finished with you,' she said, and would have continued had my uncle not reappeared. He handed me the bag with the football and the annual, then extended his hand to Mother Paul and said goodbye. As he walked towards the door I heard her apologise to him once again.

'Go over to the assembly hall and give Mother Michael all the news, I'll be over as soon as your uncle is gone,' she said.

Thirty years later, as I sat beside my uncle's hospital bed, I wondered if he could remember that day in 1958 as well as I could. As soon as the old man saw me he began to weep and every time I asked a question about my mother, his sister, or my father he avoided answering, saying simply that I would be alright. The conspiracy of silence had gone on so long that this frail old man would not break it. From whatever tiny answers I could coax from him it is only possible to sketch in the conversation he had with Mother Paul that day.

Mother Paul had questioned him about whether my aunt had said anything about me having nightmares. She told him that they were having a lot of difficulty with me talking constantly about my father's death, but assured him that they were doing everything possible to convince me that the nightmares I was having were nothing more than bad dreams.

My uncle tried to stand up but slumped back into the chair. He buried his wrinkled face in his weather-beaten hands and wept.

'I don't know in the name of God what I'll do when the boy is older,' he said.

She reminded my uncle of the resilience of children and how they eventually forget even the most traumatic events and that in a few years it would be as though nothing had ever happened.

When he was with me in the parlour he had been clutching a brown five pound note. If I am still uncertain about everything that passed between them, I know for certain that as he began the lonely journey back to Wexford it was no longer in his possession.

In the assembly hall I was busy telling the other boys about my shortened holiday. I said that my aunt got sick which was why I had to come back. A small group of us looked through the coloured pictures of the annual. Cowboys on magnificent horses, driving herds of cattle or gunning each other down.

'Is he telling you all about his holiday?' Mother Michael asked.

'I hope he's not telling any lies,' Mother Paul added sarcastically as she arrived. She asked one of the boys what I'd told them.

'He said that his aunt got sick and that was why he had to come back, Mother.'

'I see,' Mother Paul said, her voice becoming more and more icy.

'Your aunt was sick alright. Sick of you! Do the honest thing and tell everyone what really happened.' She grabbed me by the ear and guided me through the boys onto the stage in the assembly hall. Threatening me with her cane, which she brought swinging through the air, she made me tell them everything. When I was finished she hit me across the legs twice or three times.

'I'm not going to give you the cane this time, at least not as much of it as you should get.'

I remembered the last time she promised not to give me the punishment I deserved and worried about what she had in mind.

'I want you to wax and polish the dormitory floor first thing on Monday morning, I would make you do it tomorrow only it's Sunday. You'll start immediately after breakfast. Do you understand?'

'Yes Mother,' I said.

'I'll take that football and the book too,' she said, stretching out her hand. 'Mark my words, it will be a long time before you see them again.' As I walked down from the stage she said, 'I don't want any more trouble from you, no more raving and ranting about hanging men. I want to see an improvement in your conduct and I also want to see you lifting that foot of yours when you walk. Any more trouble and you can expect to feel the full brunt of the cane.'

I attended Mass next morning but, now that I was no longer allowed to serve, I had little interest in what happened inside the altar rails, though I always gave the impression of being in a state of deep meditation and prayer. I kept my head bowed, not out of reverence, but out of fear of being recognized by the townspeople. I envied the boys who were serving for I always regarded it as the ultimate accolade. Now I was just another one of the orphans. Not all the children inside St Michael's were orphaned, many came from broken homes or domestic situations into which they simply didn't fit. Inside the school there was a clear distinction between those who had parents and those who had not. Those who did have a father or mother alive who was an alcoholic were often berated by the nuns. 'Is it any wonder your poor father took to drinking. The poor man must have been at his wits end trying to manage you.' I don't know if any of the other children there had parents who had committed the mortal sin of suicide. If there were, then like me, they were probably kept in ignorance.

CHAPTER SEVEN

After breakfast on Monday morning, Mother Paul reminded me I had a job to do, not that I had forgotten. I was allowed help in moving the beds but not polishing the floor. Another boy and myself moved two rows of beds to one side of the dormitory before he left me alone. I got the tin of wax polish and, with a piece of wood that was with it, splattered lumps of wax onto the floor at intervals of a few feet, before spreading the orange coloured paste with pieces of an old sheet, too worn to be used on a bed and barely adequate for polishing a floor.

Spreading the wax was difficult. First I covered the area and, when I had finished, went back to where I had started and began polishing. It was hard, heavy work, demanding a lot of energy. I used a polishing block which was a large piece of wood, with felt tacked to its base. By pushing this back and forth and leaning heavily on it the floor began to shine. It took me many hours to finish the entire dormitory and by the time I had I was exhausted and sweating heavily. I got help to put the beds back, ensuring they were in a straight line, and sat down on the edge of my own, waiting for Mother Paul to inspect my work. I was dozing when I heard her footsteps and immediately got to my feet, pretending to be fixing the lid firmly on the tin of wax. She walked slowly up and down the dormitory between the rows of beds not lifting her eyes from the floor. I stood and waited for her to complete the inspection, hoping she would find nothing to complain about.

'What is this?' she demanded.

She held her finger so close to my eyes I had to back away to see properly.

'Dust, Mother,' I answered.

'Why is it there?' she asked sharply.

'I don't know Mother. I didn't see it Mother,' I answered.

'If you used the eyes God gave you, you would have seen it. Get the dustpan this minute and clean out that corner properly.'

She stood over me checking and double checking until she was satisfied the floor was clean. I told her that I had missed dinner because I was working.

'It's a pity about you,' she said. Then she pointed to the dormitory door saying that I would go without supper too if I didn't hurry.

It was during the following winter when we were all walking around the schoolyard in the cold under the supervision of Mother Paul and Mother Michael, that they called me over. I listened to them discuss how I was dragging my left foot and heard Mother Paul say I was bright enough to be acting the fool, and her guess was that there was nothing wrong with me at all.

'Walk over to the other side of the yard,' she ordered.

I could feel their eyes on me as I looked down at my foot, trying to ensure it was not turned in. Mother Paul spoke.

'Take him to the bathroom, give him a good washing and see that he has underwear on him. I want to take him to see Doctor Black and God help him if he's acting the fool, just God help him.'

'Why have I to go to the doctor?' I asked nervously.

'Because you refuse to walk properly.'

'I can't help it Mother, honestly,' I pleaded.

Mother Michael ran the bath while I undressed slowly.

'Hurry up,' she demanded.

There was a lot of steam coming off the water and before getting into it I told her it was too hot.

'In the name of God child, how do you know when you haven't put a finger into it.'

The unfamiliar steam rising from the water scared me. I put one leg over the edge so that just the tips of my toes touched the water, withdrew it quickly and told Mother Michael again that the water was too hot. She took no notice. Using all her strength, she pressed me down until I was up to my armpits in it.

'It's burning me,' I screamed.

She hit me with a wet flannel across the back of the head and told me to be quiet. Only when I persisted crying did she eventually run cold water into the bath, stirring it with circular sweeping movements of her arm. She scrubbed my back with carbolic soap and a rough piece of cloth. I stood up in the bath to allow her to wash my legs. She lost her temper with me when I said that she was hurting me and hit me across the thighs with the cloth. 'You're worse than any two year old. Now get out,' she commanded.

She dried me quickly and gave me a white vest and underpants to wear, all the time urging me to hurry. I was given the suit I wore for my First Communion and a clean pair of socks. She fine-combed my hair with a steel comb which dug into my scalp and when I protested she dug in even harder saying that I probably had a head full of lice.

'Wait here,' Mother Paul ordered, putting her head out the front door to see if the convent car had arrived. Mr O'Rourke was driving. He opened the door and pushed the seat forward to allow me in followed by Mother Paul. The drive was only about two or three minutes and when we got to the house the nun asked the driver to wait. When she wasn't looking the old man winked at me through the open window of the car.

In the doctor's waiting room a man was contentedly puffing his pipe, sending great clouds of smoke towards the low ceiling. When he saw the nun he took off his hat and saluted her, suggesting that she should see the doctor before he did. She accepted the offer and thanked him, before sitting upright in her chair and crossing her hands on her lap. The old man took a newspaper from his coat pocket and unfolded it.

'You don't mind if I read Mother?' he asked.

'Not at all,' she said.

'I see there's talk of putting dogs into outer space,' he said, 'I wonder what they'll be thinking of next?'

'God only knows,' she replied.

'I just hope they know what they're at,' the man said before relighting his pipe.

The surgery door opened and a woman came out bidding the nun good evening as she walked quickly past.

Mother Paul got to her feet and led me in. The doctor was a white haired woman in her mid fifties who wore glasses which she carried around her neck on a golden chain. She had a friendly face and gentle voice. She greeted Mother Paul and then looked at me closely.

'I've often seen this little man serving mass,' she said. 'Isn't that right?'

'Yes,' I replied.

'He's one of the finest altar boys I've seen in the church and a great credit to you. You must be very proud of him Mother.'

'Indeed we are doctor,' the nun replied.

The doctor sat down behind her desk and began to write on a sheet of paper, asking the nun my name and age.

'And what is the problem?' she asked, removing her glasses and allowing them to hang from her neck.

'He's walking with his foot turned in, and he seems to be dragging it along the ground,' Mother Paul said.

'When did you first notice this Mother?'

The nun thought for a minute before replying that she couldn't say for sure, but it had been going on for a good while.

'Can I have a look at your foot Patrick?' the doctor asked. Her voice was gentle and kind.

It took me some time to undo the laces and I could sense the impatience of the nun as the doctor told me to 'take it easy', before she eventually helped me to undo both boots.

'Which foot is it?' she asked.

'This one,' I said, pointing to the left.

Taking my bare foot in her hand she moved it up and down, then in a circular motion, all the time inquiring whether I was experiencing any pain. She checked the right foot, manipulating it in the same manner, asking if I could feel any soreness or discomfort. During the examination my fear and tension must have been obvious to her because I was being constantly reassured.

'Will you walk down the room and back towards me please Patrick?' she asked, watching closely as I did so, then asked me to sit on the couch and let my legs hang over the edge to check my reflexes. She tapped my knee gently with her black rubber triangular hammer and the lower part of my leg shot outwards involuntarily. It was a funny sensation and I laughed. With the same instrument she checked my ankles before instructing me to put my boots and socks on again. As I did I listened to her question Mother Paul.

'How is his health generally?' she asked.

'Fine,' the nun replied, 'He eats well and gets plenty of sleep.'

'Is there any history of disability in his family, anything that you think I should know?'

'No.'

The doctor put her glasses on again and looked over the notes she had written. Then told Mother Paul that she could find nothing wrong. I trembled when I heard this because I knew that my punishment would be severe.

'There is the possibility, Mother, that the child is imitating someone with a limp, perhaps his father or mother, and this is his way of bringing attention to himself. I presume his parents are dead if he is in the orphanage?'

'Yes,' the nun said attentively.

'I think the child is suffering some form of trauma and time will put this matter right. It may well be that he needs reassurance and a great deal of kindness. If either of his parents or someone else close to him had a limp it is quite likely he would imitate that, not out of any sense of mockery or anything.'

'I understand,' Mother Paul said.

She asked was I a nervous child and the nun mentioned my fear of dogs.

'Has he had any bad experience with dogs? Has he been bitten or frightened by a dog?'

'Not that I am aware.'

'Does he have nightmares? Has he ever mentioned his parents?'

'No,' the nun replied, 'but we do encourage the children to pray for their parents every night.'

'I see,' the doctor said. There was a brief silence before she spoke again.

'Just one final question. What did the child's parents die from?'

'An accident,' the nun answered.

'A road accident was it?'

'Yes, doctor.'

This story was different from what I had overheard my aunt saying, but again it made little impact on me at the time.

'Thank you very much Mother, I'd like you to keep a close eye on this little man and bring him back to see me in about a fortnight. We can review the position then.'

The doctor handed me a sweet, wrapped in paper, which she took from the pocket of her white coat. I held it in my hand.

'That's not the place for it, is it?' she asked kindly. 'Are you not going to eat it?'

I undid the wrapper and put the sweet into my mouth, aware that Mother Paul was watching.

'Do you like school?' the doctor asked me.

'Yes,' I replied.

'Are you happy there?'

'Yes.'

She took both my hands in hers and asked me if anyone had ever frightened me, or if I could remember anything terrible ever happening to me. She wondered if anyone had ever beaten or locked me up. I wanted to talk to the doctor, to tell her about the beatings and other punishments given to me by the nuns and about the image of the man hanging that I linked somehow in my mind with my father. I was sure she would believe me but because of the presence of Mother Paul I couldn't speak. Since my parents' death I had been surrounded by a conspiracy of silence. That evening in the doctor's room fear made me an accomplice in it. Looking back I see it as one of the turning points of my life.

Back in St Michael's I played in the yard while the two nuns discussed what had happened at the doctor's. I remember Mother Paul towering over the smaller figure of Mother Michael as they talked. I can only assume that Mother Michael agreed that she was right in lying to the doctor. They must have realized too, that the caretaker, Tom O'Rourke limped, and that it was probably him I was imitating. I think they resolved that day to make a greater effort to ensure I would eliminate from my mind the image of a hanged man because any time I mentioned him now I was caned severely. My constant talking of him turned to a frightened silence.

For a week neither of the nuns took their eyes off me. I was constantly reminded to walk properly by a shout or the threat of being beaten.

As I became more aware of being watched I became more tense and my manner of walking grew distinctly awkward. I was constantly conscious of my foot and nervous of being beaten. My limp got worse.

The nuns decided to seek a second opinion and brought me to another doctor. As I walked towards his surgery Mother Paul grabbed me by the back of my jumper and, in a sharp tempered voice, warned me about walking with my head down, adding that I was bad enough as I was.

The doctor was an elderly man with a red face and a completely bald head. His manner was abrupt and he lacked the sensitivity of the female doctor. After he had inquired from the nun what was wrong with me he made me take off my boots and stockings and walk across the floor.

He inquired whether I had any illness recently and Mother Paul mentioned the measles and the earaches. The doctor spoke to her about polio, reminding her that the country was in the middle of an epidemic of the disease. She assured him that the nuns had warned all the children to keep away from rivers and sewers. The doctor considered for a moment, then told Mother Paul he wanted me admitted to hospital immediately as a precaution. My heart pounded, my breath raced and I could feel tears coming to my eyes. I wanted to plead with him not to send me away, that if he didn't I would do my best to make sure I walked properly.

He wrote a short note which he handed to Mother Paul, instructing her to take me to Cork that evening. Then he telephoned the hospital.

From the doctor's house I was driven back to St Michael's and when we arrived Mother Paul ordered me to stay where I was until she came back. Tom O'Rourke noticed I was crying and he did his best to comfort me by just talking. He took out his pipe and lit it, saying that he didn't like to smoke when the nuns were in the car. As he drew on the pipe I could hear the moisture make a sizzling sound in its stem. After every few pulls he coughed and waved his arm to disperse the smoke.

'I do have to do that,' he said, 'in case the nuns might think the car was on fire.' Then he laughed loudly.

'Begob and d'ye know what it is, I don't think the ould hospital would be all that bad all the same, and sure didn't I hear the nun sayin' that it would be only a week before I'd be going to collect you to bring you back.' I looked deep into the jaundiced eyes of the old man and through my own tears could see he didn't really believe what he was saying. I sobbed and still he tried to comfort me. He looked out the car window to see if Mother Paul was coming.

'Begob they must be having a party in there, she's a good while gone now.'

I drew a deep breath in an effort to stop myself crying and asked him how far away Cork was. He thought for a minute before answering.

'Well I suppose it'll be around the seventy or eighty mile mark,' he answered. 'Sure it could happen that I wouldn't be able to find the hospital at all and then we'd have to come back.'

'How long will it take us to get there?' I asked.

'Three or four hours,' he answered as he looked at his watch. It was getting dark and rain began to fall in tiny droplets on the windscreen. I saw the convent door open and the figure of Mother Paul come out into the grey evening light. Tom O'Rourke noticed her too and pressed his thumb into the bowl of his pipe and put it into his breast pocket then waved his hand towards the open window, urging the smoke to go out.

'Whist,' he said, 'I see herself coming and she has company with her for the prayers. You'd think I was going to kill them on the road.' He got out and opened the door. Mother Paul sat in the back seat beside me while the other nun took the passenger seat. As soon as we moved away, the nun in the front began to say the rosary. Mother Paul responded and encouraged me to join in. I did make an effort, but the sorrow I felt at being taken away from St Michael's would not allow me to.

As it got dark the lights of oncoming cars dazzled me, and the heavy rain made it difficult to see out. The wipers swished from side to side, but the rain was so heavy, they were of little use in keeping the windscreen clear. Halfway through a Hail Mary Mother Paul nudged me in the ribs.

'What are you crying for?' she asked.

'I don't want to go to hospital,' I answered.

'Don't be stupid, thousands of children your age go into hospital every day of the week – most of them much worse off than you are. You should be thanking God that your complaint is just a simple one that will take no time to put right. Now join in the prayers.'

I did my best to join the nuns as they went from one decade of the Rosary to the next and on to the Litany of Saints. Only when the car stopped and they got out to go into a big store did the prayers stop. When they got back in and the engine started they resumed praying.

Coming into Cork city I was amazed by the different colours of lights flashing on advertising boards, particularly by an advertisement for Donnellys Sausages, a neon Don tossing a neon sausage to a neon Nelly. Reading the advertisements and listening to the lilting voices of newspaper sellers distracted me from what was happening and I stopped crying. I had never been outside the Industrial School after dark except to go to the local church to serve at Benediction when the missionary priests were conducting their annual retreat for the local people. Now I was in a city, buses, cars and people. Brightly lit streets and illuminated shop windows with shop models dressed in the latest fashions. Despite the noise of traffic, the voices of the newspaper sellers could be heard through the streets urging people to buy an evening paper.

'Would ye mind if I stopped for a minute Mother?' Tom O'Rourke asked. 'I just want to go into one of the shops to get something.'

'You won't be too long Tom, will you?' Mother Paul said.

He pulled the car in to the edge of the pavement and limped into a shop that had its window and interior brightly lit. I could see him talking to the shop assistant, indicating with his finger that he wanted something from one of the high shelves behind the counter. The girl stood on a small step-ladder and took down a large box which she handed to him. He looked at it for a few seconds before handing it back to her to be wrapped. When he came out of the shop he was carrying a parcel wrapped in brown paper which he put into the car behind his seat and in front of me. He got in and remarked that 'the next problem would be to find the hospital.' He laughed, the nuns didn't.

The Morris Minor stopped outside a red-bricked building with tall Georgian type windows. Light was shining from each of them. A light over the front door shone onto a large brass plate with the words 'Mercy Hospital' etched onto it. Mother Paul stepped from the car and coaxed me out. I hesitated, but eventually followed her.

Going up the rain soaked steps to the entrance of the hospital, I stopped and pleaded with her not to allow them to keep me in but to bring me back to the other boys. Embarrassed by the commotion I was causing she grabbed me firmly by the arm and tried to force me up the steps. I stood absolutely still and I would have run but for the tightness of her grip. Her lips puckered as she became annoyed but it didn't worry me. I knew she couldn't hit me now.

'You are only going to have to stay a couple of days,' she said, stressing each word.

'I don't want to go in there,' I screamed.

'In one week, maybe even less, you'll be coming home to us again,' she promised.

Because I believed that nuns never told lies, I stopped crying and walked slowly up the steps with her holding my arm.

A bespectacled, sharp-featured lady took details from Mother Paul before ringing for a nurse to take me to one of the wards. As she arrived I held onto the nun's black habit and pleaded with her not to leave me there. My knuckles were white as she tried to prise my fingers loose. The nurse bent down to try and lift me into her arms.

'No,' I screamed as loud as I could. 'I don't want to stay here, I want to go home. I don't like this place.'

As the nurse tried to talk to me I shook my head violently from side to side, screaming at her to 'go away', but she persisted and eventually succeeded in lifting me into her arms, telling Mother Paul that I would settle in once she was gone. I watched as the nun opened the main door to walk out. As she did so, Tom O'Rourke walked quickly past her, carrying the parcel he had earlier bought and came towards me. He gave me the present, telling me it would pass the time. I dropped it and put my arms out to him, begging him to take me back to St Michael's with him. Looking him straight in the face, I realized that I loved this man, like a son would love his father. He held my hand tightly in his, and told me that he would probably be staying in Cork for the night because it was too late to return to Waterford. He would be back first thing in the morning to check with the doctors if I could go back with him.

'I want you to be a good lad, I'll be praying for ye and the minute I get the word I will be here to collect ye.'

I was greatly reassured by his words and calmed down considerably. He looked sad as he released my hand, and though I was no longer screaming I still wept uncontrollably. He walked away and stood for a moment at the door with Mother Paul at his side. They waved to me and the nurse tried to get me to wave back, but I couldn't. The heavy doors closed behind them, I shouted after them a last time not to leave me. They did, and though I couldn't have known it at the time and, more importantly, though I was still legally in the nuns' care for the next seven years, I was never to see either of them again nor was I to return to St Michael's School.

A nurse carried me into a ward of about twenty beds. A nun followed dressed in a white habit of the same design as the black ones I had become so used to at St Michael's. In the brightly lit ward I noticed a smell of disinfectant and the chesty coughing of old men, most of whom were watching me curiously. I stood beside my bed waiting for the nurse to get screens so that she could undress me. The castors of the screens made a rattling sound as they were wheeled across the wooden floor. There was a metallic tapping as one section of the tubular steel frame hit against the next. The nun looked crossly at the nurse and said something to her which I could not quite hear. With my view of the ward blocked by the floral patterned screens I got undressed and, with help from the nurse, got into a new pair of pyjamas Mother Paul had bought specifically because I was going into hospital. Once I was in bed the screens were taken away and the bedcovers tightly tucked in. The coughing of old men surrounded me like a besieging army.

CHAPTER EIGHT

After the nurse left I sat up and looked around the ward. Some of the old men slept with their mouths open and snored heavily, others were busy reading their newspapers and smoking cigarettes or pipes. As they smoked, they coughed and spat into stainless steel mugs on top of their bedside lockers, oblivious to the sickening effect it was having on me.

Meals were being served by three girls in deep pink striped uniforms with white starched caps. They pushed trolleys laden with trays each of which had a cup and saucer, a plate and an egg cup. In a rotation system they went around the beds, the first pouring tea, the second bringing milk and sugar and the third carrying buttered bread and a boiled egg. Only by watching the other patients did I know how to manage the egg because I never had one from the shell before.

After the meal one of the nurses went around and asked the patients whether they wanted a bedpan or a bottle. The ones who needed bedpans quickly had their beds screened off while those who wanted a bottle were handed stainless steel receptacles that looked like wine jugs I had seen in a picture bible. I had no idea how to use a bed bottle and when I was offered one I refused, though I did want to go to the toilet. The air filled with the stench of bowel movements and strong urine and took a long time to clear.

As the patients were beginning to settle down for the night and the ward lights had been switched off, I heard the low murmur of a male voice. A doctor stood at the end of my bed, his white coat open and a stethoscope hanging from his neck.

'Is this the boy?' he asked the nurse.

'Yes doctor,' she answered.

He asked that screens be brought to the bed as he held my wrist to take my pulse, glancing occasionally at his watch until he was satisfied that sufficient time had elapsed, before letting go my hand and moving to the end of my bed to write something on a chart that hung there.

Without warning he threw back the bedcovers and, with the assistance of the nurse, removed my pyjamas so that I was completely naked. I was cold, embarrassed and very nervous as his hands probed various parts of my body in search of any area that was sore. He first tapped my chest with his fingers asking me to say 'ninety-nine'. I felt stupid when he asked me to continue repeating this as he tapped on my back. Through his stethoscope he listened to my chest and back, asking me to take deep breaths, hold them and let them out slowly. Next he checked all my reflex points, never speaking as each of my limbs jumped involuntarily at the very light impact of his triangular rubber hammer. He pressed the glands around my throat and under my arms inquiring if I was feeling any soreness, then checked between my legs for swelling which would indicate the presence of infection. He rotated each of my feet and, asking me to relax, moved them up and down, before holding them firmly and asking me to push against him. After each check, he wrote on my chart.

'Do you feel sore anywhere?' he asked.

'Just a little bit here,' I said, pointing to my stomach.

As soon as his hand pressed on my abdomen I squirmed in discomfort.

'Have you been to the toilet lately?' he asked.

'Before I left St Michael's,' I answered.

He cast his eyes upward and asked the nurse to bring a bottle to me before leaving. I looked down on my nakedness and at the screens surrounding me and wished I could have been polishing boots in the Industrial School.

I was crying when the screen squeaked open and the nurse

returned, carrying a stainless steel bottle covered with a cloth.

'I want you to use this for me,' she said and handed me the bottle. I looked from her to it and wondered what I was supposed to do.

'Have you ever used one of these before?' she asked.

'No,' I answered.

'Put it down between your legs and pass water into it.'

When I did get to put the bottle between my bare legs it was freezing cold. I shivered and though I managed to get my penis into it, I could not relax enough to use it. When she realized nothing was happening, the nurse became impatient and raised her voice slightly.

'Concentrate hard on what you are supposed to be doing,' she said.

Eventually I began to urinate, at first only in a trickle but then more forcefully as I relaxed. My penis slipped from the bottle and soaked the bed despite my own best efforts to control it. She grabbed it and stuck it quickly back into the bottle, annoyed that she would have to change the sheets and, as she left to get dry ones, told me to put my pyjamas back on.

She remade the bed and tucked me in tightly suggesting that I get off to sleep after my long journey. 'You'll be feeling much better in the morning,' she said as she took away the screens. She noticed I was crying and had taken my arms out from under the covers to cross them on my chest.

'What's the matter?' she asked.

'I don't want to go to sleep with my hands under the covers.' I answered.

'Why not?'

'Because the nuns said it was a sin.'

She smiled and told me that she always slept with her hands under her bedclothes and never committed a sin.

'What other nonsense did those nuns tell you?' she asked.

'They said I had to sleep with my hands crossed, because I might die while I was asleep.'

'Put your hands under the covers. I promise you won't

commit a sin, and you definitely won't die. Everyone sleeps with their hands inside the bedclothes and they're not dead, are they?' she said, smiling.

'No,' I replied, as she tucked me in again. I kept my hands covered until I was sure she was gone. Then I took them out and crossed them as I had done for so many nights of my life. Eventually I went to sleep.

On the first morning of my stay in Cork breakfast was served early and immediately afterwards the nurses began to rush about tidying beds. Some patients complained that they only had a few hours sleep. One man who was particularly contrary remarked: 'You'd swear it was the Pope of Rome himself that was coming.'

'Now, Mr O'Brien, there's no need for that,' a nurse said good humouredly.

'Consultants be damned,' the patient retorted.

'You'd be in a bit of a mess if there weren't any.'

'Bejasus, I wonder about that,' he said acidly.

'Watch the language, Mr O'Brien. We have a young child in the ward now.'

He grunted and turned on his side in an attempt to ignore what was happening.

The bustle that went on before a consultant visited a ward was something that I was to become used to as my time in hospital progressed. Floors were swept, ashtrays removed from bedside locker tops and cleaned. Every bed was freshly made up so that it would be easy to turn back the covers should the doctor require it. Charts, medical notes and x-rays were left on bedtables, carefully positioned at the foot of each bed. Outside the ward I heard the shuffling of feet and the muffled sound of voices. A senior nurse opened the doors and a tall good looking man in his mid fifties came in followed by a group of about twelve students. I watched as he walked around the beds, his voice deep and loud as he inquired from a patient about his health, then muted slightly as he discussed something with the nurse in charge of the ward.

The consultant and his students came to my bedside. He asked the nurse when I had been admitted and where

I had come from and read the letter of referral brought to the hospital by Mother Paul. Then he invited one of the students to examine me and offer a diagnosis. The other students formed a semi-circle with the consultant behind them, watching closely. My pyjamas were removed and the student checked my reflexes, pulse and breathing. He took a pin from the lapel of his white coat and told me to close my eyes. As he touched me with it, I had to say whether he was using the pointed or the blunt end. Next, I had to stretch out each arm and, with my eyes shut, bring my index finger to touch the tip of my nose. He asked which was 'the bad foot' then took a bunch of keys from his pocket and dragged one of them along my left sole, causing my toes to turn down.

'Do you have any pain?' he asked.

'No,' I said.

'Do you remember ever twisting your foot while playing?'

'No.'

'Did you ever have a bad fall?'

'No.'

'What about pins and needles, did you ever have them?'

'No,' I answered again.

The consultant came to the bedside and squeezed the calf muscles of each leg, before asking his student for a diagnosis.

I vividly recall him saying 'Post Polio'. The consultant and the students discussed whether the diagnosis was accurate, and though there appeared to be some disagreement among them initially, the consultant agreed with the student. He did say it was nothing serious, and that physiotherapy would help. Before moving away he said he expected I would be able to go home within a month. A nurse helped me back into my pyjamas, and remade my bed. Though I was not being allowed home at once, I was comforted by the fact that I would be out of the hospital within four weeks, having no reason to doubt the word of a doctor.

I unwrapped the parcel Tom O'Rourke had given me. It was a jigsaw of over a thousand pieces. The picture on the box was of a tall ship sailing through enormous waves with its sails fully blown. One of the nurses brought me a table which she felt would be big enough to accommodate its size. I opened the box and spilled all the pieces out, fumbling through them for any two that would fit together. I was becoming frustrated and was just about to put it all back in its box, when another nurse offered to help. First, she said, I should find all the pieces with a straight edge, and demonstrated what she meant. Then when I had all these together I could start to make up the jigsaw.

I did as she said and was delighted when I had a string of more than ten pieces. Whenever any of the staff had time they would add a few more pieces, until eventually the picture began to form. The blue and white of the clouds, and the deeper blue of the sea. Huge foaming waves beating off the side of the ship. Working for hours each day on the jigsaw passed the time, and after three weeks it was eventually finished. I was proud of it and took great care to ensure it would not be accidently broken. Staff who helped boasted about the part they played in its assembly.

It was at night that I missed St Michael's most. I missed the sounds of the other children sleeping, the jangle of the nuns' bell ringing to get me out of bed to use the pot. The sounds in the ward were totally different to what I had been used to. Eerie groans of men in pain or snoring loudly. The familiar red glow from the perpetually burning bulb at the feet of the Sacred Heart statue was replaced by a cold white fluorescent light shining through the glass partition between the corridor and the ward. When I could not sleep I prayed. Not the prayers I had been taught in Industrial School, but prayers I made up. I begged God to make me better so I could leave hospital, promising that I would never sin again if he granted my prayer. Because I had associated hospital with death I also begged to be allowed to live. The first thing I did every morning was to thank God for not allowing me to die during the night.

I hated Sundays in hospital. They began with the night

nurses waking the patients very early to prepare them for receiving holy communion. Beds had to be made, patients washed and shaved. Anything on top of a locker was either removed from the ward altogether or placed inside it. Despite protests from some of the men, old newspapers were thrown out. A nun prayed loudly, as she moved up and down the ward, prodding anyone who appeared to be drifting off to sleep. 'Lord Jesus,' she intoned, in a manner designed more to keep people awake than to pray, 'make us worthy to receive you.' Despite this, it was not unusual for someone to snore loudly during prayers, a source of embarrassment to the nun and the man who had to be woken by her. The arrival of the priest was heralded by the gentle ringing of a bell carried by a nun who walked some twenty or thirty feet ahead of him. Again anyone verging on sleep was quickly woken to take communion.

After breakfast, silence had to be maintained as the patients waited for Mass to be broadcast on Radio Eireann. The voice of a priest came from a large wooden radio on a shelf in a corner of the ward. Many of the men fixed their eyes on its illuminated circular dial as the priest reminded his listeners that the Mass they were about to hear was for those who were sick in hospital, and for those who through no fault of their own, could not attend church for the Holy Sacrifice. They took well-worn black covered missals from their bedside lockers and followed the Mass reverently. On one occasion, I remember someone turned on the radio thinking they were listening to Mass. It was a Protestant service being broadcast on the BBC, at which the nun in charge took great exception, saying that we shouldn't be listening to it at all before abruptly turning it off.

For an hour in the afternoon relatives and friends of the patients came to visit them. Nearly all carried paper bags filled with fruit or biscuits, as well as Lucozade or orange to drink. I watched the visitors and often eavesdropped on their conversations. Children were strictly forbidden to enter the wards as visitors, they had to wait down in the hall or out in a car. It was not unusual to see a man in bed pleading with the sister in charge to allow his sons or daughters in to see him. Rules were rules, and such demands were very seldom granted. Some people took a chance on 'smuggling' children in to see their fathers or grandfathers. Once caught, they were ushered from the ward by an orderly. Wives dutifully went through their husbands bedside lockers, removing fruit that was beginning to rot. Pyjamas for washing were taken away and replaced by freshly ironed ones, and a check was made on the toilet bags to ensure there was enough soap and sharp razor blades. The absence of visitors around my bed aroused curiosity among the patients and their visitors. They would come and talk to me, bringing a bar of chocolate or a packet of crisps before they inquired where I was from and what I was in the hospital for.

'It's a long way for your poor mother and father to have to come,' one lady said.

'They're dead,' I said, not realizing the impact it would have on her. After a momentary silence she asked me where I lived.

'In an Industrial School.'

She left my bedside and returned to the person she had come to visit. I knew they were talking about me because they stared in unison, with shocked expressions. When they noticed me looking at them, they smiled and I smiled back. Whenever people asked what had happened to me, I told them confidently that I had Post Polio.

'Are you getting better?' they would ask.

'Yes,' I always replied, though I was unsure if I was or not. Their advice was always the same.

'Don't forget to say your prayers and remember that God is good.'

The end of visiting hour was signalled by a nurse walking through the ward ringing a heavy brass bell and smiling at people as she told them politely that 'time was up'. Many took no notice until a more senior nurse came in and virtually ordered them out. Gradually they left. I often saw a weeping wife holding onto her husband's hand for as long as she could, wondering out loud when would he be 'right'.

As she'd leave she'd pull a white handkerchief from her coat pocket and wipe her eyes, her sorrow infectious. Her husband's eyes would also fill with tears as he urged her to go with a wave of his hand.

During my third week in hospital, I wrote to Mother Paul and told her I was looking forward to coming home. I asked her to tell all the boys that I was asking for them and mentioned that I was praying for her and the other nuns every night and looking forward to seeing them all soon again. One of the nurses posted the letter for me and every morning when the letters were given out to the other patients on the ward I waited for a reply. None ever came.

Three weeks became four and I had settled into the routine of the hospital. I became accustomed to bedpans and bottles and had even grown used to the doctors as they went on their 'rounds', although I did worry that one day they might decide to do surgery on me. The idea of having an operation terrified me, and I hoped I would never be taken to theatre. Too often I had seen screens being drawn around a bed or a 'fasting' sign hung up. Whenever there was someone for an operation, an air of tension gripped the ward. A sense of fear among the other patients. The radio was turned down so low it was almost impossible to hear. There was a sense of urgency in the manner the nurses came and went from behind the cordoned-off bed. No sooner had someone been told that they were being 'taken down', than a nun rushed to his bedside wondering if he would like the hospital chaplain to hear his confession. I never knew anyone who refused. As I grew older in hospital, I came to know these nuns as The God Squad.

Despite intensive physiotherapy there was no real improvement in the way I walked. When the consultant asked me to walk across the ward after four weeks I did my utmost to get my foot into its proper position. He expressed openly his disappointment at the failure of the exercises he had been so confident of bringing success, and looked at me apologetically before writing a short note which the ward sister put into an envelope.

Later that day when a nurse came to my bedside and told me to get dressed, I sensed something was about to happen. I wanted to be told that I was going back to St Michael's but my instincts told me otherwise. A nun approached me as I sat dressed on a wooden chair beside the bed and remarked on how nice I looked in my suit. I wanted to ask where I was going and yet didn't want to know. She smiled broadly and told me that I was being sent to a hospital nearer the school.

I immediately broke down and in desperation asked why I had to be moved. I had settled into the hospital. It had taken the place of St Michael's in my life. I was becoming used to its routine, its sounds and its smells. It had become my home. As I wept the nun tried to persuade me I would be much happier, before telling me that I would only be in the other hospital for a week. When I asked what would happen if my foot didn't get better then, she replied confidently that it would.

For the first time in almost four weeks I walked with my boots and socks on. I went to the table where my jigsaw had been since it was completed. I began to take it apart, first piece by piece, then in bigger chunks, before eventually scooping the remainder into its box. Then I put the box into a bag given to me by one of the patients. I sat by my bed waiting for the ambulance to arrive.

In the heat of the ward my grey suit was too warm and my black boots felt heavy and tight on my feet. I opened the laces and did not tie them again until it was time to leave.

An elderly woman wearing a heavy blue cape with red straps criss-crossed over the front of her striped uniform entered the ward and spoke to the nurse on duty. They both walked to where I was seated and the nurse handed her a paper bag containing my pyjamas and toiletries.

'What about his chart?' the older woman asked.

The nurse had forgotten it and followed us down to the ambulance with the record of my stay in the Mercy Hospital.

I began my journey in the ambulance seated on what appeared to be a stretcher. The small panes of frosted glass allowed little light in and the air was still and stuffy. An opaque sliding glass panel separated the interior of the ambulance from the driver and there were two small windows in the back with a red letter 'A' stenciled to them. The elderly nurse sat opposite me and tapped on the window behind the driver to start up. It was not possible to see through the windows and the only sense of movement was the motion of the ambulance over the rough road. Not long into the journey I began to feel sick and told her so.

'Take some deep breaths,' she said.

I did. But to no avail. As I retched and began to vomit, she banged on the glass shouting at the driver to stop. She stooped under the stretcher to get a bowl and I got sick on her cape. She was furious and referred to me as stupid. When the driver opened the back doors to let me out she shouted at him for not stopping sooner. She stepped out onto the country road, brushing her cape down with a towel she had taken from the ambulance.

'Get out child,' she said to me, angrily.

As soon as she set foot on the road she made me turn towards the ditch and told me to get sick into it. I became very distressed at being unable to control the vomiting and at being referred to as stupid and silly.

'Take plenty of deep breaths,' she said.

I opened my mouth and sucked in the fresh country air. She hit me across the back of the head.

'You're not supposed to breath in through your mouth, you eejit,' she said. 'It's in through your nose and out through your mouth.'

She demonstrated what she meant and after a few minutes I felt much better though I was shivering from the cold.

'I have a good mind to belt him again,' she said to the driver, 'just look at the state of me and he's no better. How are we supposed to put up with this all the way to Waterford? Are you finished?' she asked me.

'I think so,' I said.

'You better be sure, because I don't want a repeat of this episode.'

Just fifteen minutes after we resumed the journey I was vomiting again and the nurse was shouting to the driver. He stopped immediately and rushed to the back doors. I was dragged from the ambulance and held with my head bent over a low wall.

'Jesus in Heaven,' she said, 'what in the name of God is wrong with this lad that he can't go more than a few yards without throwing up all over the place?'

'Maybe he'd be better in the front with me, it's not as stuffy and he would have something to look out at. That would keep him occupied and maybe prevent him being sick.'

'You know well,' she said to the driver, 'that I am not allowed to have patients in the front.'

'Well, please yourself,' he retorted. 'But it's either that or carry on as we are.'

When the journey resumed, I was put into the front of the ambulance with the driver and nurse. He had the window open and the fresh air made me feel a lot better than I had in the back. I was able to see the fields and the houses in the small villages we sped through. The hedges on either side of the road rushed by occasionally giving way to flat green fields where cattle grazed. In the distance I could see the spire of a church and I asked the driver where it was.

'It's beside the hospital that we have to get to,' he answered, the nurse adding that it wasn't a minute too soon. As the ambulance drove through the town, it appeared to me that everyone was staring at me through the windscreen. I felt as if I was doing something wrong.

The hospital in Waterford was clealy visible from the town. Its stoney grey colour and shape stood drearily against the half light of evening, and its large black barred windows gave it the appearance of a prison. Hurriedly, the nurse got me out of the ambulance and left me at the admissions section of the hospital without even saying goodbye. Inside, the hospital was as drab and dreary as it appeared from outside. The corridors were high, narrow and dimly lit. Ancient people sat in rows on wooden benches along the sides of the corridors, many of them muttering to themselves while others rocked back and forth in their chairs, totally oblivious to anything happening around them. A few shouted obscenities at passing nurses who didn't take the slightest notice. But it was the appearances of these old people that frightened me most. They held cigarettes between feeble, gnarled fingers and, when they inhaled, coughed weak chesty coughs. Some sat slumped in chairs, their heads to one side and their mouths wide open, revealing toothless gums. The only evidence of life was a continuous dribble onto their dark brown dressing gowns.

A nurse came to take me to the ward, and as she took my hand, I protested, saying I didn't want to stay in the hospital. She ignored me and led me into a ward of ten beds. All the patients there were over sixty and probably much older. Like those I had seen on the benches of the corridors some coughed, some slept and others spoke out loud to no one in particular. Most of them were unshaven and looked dirty. One man smiled at me, saying that I was the youngest old man he had ever seen, before he broke down into a horrible chesty laugh that I was frightened by.

The nurse gave me a pair of oversized pyjamas but I didn't protest. She rolled up the sleeves and the legs until she was satisfied that they were a reasonable fit. Then she folded my own clothes and told me that she was going to put them away in a locker until I needed them again. I asked her when that would be, seeking reassurance that I would not be kept too long in this geriatric environment, but she didn't reply.

Beside me an unshaven man complained bitterly about the pain he was in and wished aloud for God to take him. When he wasn't praying for deliverance he used to talk to me about when he was my age, all the running, the jumping and the climbing of trees. He looked sad and pathetic there, barely able to breathe and unable to sit up in bed without the aid of many pillows pushed under his back and sometimes two or three nurses to hold him.

'Where is it ye hail from?' he asked and became impatient when I didn't answer immediately.

'What part of the country are ye from?' he asked again.

113

'Cappoquin,' I answered.

'I know it well, I used to sell cattle at the market there and many's the pig I brought to the bacon factory. What about the big school that's there? D'ye know that?'

'I live there,' I said.

'All belonging to ye must be dead so, are they?'

'I have an uncle and he lives in Wexford.'

'What part?'

'I don't really know.'

'What was it they died from?' he asked.

'A car crash,' I answered.

'It's not so bad when ye have someone all the same. Will ye be in long?' he asked.

'They told me I'd be staying a week.'

He laughed. 'That's what they told me twelve months ago when I came in and there isn't a sight of me getting out.'

Then he sighed deeply and turned his head away saying that the only way he would get out of hospital would be feet first, 'in a wooden suit'.

It was difficult to sleep at night. The coughing, the ravings of a man out of his mind or the sound of a priest imparting the last rites broke the stillness. It was the regularity of death in the hospital which had the most profound and frightening effect on me. I spent a week there, and during it I experienced what death meant for the first time in my life. In seven days, five or six people died. The ritual became familiar, silence in the ward, the radio turned off, the deep voice of a priest invoking God's blessing on the soul of the dead person and a plea to God that he would see fit to take that patient, who had suffered in pain, to his right hand in Heaven where he would live for ever and ever.

Once the corpse had been taken from the ward the other beds were shifted around. The men joked with whoever was nearest the door, that it was their turn next. They referred to it as 'Death's Door'. For some reason I decided that what they were joking about was in fact true and became increasingly worried as I moved closer to the door. I prayed hard remembering the words of the nuns in the dormitory each night before I went to sleep: 'You never know the day or the hour when God will call, and you must always be ready with your soul as white as white can be.' Any black marks would mean eternal damnation.

The way nurses and doctors reacted to death was a source of confusion to me, I could not come to terms with their laughter from behind the screened-off bed, it all seemed so irreverent and disrespectful, and it was not until I was older that I realized that this was to hide how they were really feeling.

While I was frightened by the death of an individual, the men in the ward didn't appear too upset. They joined in the prayers for the soul departed and remained silent until the dead body had been removed from the ward. Once that was done, one of them would pull a bottle of Guinness out of his locker and uncork it while the others gathered around his bed like a bunch of children planning a mischievous deed. In turn they put the neck of the brown bottle to their wrinkled lips and swallowed hard, gasping pleasurably. If a nurse appeared, the bottle quickly disappeared beneath the bedcovers until she was gone. When it was empty they rolled it in as many sheets of newspaper as they could find and left it in a bin at one end of the ward.

In the mornings a man came around the wards selling newspapers and almost all of the men took one from him, even those who looked so frail that it was hard to imagine that they could read at all. They studied the racing page and discussed among themselves the form of the horses and what kind of money they were prepared to bet on them. Heated discussions took place about how good or bad jockeys and horses were. After all the debate the bets were written out on pieces of paper and given to the porter in charge of the ward who would place them when going to the shops to get messages for the patients. When the money for the bets had been added up, a few shillings was added for him as a token of appreciation. In the evening they listened attentively to the radio waiting for the results and, as they came through, marked their newspapers. Those who lost cursed the horse or the jockey, though usually the horse, describing it as a 'three legged ould nag only fit for the knackers yard'.

One week after I arrived in St Joseph's I was told to be ready for the ambulance which was to take me to a hospital in Kilkenny. It was another upset in my life but I was becoming used to it, resigned to moving from place to place, not even bothering to ask nurse or doctor whether I was ever going to come back. I shook the hands of each of the patients before I left and they wished me well. As I was saying goodbye to one of the nurses, she told me that the new hospital I was going to would be much nicer than the one I was leaving. There would be children there. As the ambulance doors were being shut she shouted to me to write to her. I said I would, then realized that I didn't know her name. I was sick many times during the journey but the nurse in attendance didn't seem to mind and by the time I reached Kilkenny I was exhausted from retching and vomiting.

The hospital in Kilkenny was of modern design and completely different to any other I had been in previously. It was a single-storey building spread out among the green fields of the countryside. I was admitted and brought down a long glass-walled corridor to the childrens' ward, where I was welcomed by a friendly faced nurse who took me to a room with just one bed. It had large glass doors looking out across fields towards the spires of Kilkenny city. Once a chart had been made out for me, I was helped to undress and put into bed. The room was quiet and from down the corridor I could hear the voices of the other children shouting and playing. I asked if I would be allowed into the childrens ward but the nurse said I would have to wait. 'The hospital is new and we have very few patients yet. When things become a bit more organized we will decide what to do with you. How is that?'

'Fine,' I told her.

I found the solitude of the room disturbing and as each day passed and I was not brought into the main ward I became more and more anxious. The only time I was moved was if the weather was fine when the big doors of the room were opened and my bed was pushed out onto the veranda.

During my first weeks in Kilkenny doctors spent a great deal of time examining me, listening to my chest and heart, moving my foot about, testing reflexes and doing the other examinations I had become used to. They asked me many questions, a lot of which, about parents, relations and brothers or sisters, I didn't understand or simply had no answers to. I became frightened that I would be operated on and, with this in mind, always answered in a way which I felt would deter them from taking me to the theatre. I dreaded the idea of being put to sleep, to me it meant certain death.

I found being alone very difficult. I was nine years old and had been used to company for as long as I could remember. Now the days were empty except for the occasional visit of a nurse, a doctor or one of the domestic staff serving meals. The company of sick and dying adults was preferable to the loneliness of my room. The isolation frightened me and convinced me more than ever that I was going to die. It is possible that I was kept separate from the other children because of the stigma attached to being an orphan, or more likely, because of the danger that my condition, as yet undiagnosed, might be contagious.

At night time, the anxiety I felt during the day turned to sheer terror. The image of the hanged man returned to torment and terrorize me. When the fear became unbearable I would scream loudly to get attention and was always greatly relieved by the presence of a nurse, even though their attitudes to me varied greatly. Some tried to find out why I was so frightened and though I wanted to tell them I felt certain they would not believe me. Others became annoyed and demanded that I stop making a racket.

I would turn and twist in bed, trying desperately to get to sleep and away from the fear, but there was no escape, no release. I sweated profusely and often sat up in bed with my knees gripped firmly in my arms. Somehow this position gave me a degree of comfort. To try and sleep I used to kneel in bed and bury my head under the covers with my forehead pressed tightly against my knees. By adopting this position I could muffle my frightened cries and relax my tense body.

Whenever I was fourd like this I was made to lie down and once I had been tucked tightly into bed I was left alone with the room door slightly ajar. With the silence, the fear returned so that I spent many nights in terror and was always greatly relieved to see the dawn break.

CHAPTER NINE

My nightly terror continued as the weeks dragged on in Kilkenny. Each night out of a deep fear of dying, I begged God's forgiveness for any sins I had committed and prayed fervently for a cure and a return to St Michael's and the nuns. The light from the corridor shone through the mottled glass of the door. Whenever I heard footsteps outside or saw a shadow pass I cried aloud hoping to be heard. I couldn't find a position that was comfortable. Finally when complete exhaustion overcame me I'd scream. I didn't care what the nurses said to me anymore, I was too terrified to, and besides even a bad tempered nurse was better than the image of the hanging man. One night, a month after I arrived, the night nurse came in.

'What's wrong with you?' she asked, trying to hide her irritation.

'I can't sleep,' I sobbed.

'If you're tired you can sleep.'

'I am tired, I am tired, but I can't sleep,' I pleaded.

'Then there must be something wrong with you?' she said, becoming more annoyed.

I wanted desperately to talk to someone who would understand the agony I was enduring and the awful fears that were my constant companions. I wanted her to understand the reality of the image I was seeing with increasing regularity. If I could do that she might understand why I was so distressed and anxious. Then I remembered the nuns and how they described what I was seeing as nonsense. Why should a nurse be any different? Because I said nothing which would have led her to understand why I had screamed the nurse told me to stop being ridiculous and to count sheep. I didn't even know what she meant and as she left the room I pressed my face down into the mattress and cried.

Later when she checked and found me still awake and distressed, she returned with a doctor. He placed his hand on my sweating forehead.

'What are you frightened of?' he asked.

'I don't like being on my own,' I said.

He told the nurse that I was hysterical about something and she agreed.

'Has he said anything?' he inquired.

'Nothing.'

He asked again what was frightening me but again I couldn't tell him. He asked the nurse for my chart, wrote on it and told her to give me two Phenobarbitone tablets immediately, and to keep me on that dosage three times a day. Within minutes the nurse returned with a tumbler of water and two capsules which she handed to me. One at a time I put them into my mouth and swallowed them with the aid of a drink.

'Now, I don't want to hear another sound out of you,' she said as she held the bedcovers aloft to allow me to get down under them before tucking me in. 'Off to sleep,' she said, leaving the room and closing the door gently behind her.

It was dinner time next day before I woke. I was groggy and didn't feel like eating the meal offered to me, but the nurses persisted until eventually I began to eat and as I did so I became more conscious of my surroundings. I felt relaxed, no longer afraid of the room or of dying. The sun shone through the large glass doors, warming the room and its brightness made it difficult for me to open my eyes properly.

When I had finished eating I asked a nurse if I could write a letter adding that I did not have either a pen or paper. She returned with a blue writing pad, matching envelopes and a biro which she said she was lending to me on condition I took good care of it and gave it back when I was finished. I addressed the letter and wrote:

Dear Mother Paul,
I hope you are well as I am myself thank God. I pray for you and all the other nuns every night and I also pray for all the boys.

I would be grateful if you would send me the anual my
uncle gave me when I was on holidays as I am in a room on
my own and I get lonely for something to do. In case you
cannot find the anual, Mother Michael left it on top of the
press in the classroom.
I remain,
Yours truly,
Patrick Doyle.

I decided to wait and show the letter to the nurse who
had given me the writing materials before putting it in the
envelope. She read it quickly and remarked that although there
were one or two mistakes, she doubted that anyone would
even notice them. Before I could say anything, she had the
letter in her pocket with a stamp affixed, ready for posting.

It was nearly a fortnight before a reply came from Sister
Paul. Her letter arrived in a brown envelope with a black harp
printed on the front. In the bottom left hand corner the words
'St Michael's Industrial School, Cappoquin', were printed in
black lettering between two thin black lines. The nurse who
had posted my letter stood by the bedside as I opened the
envelope. The reply was short.

Dear Pat,
I got your recent letter and I am glad to know that you are
praying for us all here. Your writing is not as good as it should
be and I expect that it will improve before you write again.
At the moment I am very busy and cannot find the book
you asked for. I am disappointed that you could not spell
annual right.
Good Bye,
God Bless,
Mother Paul.

I showed the letter to the nurse and I'm certain she said
'bitch' as she read it. It was the last time I was to hear
anything from St Michael's Industrial School or from any of
the nuns in it, although, their legal responsibility for me as
ordered by the courts did not end until the 19th of May, 1967.

I had spent a long time, perhaps a year, in a room on my own before I was eventually moved out into a ward with other children. It was a move I had looked forward to, but one I was to deeply regret. This was the period in my life when I felt most alone and came to realize fully the stigma of being orphaned. Some of the children delighted in my never having visitors, and jeered me about being an orphan, and about how my ears stuck out. When I cried they used to throw wet face cloths at me. Isolation was better than almost constant taunting. I'd scream at them to leave me alone, but they continued until a nurse reprimanded them, and told me I was worse to be taking any notice of them.

I hated night time, the drugs I had become dependant on no longer had the effect they used to. Death figured again in my life, and though I didn't actually see any images of a hanged man this time, I was always terrified they would appear and I realized that this fear would be another cause for the children to mock me. I used to sleep hunched in a ball, my knees flexed under me, my head bent down with my forehead resting on them and my face pressed tightly to my thighs to muffle my crying. Nurses repeatedly reminded me that I was nine years old, no different from any other child, and that I should act my age. When I complained about being pelted with wet cloths and called names, they paid little attention. As the dosage of medication I received was increased it became easier to cope with what was happening around me. The price was addiction to drugs, an addiction that would cause me much suffering and take years to overcome.

For an hour every Wednesday the ward was quiet while 'Hospitals' Requests' was on Radio Eireann, with each patient hoping to have a request played for them. When one was played and the names of parents and relatives read out, there was always some jeering. Good natured banter about the name of a father or an uncle often turned into a vicious row with things being thrown across the ward by two combatants. I remember one boy having a request played from his mother, father, his uncle Dick and aunt Mary, which immediately brought a chorus of; 'Mammy, Daddy, Uncle Dick, went to

London on a stick, the stick broke, what a joke, Mammy, Daddy, Uncle Dick.' It was strange events like this that brought a sense of reality to the sterile atmosphere of the hospital. Children would act as they might in normal circumstances, physical barriers such as plaster of paris on broken arms or fractured legs could not restrain anger or dampen furious tempers. One evening as two boys, both almost completely paralysed, were having a game of chess, one accused the other of cheating. Both had only the slightest use of their arms, and as they threatened to kill each other, they moved their wheelchairs as close together as they could. Then slowly, each managed to get his hand to his head, by using his fingers to make it 'walk' up his body. With a swear, each allowed their paralysed arms to fall, as a dead weight, on the other. There was never the slightest chance of injury being inflicted and the physical effect of receiving a blow was nothing like as exhausting as that of raising a limb.

The chief consultant in the hospital, was a small, chubby, sallow-skinned man with steel-grey hair neatly combed in waves back from his forehead. His hands were said to have been blessed by Pope Pious XII. I often heard adults talking of the great healing powers he had in those hands. When he did his 'rounds' and came to my bed I was always afraid, certain that one day he would decide that an operation was the only way to straighten my foot. My nervousness was obvious, I became tense and fidgety, my breath came fast and I sweated a lot. Whenever he examined me he always did his best to relax me. In my early days at that hospital his examinations were never intense, the most he did was to hold my foot in his hand and move it about gently, but as time went on and he became less and less satisfied with my rate of progress, he became more thorough in his effort to discover what could be wrong.

One Thursday, he examined me in a manner he had not done before. He pricked my foot with a pin, asking me to close my eyes and tell him if I could feel its point. He checked my breathing, and made me follow his finger with my eyes as he moved it slowly across my line of vision. 'Good,' he said as I managed all the tests put to me. Then he asked me to stand out on the floor. The parquet wood felt cool beneath my feet and momentarily I was reminded of the times I used to throw off my boots and socks in St Michael's and run across the field that separated the convent from nearby agricultural land. As I stood, he said he was going to push me and I was to do my best not to let him knock me down. With his first push on my chest, I rocked back on my heels and it required the swift movement of a nurse to prevent me falling. I was caught unaware by the suddenness of the move and I said so. Before he attempted the same thing again, he asked if I was ready. I was. Putting both feet firmly on the floor, I hardly moved, except for a slight swaying initially. Back in bed, he asked me to perform tasks I had done before. I experienced no difficulty in doing anything asked of me and the consultant praised me for that. I was so anxious to impress that when he asked me to walk across the ward, I tripped and almost fell. I steadied myself and slowly began to walk across the room looking down at my feet as I went along, each step being taken slowly and deliberately.

'Don't look down at your feet as you walk,' he said as I returned to where he was standing, adding, 'don't be afraid to walk, you won't fall, try moving a bit faster.'

Standing back from the bed he spoke to those around him, junior doctors, nurses and the ward sister. He could find nothing physically wrong, no evidence of paralysis or muscle wastage. Yes, there was a slight inversion of the foot but it was nothing serious as far as he was concerned. He asked the nurse in charge to have me measured for a splint, a steel bar that would be strapped around my leg below the knee and run down the outside of the lower leg into a hole in the heel of a new pair of boots which were also to be ordered. This he hoped would pull my foot outward and eventually rectify the problem. As the consultant wrote on my chart I heard him inquiring about my parents. The most senior nurse pointed to a piece of paper and said that I was a 'Ward of the State'. It was the first time I had been referred to as such. He wondered how my parents died, adding that he presumed they were dead.

He was assured they were, but the circumstances were not

altogether clear, though she presumed 'natural causes'. The consultant wondered at what age the deaths occurred and he was given my date of birth and the date I was committed to the Industrial School. He remained silent as the nurse told him that I cried a lot and had great difficulty in getting to sleep at night. When she was asked if I had ever spoken about what was distressing me, she replied that I had not. He then asked what medication I was on.

'Phenobarbitone,' the nurse said, 'it has calmed him a great deal.' He thought for a while, expressed his dislike of Phenobarbitone, but added that if it was helping it should be continued. Before moving away, he requested the nurse to try and obtain whatever information there was on myself and my family. She made a note of it and slipped it into the brown folder containing my medical records. He pinched me gently on the cheek and told me not to worry about anything. 'We'll have you right in no time at all.' I felt confident enough to ask him if I would have to have an operation.

'Why?' he asked.

I hesitated for a moment before telling him I was afraid of operations.

'You don't worry about operations, you won't have to have one.'

I felt so happy that day that I decided to write to my uncle, telling him I was in hospital and asking him to come and see me or to send something I could play with. If he wasn't able to get a game, I asked him to send some money, saying that I would buy something myself. No sooner had I given the letter to a nurse to post than I was sorry for writing it. My uncle had not been a part of my life since I last saw him on the day he left me back to the school from my aunt's. I worried about him writing to the nuns to tell them I was begging.

I had become particularly friendly with a fat round faced boy from Kilkenny, whom some of the others called 'Fatso', a name he hated and which caused him to issue the fiercest of threats to those guilty.

'I'll break your fucking neck,' he used to say, 'as soon as I can get out of this plaster.'

He was older than most of the other boys by about two years

125

and was in hospital to have his leg straightened at the knee. He had had surgery and was in plaster of paris. He liked to read and chew sweets or gum, if he could get it without the nurses knowing. He was an avid radio listener and, with his guitar, used to mimic Cliff Richard or Elvis Presley. Occasionally he tried to play some of the instrumentals which the Shadows had made popular at that time. 'Apache' was his favourite. He hated anyone to touch the instrument, anyone who did was warned that they would end up with their necks in plaster. Somehow, I looked on him as the one person who would take my side when all the others were jeering me, and though he was immobile I was satisfied that he would one day carry out the threats he was issuing from his bed.

'You leave him alone, you little bastard,' he'd say and anyone who was teasing me stopped immediately out of fear of him. I was afraid of him too, and because of that, I never did anything to turn him against me.

I was careful to agree with him when he said that Cliff Richard was better than Elvis Presley, though I hardly knew the difference between the two. He used to buy chewing gum with pictures of various stars in the packet and keep them in his locker in a scrap book. He spent a good deal of time doing his hair to look like Cliff. He had his own large jar of Brylcream which he applied liberally and with the aid of a double-sided mirror he combed it back with a coiff at the front.

'What's that like?' he'd ask.

'Grand,' I'd reply.

'Is it like that?' he'd say, holding up Cliff's picture.

'Yeah, very like it.'

Then he would pick up his guitar and play the first few chords of 'Travellin' Light' or 'Livin' Doll' before beginning to sing, doing his utmost to sound like his idol.

'When I get out of here,' he said, 'I am going to start a band.'

At night after I had been given my tablets, John Gorman and I used to pull our beds as close together as we could. He had a cage in his bed to keep the weight of the bedcovers off his plastered leg and from the bars of this he'd hang a small transistor radio tuned to Radio Luxembourg. He also had a torch which he hung beside the radio so he could read when the lights had been put off. He was curious to know why I never had visitors. Because I wanted him as a friend I didn't hesitate to answer anything he asked. As I was not exactly sure of how my parents had died, I told him they were killed in a car crash and that I was in the back at the time. It seemed the easiest thing to say and avoided the necessity for further awkward questions. He wanted to know where I lived and who looked after me.

'A school, with a whole lot of other boys. Nuns look after us.'

'I hate nuns,' he said.

I repeated what he said, and then realized that for the first time I was expressing how I really felt about Mother Paul and Mother Michael, finally admitting my real hatred of them to somebody. I was about to ask him what it was like to have parents when we heard a nurse approaching. He turned off the radio and the torch and pretended to be asleep.

Everything was quiet for a while then he whispered to me that his mother and father slept in the same bed. I said I didn't believe him and repeated what my aunt had told me about men being naked in front of women.

'Cross my heart,' he said making the sign of the cross over the pocket of his pyjamas top.

'Do you know the difference between men and women?' he asked.

'No,' I said.

He made me swear on the bible that if he told me I would not tell anyone else, ever. I promised.

He said that one Sunday morning he had rushed into his parents' bedroom without knocking and his mother was standing on the floor with no clothes on her. He described her breasts as 'diddies' and said that she had no 'mickey' like a man, just a big bunch of hair with a slit in it. His father had roared at him to get out and never to enter the room again without knocking. Then he asked if I knew how babies were made.

'No,' I answered, sensing that there was something wrong

127

with the conversation taking place, and yet wanting to know. Again I had to swear never to tell before he would continue. He said it was a bit dirty and wondered if I really wanted to hear it.

'Yes,' I said.

'You know sometimes,' he said, with a tremble in his voice and hesitated, 'when your mickey gets hard and stands up?'

'Yes.'

'Well the man puts his mickey up into the woman's bum and pisses into her.'

'How do you know?' I asked.

'I just do,' he replied, before saying that another boy had told him. I was gripped by a strange, inexplicable sensation that made me want to hear more, even though I was feeling guilty as if doing something wrong.

'You can only do it at night,' he said, 'because that's when your mickey gets hardest and that's when you have the most piss saved up inside you.'

He kept silent for a short while and then asked 'Did you not know that.'

'No,' I replied.

I was becoming sleepy as John Gorman asked me again to keep what he said a secret. I agreed and said I was going to sleep. Without thinking, I put my hands under the covers and was surprised and a little frightened by the pleasure I was getting from feeling my own erect penis.

'There's a letter for you,' a nurse said as she tossed an envelope onto my bed next morning. I was surprised that the envelope was white and knew immediately that it had not come from St Michael's. I opened it and unfolded a single sheet of notepaper, out of which a ten pound note fluttered down onto my bedcovers. In my excitement I grabbed the money in case anyone saw it and stuffed it under the mattress before reading the letter from my Uncle. He didn't say much except that he was enclosing money and hoped that I would be able to buy whatever I wanted. He signed the letter, 'Uncle Con'.

I couldn't wait to tell John Gorman but before I did, I made him swear not to tell anyone. He suggested that if he said anything about the money I could tell what he told me about babies and the difference between men and women. Slowly and with great caution, I took the money from under my mattress and showed it to him. He gasped and asked who sent it to me.

'My Uncle,' I said.

'Jesus,' he responded, 'he must be awful rich.'

'He is,' I said, jumping at the chance to give him a better impression of me. I said that my uncle was living in the house my parents used to live in, that it was a big house and there was a farm with it.

'When I'm twenty one,' I said, 'I'll be getting it all as well as the money my mother and father left me.'

I don't know how I came out with that tale but it was obvious that John was impressed and, from that day, his attitude to me changed. I even somehow managed to convince myself that there was a house, a farm and money waiting for me. One day, I would be rich.

'Jesus!' Gorman exclaimed again, 'Ten pounds is an awful lot of money, you could buy loads of things with it. All you have to do is hide it until your new boots and splint come, then you can go to the shop and get ice-cream and lemonade and sweets and cigarettes.'

'What would we do with cigarettes?' I asked.

'Smoke them of course.'

It was a hospital rule that patients couldn't keep money, it had to be handed up to the sister in charge of the ward. Gorman got annoyed when I told him so, and said that I would be mad to give it up because the most I would get at any one time would be sixpence or a shilling, which he described as being 'fuck all use'.

'Hide it,' he urged.

'What happens if I'm caught?' I asked nervously.

'Nobody is going to know you have it as long as the two of us keep our mouths shut,' he said.

'Suppose,' I said, 'that someone asks where I got the money when I go to the shop?'

'All you have to do is say you're getting messages for a patient in the men's ward.'

Later, when a nurse came around asking if anyone had money to be 'handed up', I remained silent.

When my splint and boots arrived a nurse fitted them on me. She tied the shining leather boots tightly and then fixed the iron splint firmly to my leg. Before being allowed to stand out of bed, I had to sit for a time with my legs hanging over the edge. As I did, I noticed the tightness of the boots on my feet and in particular the pulling effect of the splint on my foot. Before I stood up, I mentioned that the leather strap just below my left knee was hurting me, and she loosened it slightly. Even though it was extremely uncomfortable I said nothing, fearing I would not be allowed up. I had spent long enough in bed, now I was anxious to be walking again. I looked forward to the freedom. There would be the opportunity to play table tennis and walk around the hospital grounds. But it was the shop I was most excited about. Having money of my own, and being able to spend it was a new experience, one I was determined to enjoy.

I felt desperately weak when I stood up and was certain that I would faint. The blood seemed to drain from me and I could almost feel my face turn white. The nurse looked at me and could see I was in difficulty.

'Are you alright?' she asked.

'Just a bit dizzy,' I answered.

She held my arm as I took a few steps and inquired how I was feeling. I felt less weak, and said so. After two or three minutes walking she suggested that I sit on the bed and only take short walks with long rests in between until I got used to being up. She warned that under no circumstances was I to leave the ward.

'Never?' I asked incredulously.

'Well not today anyway.'

Later that day as I was walking along the corridor with the nurse, the consultant approached and recognized me. He gestured to her that he wanted me to keep walking and, having watched, said that he would like to see me the following week, 'after he has had some time in the caliper'.

As I became stronger my walking improved and I was free

130

to move around the ward and the grounds outside as I wished. John Gorman watched my progress and eventually suggested that I go to the shop. The ten pound note which had been hidden for almost three weeks was withdrawn from under the mattress.

'What will I get?' I asked.

'Lucozade, biscuits, twenty 'Players' and a box of matches.'

'How am I going to get cigarettes?' I asked.

'Just ask for them.'

'What if I get caught?'

'Say they're for one of the men.'

Nervously, I left the ward and walked up the long corridor to the shop which was situated in a room adjacent to the mens' ward. A small group of men had gathered outside it, all in dressing gowns. As they chatted among themselves I stood at the end of the queue and rehearsed over and over in my head what I was going to ask for when my turn came to be served. I wanted to sound confident.

'Are you new here?' one of them asked.

'No. It's just that I was in bed until I got this,' I said, pointing to the splint.

'Now that you're up and around, it won't be too long before you'll be heading home.'

'I don't know,' I answered.

I never expected to find a nun serving in the shop, and if John Gorman knew, he said nothing. She looked to me and asked what I wanted.

I drew a deep breath and quickly told her. I was going to add that they were for one of the men but decided against it. To my surprise she put everything into a brown paper bag, took the money and asked me to wait a minute for the change. I took it, and without checking stuffed it into my trousers pocket and walked as quickly as I could back to the ward.

Just as I left the bag on John Gorman's bed the sister in charge of the ward appeared, demanding to know what was in the bag and who gave me permission to leave the ward. 'I don't know,' Gorman said, 'Pat Doyle bought them and he was leaving them on my bed because he was tired.'

I glared at him and felt cheated.

She emptied the bag and held the cigarettes aloft. 'I don't suppose,' she said, 'either of you had the slightest notion of smoking these.'

'No sister,' I said, and John agreed.

I had thought of telling her they were for one of the men and that I was going to bring them to him later, but I realized she wouldn't believe me. I admitted having bought them for myself and John Gorman. He was furious and denied any knowledge of the cigarettes.

Then the question of where the money came from arose. Because it was such a large amount of money I was convinced she would think I had stolen it.

'I got ten pounds from my uncle in a letter.'

'You know the rules regarding money,' she said.

'Yes sister.'

She held her hand out and I dug deep into my pocket and took out what money I had. She left the ward with it and the messages.

'You're a pig,' I said to Gorman, furious with him.

'Don't call me a fucking pig,' he replied angrily.

'You made a promise and you broke it.'

'Did I say anything about the money?' he said, 'Did I?'

I threatened to tell the ward sister what he told me about babies. He sat upright in bed, pointed his finger, then squinted his eyes and swore to break every bone in my body if I opened my mouth.

'You're a bastard,' he said, after a brief silence.

'I'm not,' I retorted.

'You don't even know what the word means,' he teased.

'I do.'

'What?' he snapped.

When he realized that I hadn't the slightest idea, he grinned and said that I was a bastard because I didn't have any parents. 'That's what a bastard is.'

I walked away from him, realizing that the friendship we had was beginning to crumble and, angry though I was, had no wish for that to happen. It was he who got me through the rough times in the hospital. I had never wanted to be on the receiving end of his anger. Despite my feelings towards him at that moment, I hoped that our relationship would not be ruined.

In time we forgot our quarrel and once John Gorman was allowed out of bed I had a companion with whom I could walk around the hospital grounds. When the weather was fine we used to sit in the fields while he pointed out the direction of various Kilkenny landmarks like Castlecomer coal mines and the steeple of the Cathedral. He could also show me where his house was. At six o'clock most evenings, both of us would go to the shop and spend any money he had been given by relatives the previous day. Anything we bought was carefully concealed as we made our way cautiously back to the ward and headed for the toilets. One evening, while we were both in one of the cubicles, John Gorman sat on the toilet bowl and carefully stood his crutches against the wall. He lit two cigarettes and handed me one. He had smoked before but I hadn't. I watched as he inhaled the smoke deep into his lungs and allowed it to stream out his nostrils. I drew on mine, filling my mouth with smoke, before taking a deep breath. I nearly choked. I could feel the smoke crushing my lungs and as I gasped I felt my face redden and my head become light. The cubicle spun as I coughed uncontrollably and tears streamed down my cheeks.

'Shut up,' Gorman said, 'or you'll get us caught.'

I tried to say something but could only cough. It was some minutes before I got my breath back and the dizziness subsided.

'Pull on it like this,' he said, holding the cigarette between the thumb and first finger with the burning end covered by the cave formation of his hand. He pulled deeply on it and asked me to do the same. I tried but couldn't and when he stood up I threw the half smoked cigarette into the toilet. I watched it sizzle and become saturated before fragmenting into tiny pieces. I knew I was going to vomit and gestured for Gorman to get out of the way before bending over and being violently ill.

'For Jesus sake,' he said.

A sudden knocking on the door startled both of us. The

familiar voice of the ward sister demanded to know who was in the toilet. I spewed out what was left in my mouth and spat into the bowl to eliminate the sour taste of sickness and tobacco.

'I want both of you out here this minute,' she said.

Slowly John Gorman slid back the chromed bolt of the toilet door, before putting a crutch under each arm and inching his way out. I followed.

'What happened to you?' she shouted at me.

'I was sick,' I replied.

'I wonder why?' she said sarcastically, asking us both to turn out our pockets. Picking up a packet of cigarettes which had fallen from my pocket she warned that we would get the severest punishment. 'Both of you will go back to your ward, get straight into bed and you will remain there for a week.'

Later that night both our beds were taken from the main ward and moved to the babies unit. The nurses pushing the beds took no notice whatever of Gorman's threats to get his father after them and that he was going to run away in the middle of the night.

There were fifteen or twenty babies in the ward, often no more than a few weeks old, who cried, demanding to be fed. Some were in plaster from the soles of their feet right up to under their arms. Nurses had difficulty in lifting them from their cots for feeding while others could not be lifted at all. They were on traction with weights on pulleys, hanging from their legs. Those that were being fed sucked contentedly on their bottles. They slept as the nurse changed the pads which had been placed at the cut-outs in the plaster at the backside and the pelvic area. In the soft light of the ward I could see babies with large heads and tiny bodies and others born without limbs or with only part of hands and legs.

As I was drifting to sleep John Gorman threatened to run away and asked if I would go with him. He said he had no intention of spending a week 'stuck in a ward full of squealing babies and shitty nappies'. He swore he would be gone by morning.

I woke early next morning to find Gorman still in his bed,

curled in a bundle beneath the sheets, oblivious to the sounds of babies demanding breakfast.

The ward sister arrived and told me that the doctor was going to see me and she wanted me 'up and out of bed immediately'. I hadn't expected to be allowed up so soon after beginning my punishment and was surprised that the doctor wanted to see me. I sat motionless until she hurried me.

As I got dressed she woke my companion and told him we were both being given a chance, provided we gave an assurance to stay in our own ward and not to smoke in the future.

I was worried about seeing the consultant, even though I felt sure he would be happy with the progress I was making. I washed my face a couple of times and brushed my teeth until the gums bled. I combed my hair and where bits of it stuck up, wet it and combed it down.

'What are you all cleaned up for?' Gorman asked.

'I have to see the doctor,' I replied.

'He'll probably want to take you down,' he jeered.

'He won't,' I said, not really convinced by my own words. 'He already said I wouldn't have to have an operation.'

'They always say that,' he replied, 'and then they change their minds.'

'You think you know everything,' I said, walking away from him.

I was brought to a room off the main ward to await the arrival of the doctor and as I sat there I prayed silently that he would not operate on me. I practiced walking, watching my feet and trying to ensure they were straight.

When he arrived he was in a cheerful mood, rubbing his hands together as he asked me to walk across the room. I stood up and took the first few steps cautiously, looking downward all the time. Halfway across the floor my leg flexed at the knee and I had difficulty in getting it back down to the floor again.

When I turned to face him, he asked me to raise my head, and ignore my feet. Again my leg flexed and the harder I tried to get it back down the worse it became, until, in a sudden

135

movement, it released like a string snapping and I walked the rest of the way.

'What happened there?' the consultant asked.

'I don't know,' I said.

'Has that ever happened to you before?'

'Only since I got the splint.'

'And does it happen often?'

'Just when I get afraid.'

'And are you afraid now?' he asked.

'Just a bit.'

'Sit down there.' He pointed to a chair and told the nurses who were with him that he didn't see any further need for the splint. 'It doesn't appear to be doing any good and in fact it may be causing harm.' He asked me to walk without it. My feet felt free and light, there was no difficulty walking and no involuntary flexing.

'Patrick,' he said, 'you've been here for a long time now, nearly two years, and we haven't been able to put your foot right.' I waited anxiously for what was coming next.

'Because you're not getting any better I want to send you to another hospital to see a specialist who will be able to help you. Once that happens you will be able to go back to your school and the friends you have there.'

I began to cry and said I didn't want to go back to the school and I didn't want to go to any other hospital either.

'It's for your own good,' one of the nurses said.

'I don't care, I like it here and I want to stay.'

The consultant intervened, 'But you don't want to spend the rest of your life in hospital. Do you?'

'No,' I said hesitantly.

'Right then, we'll get this other man to have a look at you, and we'll see what happens from there.'

'Will I have to stay in the other hospital?'

'Just for a little while, until they do some tests. Once they have been done we should be able to get that foot right for you.'

He wrote a letter on a piece of hospital headed notepaper and put it into a long white envelope which he sealed and addressed to 'Professor E.D. Casey, Consultant Neurologist'.

'What does it say on the envelope?' I asked.

He held it up for me to read. I read the name and then stopped.

'Consultant Neurologist,' he said.

'What's a neurologist?' I asked.

'Just another type of doctor that's all, nothing to worry about.'

CHAPTER TEN

For two days I roamed around the hospital stunned and unable to believe that I had to leave. I had made it my home, I had friends there, I liked the way I was treated and had come to enjoy the companionship of the other boys. The initial stress-filled weeks of being teased and tormented seemed a long time ago and irrelevant now. I wanted to stay. John Gorman tried to be consoling, and said that he would visit me when he went home.

'But it's in Dublin,' I said.

'How do you know?' he asked.

'I heard the nurses saying so.'

'That doesn't matter, I can get my father to take me. Anyway you won't be staying there for long.'

I wanted to agree with him, but I knew I wouldn't see that hospital or John Gorman again. Promises made by nurses and doctors were something I had learned to mistrust. I had heard them all before and things never worked out the way they said they would.

On the day I was leaving, after I had said goodbye to the patients and nurses, the sister in charge took me by the hand and led me from the ward. I cried bitterly, pleading with her not to send me away. I dug my feet into the floor to prevent her dragging me further.

'I'm not going to any new hospital,' I screamed at the top of my voice and as we were nearing the top of the long sloping corridor I gripped a radiator and held it until my knuckles turned white. She pulled at my arm but I was determined not to budge. I kicked out, attempting to catch one of the nurses across the shins and threatened to kill them if they didn't leave me alone. I was so determined not to leave that it took three nurses to make me release my grip on the radiator.

Though my vision was clouded by tears I could see the senior nurse talking to a doctor. I couldn't hear what they were saying and I didn't care. They stopped dragging at me and for a moment I thought I was going to be returned to the ward, then I saw the doctor return. He had a needle and syringe prepared in the kidney dish he was carrying.

'Now Pat,' he said gently, 'this will make you feel better.'

'I don't want that needle,' I protested.

He inserted the needle into a vein in my right arm which was held in an outright position. I felt it puncture my skin and I screamed again. Within minutes my screaming and protestations stopped, my vision became clouded and my mouth felt dry. I was so light-headed that I could no longer walk. I had to be lifted and carried to a waiting ambulance where I was put lying on one of its two stretchers. The nurse who was travelling woke me when we reached Dublin. I was thirsty and she gave me some water from a plastic bottle.

'How far is it now?' I asked.

'Just a couple of minutes,' she replied and suggested that I sit up and fix my clothes. She wiped my face with a cool damp towel, which made me feel more alert. I began to worry again.

I felt very weak walking up the granite steps of the Dublin hospital, with its tall Georgian facade and massive hall door. The nurse greeted the porter who directed her to the admissions office. She sat me down on a long bench and gave me my chart to keep on my lap. The waiting area was dark and quiet; the only light available came from the sliding glass panels of the admissions office itself.

'Someone will look after you in a minute or two,' she said and prepared to leave.

She brushed my fringe off my forehead with her hand and said that she would see me soon again. I looked at her but didn't speak, then I bowed my head as she walked away.

An attractive, dark-haired young woman came to the window of the admissions office and asked me to come in. She wore bright red lipstick and I couldn't help noticing the length of her fingernails and the fact they were painted to match her lips. I handed her my chart and she copied down the information from it. Every time she smiled, she revealed two rows of pure white, straight teeth slightly stained by her lipstick.

'And you're just nine years of age, Patrick, is that right?' she asked in a refined accent.

'Yes,' I said.

'You're a very big man for nine, and very brave too.'

I forced a smile. I knew I was very small and slight for my age. Then she said I was making a bit of history, as I was the only child in the hospital. She couldn't remember if anyone so young had been admitted before. Because I was the youngest person there, she suggested that I should receive special treatment.

'You don't have any brothers, do you?'

'No.'

'Well I have three brothers who are a little bigger than you. They have lots and lots of comics and I think you should have some of them to read while you're with us. Isn't that a good idea?' she asked.

'I don't know,' I replied.

She telephoned to tell a nurse that the patient they were expecting was now ready to go to the ward. I became nervous and began to cry. The receptionist did her best to comfort me with assurances that she would be calling with the comics and that I would get to like the hospital after the first few days.

A nurse came and brought me the short distance to the lift. She slammed its criss-crossed iron gate and pressed the button numbered three. Its sudden movement frightened me and I held her hand tightly until it stopped with a jolt. When the gates opened, I stepped out quickly.

St Patrick's ward was bigger than any ward I had ever been in. Its high walls were painted two different shades of green with a grey dividing line. The windows were very tall and had ropes to open the top sections. The amount of light getting into the ward during the day was restricted because of shadows cast by other parts of the building which jutted out from the ward I was in. The view from the windows consisted of the back of other buildings, and, looking down, I could see the felted roof of what was obviously a new extension to the hospital. Large fluorescent lights hung from the ceiling, suspended with chains and covered by wide metal shades. They were only switched off on the brightest days and then only for a very short time. The patients were mainly elderly, though there were a few who were probably in their twenties. The coughing and discharging of phlegm into stainless steel cups were sounds I had experienced before; so was the smell of stale urine from uncovered bottles on the floor under some of the beds. What scared me were the painful groans of a man whose bed had been screened off, his voice feeble and tired as he tried to get the attention of one of the nurses. The only evidence of his existence, apart from the groaning, was the sight of a circular glass bottle, inverted and discharging blood into his arm from a T-shaped stand. Patients like him were screened off most of the time, though whenever a nurse went inside their curtains to adjust the flow rate of the drip, I made a point of peeping through gaps to see as much as I could. I was always frightened by what I'd see – a sickly looking man propped up on many pillows, his arm strapped to a plastic-covered splint to prevent him flexing it where a needle with its tube attached entered his skin. His face would be grey and lifeless, his cheeks sunken and his dull eyes stared from deep caverns framed by black circular lines. Inevitably they died. The entire ward joined the hospital chaplain as he recited a decade of the rosary for the departed soul.

'He has left this world,' the priest would say, 'and gone to a place where he will experience no more pain, only joy and happiness, eternal life with God and his angels.'

Whenever a death occurred those men who were allowed out of bed took it in turns to pray beside the corpse. They opened and closed the screens gently to avoid making unnecessary noise. Distraught relatives arrived, crying wearily despite the best efforts of nurses and nuns to comfort them. Often wives, their faces distorted with grief, wailed openly and pleaded with the Almighty to give them back their husbands. Grieving sons and daughters tried to console them only to find that they too were angry with the compassionate God who had taken their father. The priest held the hands of the people overcome with pain and grief and reminded them that it was the will of God that their loved one had been taken. During my stay in that hospital I was to witness the heartbreak and the agony of death many times, I was also to become less afraid of it than I had previously been.

Because I was so young, nurses and patients tried to protect me from these scenes. I was given comics to occupy my mind and distract me from what was happening. This practice served only to make me more curious about the subject, and even though I was terrified of dying, I wanted to know what a dead person looked like.

A man died and I asked a nurse if I could go behind the screens and see him, saying that I wanted to say a prayer for him.

She hesitated and then said she would carry me as long as I was sure that I wouldn't be frightened.

'I can walk over,' I said.

'No,' she insisted, 'I'll carry you.'

She lifted me into her arms, asking me not to squash her white triangular veil. I carefully put my hands underneath it and she asked me to make sure I didn't pull it off altogether. I grew tense as I got near to the dead man, and wondered if she could feel me trembling. She opened the screens and from her arms I looked directly down on the man's sunken, marble-like face.

'He's just like he's asleep,' I whispered, somehow realizing that to speak out loud would be wrong.

'Yes,' she said, 'it's like going asleep and never waking again.'

His hands were crossed on his chest and there was a rosary beads and brown scapular entwined in his fingers. Beside the bed a small table was covered by a white cloth embroidered with a gold cross. A candle burned in its brass holder beside holy water in a brass bowl.

'How do you die?' I asked her as she carried me back to bed.

'Your heart stops,' she said, putting her hand inside my

pyjamas top and holding it gently over my heart. 'Your heart is beating away in there and it will beat for many, many years to come.'

She tucked in the covers tightly over me, then took my face in her hands and kissed me lightly on the forehead before walking away. The tenderness of that moment is something I will never forget.

During my first weeks there I was examined by many students. Mostly they were in groups accompanied by a senior doctor, but sometimes by themselves. At other times it would be one or two students. Such experiences were always embarrassing and seemed devoid of any consideration of how I felt. Bedcovers were literally thrown back, and my clothes removed without anyone ever asking whether I objected. A group of staring eyes pierced my naked body while first one, then a second, third and fourth tried out various examinations, from simply listening to my heart and lungs to holding their hands beneath my testicles and asking me to cough. There was the usual barrage of questions about whether either my father or mother had any form of illness. I didn't know and said so. Brothers and sisters, what about them? I had a sister and told them that she was alright. Foreign students were the most difficult to deal with. Their accents were strange and I had the greatest difficulty understanding their questions. When I did answer, I often had to repeat myself as they didn't appear to understand me. Group examinations often lasted an hour, after which there was practically no part of me left untouched. When they were finished they simply left me behind the screens where I put back on my pyjamas and waited for a nurse to remake the bed.

While in St Patrick's Ward, I was under the care of Professor Casey, an elderly bespectacled man with a deeply wrinkled, kind face. He always smiled at me as he approached my bed flanked by an entourage of students and other doctors, seeking a diagnosis from the students after they had examined me.

He'd pointed out that I had been in three hospitals before this one and that so far there was no positive diagnosis of my condition made. He'd refer briefly to post polio before dismissing it on the grounds that there were none of the symptoms associated with that condition, such as muscle wastage or paralysis.

One morning as his students listened attentively he suggested that there might be some neurological disorder which would take time to ascertain. A biopsy would have to be done and the results closely looked at. He finally said the words I feared most. 'I will be taking him down to theatre in the morning.' As I shivered with fright, he suggested that those interested in furthering their medical careers should be present. Having spoken briefly to the ward sister, the Professor came to my bedside and told me he would see me in the morning.

The greatest fear I had, that of being operated on, was about to become a reality. I wanted to scream but was too terrified to do so. I thought of dying and when asked about going to confession I readily accepted. My old fear of dying returned as I confessed to telling lies and being disobedient to the hospital chaplain. While he was imparting absolution, I wondered if I had told him everything. Somehow surgery and death had become inextricably linked in my mind. I was certain I would die. The years of giving answers which I thought would prevent an operation were gone. The worst thing that could ever happen to me was less than twenty four hours away.

In the afternoon a nurse came to my bed to prepare me for the operation. She removed my pyjamas bottom and shaved all the fine hair from my left thigh. As the razor glided over my soapy skin I was trembling so much she had to repeatedly warn me of the danger of being cut. She looked closely at my pubic area and decided it did not require shaving.

There was an elderly man in the bed next to mine who was also going to theatre. More than anything else, he convinced me that not only was I likely to die, but so was he. He dragged out his words as he spoke in a loud thick country accent which I found difficult to understand. He insisted that I join him in saying the rosary and when he started I had no choice but to answer the prayers.

144

After tea, signs were hung on our beds indicating that we were fasting.

'Oh 'tis a bad sign when ye have to see the like of that thing being hung on the bed. They starve ye first and then they set about cutting ye up while ye'r asleep.'

'They're not going to have to put me asleep,' I said.

'Sure how can ye have an operation without them knocking ye out? Who told ye that?'

'The nurse did.'

'God bless yer innocence son, but I'd not believe a word that'd come out of the mouth of them people. They mean well I know, but they don't be telling the truth all the bloody time. They'd say anything to keep ye from asking questions.'

I tried to ignore him, to block out what he was saying. I mistrusted doctors and nurses enough without him adding to it. He kept talking, dragging out the words he wanted to stress.

'Sure they can't go cuttin' anyone open without having them asleep and once they have ye asleep, there's no knowing whether ye'll ever come out of it.'

By that night I was in a terrible state of panic, sweating profusely and crying. I didn't want to believe anything he was saying, yet neither could I believe the nurses, despite their sincerity. When I could not get to sleep on my usual dosage of medication, I was given another dose equal to the first. Despite reproaches from the nurses and protests from other patients, the man beside me continued to pray aloud.

When I woke the following morning my bed was screened off. A nun recited the 'Morning Offering' and the baritone voices of the men responded wearily to her various invocations. Breakfast was being served, I could hear the domestic staff asking patients how much sugar they wanted in their tea and when to stop adding milk. Spoons tapped on egg shells or rang around the sides of cups being stirred. A nurse came through the screens to my bedside carrying a steel dish with a needle and syringe in it. She had cotton wool and a bottle labeled 'ether'.

She helped me to change from my pyjamas into a long white cape which she tied at the back.

145

'Lie on your side,' she said, 'I just want to give you a little injection.' I lay with the gown up around my waist, tensely waiting for the needle.

'Relax,' she said as she swabbed the area with ether, 'if you relax a bit you won't feel a thing, it's just a little prick.'

She administered the injection and I screamed, feeling the liquid in the syringe penetrate through the muscle in my backside before the needle was withdrawn and the area rubbed again with cold ether.

She asked me to allow her to wipe my face and to see me smiling. I was in no humour to oblige and buried my head deep into the pillow and wept.

The injection had the effect of making me drowsy and my mouth began to dry up. By swirling my tongue about I thought I might be able to create the moisture I so desperately craved. I drifted in and out of frighteningly colourful sleep, hallucinations and nightmares, blue rivers and green skies. Enormous spiders and ants crawled across my body. There was a sense of falling from a great height and being unable to stop.

'Can I have a drink of water?' I asked the nurse who came to check on me.

'You can't have any now, but you can have as much as you want when you come back.'

The fears I held were numbed by drugs, and when the trolley arrived to take me from the ward, I was too doped to be frightened. Two men dressed in light green cotton suits, wearing white cotton caps, and masks over their mouths, lifted me onto the trolley and pushed it to the lift. I heard the gates open and felt the wheels roll across the gap between the floor and the lift. I kept my eyes fixed on the ceiling as I was being wheeled to the operating room.

By the time I reached the theatre, the numbing effect of the drugs had given way to fear. I was alert, frightened and acutely aware of what was happening and being said. By contrast with the corridors outside, the theatre was brightly lit and smelt heavily of disinfectant and ether.

The consultant who was to perform the biopsy came to the side of the trolley and checked my pulse.

'How are you?' he asked.

'Alright,' I said, my voice trembling.

'There is nothing to worry about. We'll be finished before we get started.' He laughed.

The intensity of the bright circular light overhead caused me to squint. Doctors and nurses gathered, one indistinguishable from the other, except by their voices, caps covering their heads and masks hiding their faces. A green cloth was draped over my face, reducing the blinding light to a dull shadow.

'Are you alright under there?' the cheerful voice of Professor Casey asked.

'Yes,' I replied.

'You're just going to feel a small injection on your thigh and that will be all. You can sing a song if you like.'

I cried as the injection was given and when I tried to reach my thigh with my hand it was pushed away.

'That's it now,' Professor Casey said, 'no more needles, and just another few minutes then we're finished.'

There was a pause while they waited for the local anesthetic to take effect before a voice asked if I could feel my thigh being pinched.

'No,' I answered.

Someone gripped my hand firmly as I perspired beneath the cloths that covered my body. I winced as the scalpel made its incision and though I couldn't feel the actual cut being made, I felt a dull pain as my skin was opened.

'That hurts,' I said.

The consultant asked that another injection be given immediately. Nurses and some of the students were encouraging me to sing.

'A person can hardly be expected to sing with a towel over his face,' Professor Casey said.

The cloth was moved just enough to enable me to see directly over my head, it still covered my nose and mouth. I wonder how many people have actually sung 'Kelly the Boy from Killane' while undergoing surgery to the great amusement of all present?

When he was finished Professor Casey held up a glass

tube containing my skin steeped in a liquid. 'That's what all the fuss was about,' he said, 'and you're still alive.'

I felt greatly relieved as covers were taken away and I was allowed to sit up and look at my leg. It was covered with a strip of plaster about four inches long and two wide. The skin around the plaster was daubed in a pink disinfectant.

'Will I have to come down here again?' I asked.

'Do you want to?'

'No,' I laughed nervously.

'In that case I won't ask you to,' the consultant said.

On the way back to the ward, I was happy that the doctors and nurses had kept their word. I had not been put to sleep as I feared and began to feel that I could trust them. When I was put back into my own bed I noticed the one beside it was empty.

Being in a ward with a lot of old men had its advantages especially when it came to disposing of fruit or sweets they had been given but didn't want. My bedside locker was a depository for all sorts of things, much of which I never ate. Once a week when the nurses cleaned out the lockers there was always rotting fruit in mine which had to be dumped. I'd remember the times I had prayed for an apple or an orange. Now I had more than I could manage to eat. The only time I refused it was when it was offered to me by the relatives of someone who had died. I was afraid to eat that.

In the evenings I was allowed out of bed for a hour. I had pyjamas that were far too big for me and wore a dressing gown more suited to a small man than a young child. One man I particularly liked was in his early thirties, dark haired, quiet, and an avid reader. He kept a chess board, with pieces in place on top of his locker. I was often amused as he played games against himself, moving the white and black pieces in turn. To me, he was a curious figure who never went to communion or confession, even before he was being taken to the theatre. When I got to know him better and he was teaching me how to play chess I asked him why.

'I'm a left footer,' he said.

'What does that mean?' I asked.

He laughed and at first seemed reluctant to tell me, but I persisted.

'I'm a Protestant,' he said casually.

I was shocked and the harder I tried to conceal it the more obvious it became. I remembered everything I had been told about Protestants not getting to heaven and never being able to see God. I even felt it was a sin to be talking to him. Yet I liked him and he was the person in the ward nearest my own age. I told him about the nun who turned off the radio in the Cork hospital because the patients were listening to a Protestant Service.

'You wouldn't want to take much notice of the nuns,' he said.

'Why?' I asked innocently.

'Because sometimes they don't exactly tell the truth.'

I couldn't imagine a nun telling lies and I told him so.

'What about a game of chess,' he suggested to get off the subject.

After just a few moves I asked him if he believed in the Blessed Virgin.

'What's the first rule of chess?' he asked and, when I didn't reply, told me.

'Silence. That's the first rule.'

I remained silent and copied each of the moves he made until the board became congested and he began to pick off my pieces and place them to one side. He suggested that if I really wanted to win, I should start making my own moves. Still utterly obsessed with the fact that this man was a Protestant I asked him if he was going to heaven or hell when he died.

'Haven't a clue and I don't care really.'

'Why don't you believe in the Blessed Virgin?' I asked.

'Because virgins can't have babies.'

'Why not?'

'It's a long story,' he said, 'and when you get older you'll understand.'

My curiosity was aroused and I persisted in trying to get him to answer. He refused and, when I asked why, just

149

said 'Because it's time for you to go back to bed.'

I waited for the nurse to come with my medication and when she did, I was given two and a half tablets, instead of the usual two. I recognized the phenobarbitone, but not the white half tablet.

'I usually only get two,' I said.

'Well you're getting two and a half now,' she replied.

'Why?' I asked.

'Because the doctor said so.'

'What's the half one?' I asked curiously and she replied that patients were not supposed to know the names of the drugs they were being given. She was becoming agitated by my constant questioning but eventually told me, before warning me to keep my mouth shut or she would get into trouble.

'What are they for?' I asked.

'What are they for? They're to make you better of course. Now will you for God's sake stop asking questions. Just lie down and go to sleep before I get mad.' As I was going to sleep, I repeated the name of my new drug to myself. I never forgot it.

The first time I actually remember celebrating Christmas was in St Patrick's Ward. I was nine years of age. In the days leading up to it many of the patients were allowed home – some for good, others for a few days. The nurses who were artistic painted seasonal pictures on the large windows of the ward and, in one corner, erected a tree which they spent hours adorning with tinsel and crepe paper streamers. For a few nights before Christmas groups of them, in uniform and capes, visited the wards singing Christmas carols.

The expected arrival of Santa Claus during the night was a new experience to me which I found difficult to believe. It was not that I had ever questioned his existence – I simply hadn't heard of him, or if I had, I couldn't remember. The patients and nurses kept reminding me to get to sleep early or otherwise I would get nothing. Every time I was asked what I hoped Santa Claus would leave for me, I answered, 'an electric train'.

There was little doubt that I was the main focus of attention. No visitor came to see any of the patients without calling to my bed and giving me a bag full of fruit or sweets.

On Christmas Eve I hung a pair of socks on the end of my bed. One of the men gave them to me because they were big and 'Santie would fit a lot more stuff into them'. I was told to clean out my locker, 'just in case he might want to put a few things in there too'. In the night, I heard the sound of shuffling and whispers. Opening my eyelids slightly I saw five or six men and a couple of nurses filling my socks. I pretended to be asleep and, all the time they were there, I never moved.

I woke early next morning and went to the end of my bed to see what had been left there. I tore open a parcel wrapped in colourful paper as patients and staff watched, revelling in my excitement, and pretending the whole business was a mystery to them. Inside I discovered a variety of things: jigsaw puzzles, dinky cars, a train engine with a key sticking out of its side and some lengths of track which, when joined together, formed a circle. I delighted in watching the train go round and round.

'Try the locker,' one of the patients said.

I opened its metal door and an avalanche tumbled onto the floor. Apples, oranges, rolls of sweets and boxes of smarties. There were boxes wrapped in cellophane paper containing cakes sprinkled with fine white sugar. Someone picked up the items that fell and put them on my bed, which by now was taking on the appearance of a shop counter.

On Christmas Day there was no restriction on visiting. Children were brought to see the parent or uncle they had not seen for months. There were great scenes of emotion and joy as a father clasped his sons and daughters to him and wept. They all brought presents and some even had things for me, colouring books and paints, packets of plastic soldiers and books. I noticed a number of patients sharing a bottle of whiskey between them and as they drank they became more and more high-spirited, singing Christmas songs and pursuing fleeing good-humoured nurses who passed. One man who managed to get his arm around a nurse's waist, sang at the top of his voice, 'Give us a kiss for Christmas' and attempted to place his lips on hers, but she turned her head and offered her cheek instead. He protested that it was a 'mean round'.

'Make the best of it,' she said, 'It's all you're going to get.'

As he continued to drink, he became more daring in his approaches to the nurses.

'What about you?' he asked another, 'any chance of a feel?'

She became angry and reminded him of my presence, and when he said I would have to learn sometime she stormed out of the ward.

'It's just a bit of fun,' he shouted after her, 'and anyway, it's Christmas.' But she ignored him. For a time there was an uneasy silence and I heard some of the men say he had 'gone a bit too far'. He blamed the whiskey. Later in the morning when the nurse returned to the ward, he called her over, saying that he wanted to apologise but she ignored him again. He sat on his bed in misery, the Christmas presents from his family unopened around him.

CHAPTER ELEVEN

At about half past twelve that afternoon, after I had been given my mid-day dose of tablets, a nurse appeared carrying a bundle of new clothes and told me I was being taken out for the day.

'Where am I going?' I asked.

'Professor Casey wants you to go to his house for Christmas dinner and to play with his children,' she said.

'I don't want to go.'

'Of course you do.'

'I don't,' I said.

'Well you're going anyway, you wouldn't want to insult him after he buying you all these new clothes.'

Realizing I didn't have any choice I allowed her to dress me in a new pair of short trousers, a white shirt and blue jumper. There was also a pair of white socks and a new pair of black shoes.

When she was putting on the socks the nurse noticed that my big toe was bent, cramped down towards the sole of the foot.

She asked me to straighten it but I couldn't, and I told her so. Because of its position it was extremely difficult to get the shoe on. I used to wait until it released and then, quickly get the nurse to push it on.

I sat on the edge of the bed for a few minutes, admiring my clothes and savouring their smell of newness. I walked across the ward amazed at how light my feet felt, having been so used to walking with heavy boots. Suddenly, my back arched and I couldn't move – then, after perhaps thirty seconds or so, it released like a spring uncoiling. I was frightened by this involuntary movement, and as I began to worry about it, it happened a second time. I didn't want the nurses to see but one did and rushed towards me. She tried to push me upright but that made matters worse, and eventually she had to carry me back to bed, where she told me to lie down and take it easy for a few minutes. Another nurse joined her as my back relaxed.

'What happened?' she asked.

'I don't know, I was just walking and I couldn't walk anymore.'

Then I asked them if I could take off my shoe because it was hurting me.

'My toe just keeps bending inside it and it's sore.'

'Well stop bending it then,' she said.

'I can't, it just keeps doing it.'

They both looked concerned and agreed to mention it to Professor Casey when he arrived to collect me.

When he came into the ward I watched him speaking to the nurses on duty. He looked concerned as one of them demonstrated with the use of her hand and forearm what was happening to my back. Before coming to my bed he was handed a brown bottle of tablets by the nurse.

'I hear you're in some difficulty?' he said to me.

'Just my toe,' I replied.

He took the chart from the end of my bed and said he was increasing the dose of my 'new tablet'. That would help ensure that my back didn't arch and prevent my toe giving me trouble. He asked if I would be able to walk from the ward to the car.

'Yes,' I said confidently.

I had only gone a short distance when I was forced to stop. Professor Casey urged me to take my time, to relax, everything would be fine. When I resumed walking, I was determined to keep going and not allow my body to be taken over by strange movements over which I had no control. Within the space of a minute, it happened again and I became terrified that this time I would not emerge from the tight grip of the spasm.

'Has this happened to you before?' he asked.

'Once or twice in Kilkenny hospital when I had the splint on my leg.'

'When did you notice it first, since you came to this hospital?' he asked.

'I don't really know,' I replied.

'Would you say it is just since you started on the new tablets?' he asked.

I thought for a moment and told him that I didn't really know.

'We won't worry about that for the moment,' he said as we walked down the hospital steps to his car and introduced me to his three children who were sitting quietly in the back. They were older than me, with probably as much as five years between his youngest child, a boy, and myself. The two girls looked about sixteen and seventeen. I sat in the front seat for the ten minute journey from the hospital, looking at the various types of houses we drove past on the way. Despite the urgings of their father, none of the children spoke to me and I said nothing to them.

I was desperately uncomfortable in the car. My toe twitched violently inside my shoe causing me to squirm. I didn't want anyone to notice, but knew they could see me sweating heavily. Professor Casey shifted his gaze from the road to me many times during the journey and each time I tried to give the impression that I was alright.

'Have we far to go?' I asked.

'Another couple of minutes.'

The car pulled up outside a Georgian house with an elegant oak halldoor, its brass fittings looking like they had just been polished. A neatly groomed woman opened the door and descended the three steps to the car. She opened the passenger door and embraced me, welcoming me to her home and hoping that I would enjoy the day. The rest of the family got out and, at their father's request, went into the house while his wife and himself inquired whether I could manage the steps.

'I think so,' I said.

I got out of the car without difficulty and waited as the Professor locked it. He walked towards the house and invited

155

me to follow. I couldn't move. His wife offered to help, but he suggested that I be left alone and given time to relax. As I urged my body to move, I noticed the children watching from a front window. This made the situation worse. My body was refusing to do what my brain was demanding. Then Mrs Casey held my hand which had a soothing effect and I relaxed sufficiently to be able to walk up the steps, through the hallway and into a large brightly lit sitting-room, decorated with Christmas lights and cards hanging from string over a magnificent white marble fireplace where a fire blazed. The Professor offered me something to drink and I accepted a large cool glass of lemonade. He and his wife had a glass of sherry and before drinking they toasted each other, their own children, and me. Whenever I looked at him he diverted his gaze. I felt uneasy, conscious of being watched, and worried that what he was observing would give him a reason to operate on me again.

The children were curious about what I did in the orphanage at Christmas. Did Santa come? Did we have a party?

There was no santa, I said, but I did have to serve three Masses and I added that all of us used to get jelly and custard. The boy, who had been silent up until now said 'that wasn't much of a Christmas.'

Then I told them about how Santa came in the hospital and they laughed at me pretending to be asleep while the nurses and patients stuffed my locker and the big pair of socks. Mrs Casey said I was right, and laughed too.

'But,' she added, 'I'm certain the real Santa did come once you were asleep.'

During the day I became increasingly uncomfortable as my toe flexed wildly inside my shoe and became sore. When I could no longer tolerate it I asked Professor Casey if I could remove my shoe.

'Certainly,' he said, asking if my toe was still giving me trouble. He reached into his pocket and took out the bottle of tablets he had taken from the hospital, then looked at his watch and remarked that it was a bit soon to take any more. Later in the afternoon when he gave me two I was embarrassed swallowing them while his children watched.

At six o'clock dinner was served. The table was covered in a white, finely embroidered table cloth and at every place there was a cracker, laid out along with an assortment of knives, forks, and spoons. The golden coloured turkey was placed on a silver tray in the centre of the table, its basted body glistening in the candle light surrounding it. Professor Casey sat at one end of the table, his wife sat opposite him. I was seated at his right, opposite his son, who offered me a cracker to pull. It broke with a sharp crack which instinctively caused me to duck as paper hats and tiny plastic toys flew into the air. I had never pulled one before and had no idea that the pieces of coloured paper wrapped tightly in elastic bands were paper hats.

The doctor and his family rose to say grace before meals and as I attempted to stand, he indicated that I could remain seated. When grace was finished he reminded his family to remember children like me who didn't have parents or a home for Christmas. I could feel my face redden but kept my head bowed so that no one would notice.

Everyone at the table wore a paper hat during dinner, and as the adults poured themselves wine, their eldest daughter asked if she could have some. Her father refused, saying she had taken the pledge and couldn't take alcohol until she was twenty one.

Throughout the meal I felt uneasy and uncomfortable. I was an intruder in a family unit, expected to fit but unable to do so. Everything that went on was alien to me, the food was unlike anything I had ever tasted before. I was confused by the variety of knives, forks and spoons around my plate, never sure which one to use. I was reluctant to try the various sauces which the children spread so liberally over their food. I was afraid to ask for anything and, as they all chatted, wondered if I would always feel so out of place in a family situation as I did that day.

My bare foot was now involuntarily either kicking one of the family or banging hard against the wooden frame of the chair. My paper hat became soggy from perspiration and its dye ran down my face. I wanted to get away from the table and to sit on the floor, where I knew I would be most comfortable.

The room lights were switched off and the candles on the table cast eerie shadows on the walls. Those members of the family still at the table whispered to each other as though some secret ritual was about to begin. I wondered what was happening. From the kitchen I heard Mrs Casey singing 'Silent Night, Holy Night,' her voice becoming clearer as she re-entered the room carrying the Christmas pudding on a plate. On top of the pudding a blue flame danced lightly and the air was filled with the rich smell of brandy. The family joined in the singing as I watched the flame flicker and begin to die away in a stream of blue rivulets running down the sides. There was silence as the flame on the pudding wavered between life and death and when it finally died, they cheered. This was obviously a family tradition to which they attached great importance.

After dinner Professor Casey and his wife sat on the big settee near the fire, drinking from magnificent bulbous glasses. I sat on the floor with their son playing a dice game. They spoke quietly to each other, not realizing I could hear parts of their conversation. She asked her husband had he any idea what I was suffering from, adding that I looked desperately uncomfortable most of the time.

'No,' he sighed, 'but it appears to be progressive.'

'What will happen to him?' she asked.

Again he sighed and said he didn't know. He stood up and reminded me it was time to go. I put away the various pieces of the game and was about to put my shoe on when he said there was no point in wearing a shoe that hurt. Asking his children to remain with their mother and assuring them he would be back soon, he lifted me into his arms and held me as I said goodbye to everyone. It felt very strange to be carried to his car. He settled me into the front seat.

'We'll go for a quick spin into town to see the lights,' he said. It was not a long journey and we didn't speak until we reached the city centre. There were few people about, mostly young couples, hand in hand, or with an arm wrapped tightly around their partner's body. They were dressed to keep out the chill of the December evening with heavy coats, gloves and scarves, yet despite these barriers, there was a sense of real intimacy between them.

O'Connell Street and Henry Street were a mass of brightly coloured lights which were reflected on the windscreen of the car. Whenever we came to a shop window with toys the doctor pulled up close to enable me to have as good a view as possible of the display.

Driving back to the hospital he chatted to me about the hospital. Did I like it? Were the nurses nice to me? What were the other hospitals like and would I like to be able to go back to the school?

'I don't really ever want to go back to that school,' I said.

'Why?' he asked inquisitively.

Without really intending to I found myself telling him about everything that had happened to me there, the beatings by the nuns, the locking up in dark rooms, even how I had fallen down the altar steps while carrying the missal during Mass. He laughed loudly at that, saying it could have happened to a Bishop.

Suddenly I was tempted to ask if he knew anything about my parents. I wanted to tell him about the recurring fears I had of hanging men and of death. I was certain he would believe me. But though I felt very much at ease with this man now, I stopped short of telling him anything about my secret fears. I wanted him to know, not to gain his sympathy, but because I was certain he would understand and believe me. Sometimes I still wonder if he too knew the facts that were hidden from me.

He carried me from the lift into the ward and when one of the nurses offered to help he would not allow her to, saying that I was no weight at all.

Before he left he looked at my chart and told the nurse he wanted the dosage of the new tablet increased immediately and the Phenobarbitone continued with one extra tablet anytime I showed signs of distress.

Perhaps it was because I had been with him over Christmas that I felt much more relaxed with him afterwards. One morning early in the new year he checked my foot and noticed the position of my toe.

'Is that the way your toe stays all the time?' he asked.

'Most of the time,' I answered.

'And when is it not like that?'

'When I'm busy doing something, like playing a game or reading.'

He asked the nurse if I was sleeping alright and if there was any movement of my foot while I was asleep. She said there was not.

'Patrick,' he said, 'I am going to have to send you to another doctor.'

I froze with fear and disbelief. This was the man who was so kind and gentle to me, who had introduced me to a family for the first time I could remember. Now he was sending me to another doctor, which to me meant a change of hospital. I didn't want him to see me cry as I told him that I didn't want to go away.

'Who said anything about going away?' he asked. 'You won't have to move hospitals, just wards. That's not so bad. Is it?'

'No.'

'And I'll be able to keep an eye on you, and no doubt some of your nurse girlfriends will come and visit you for the time you are there.'

He pressed his hand firmly down on my head and remarked on the length of my hair. 'We'll have to get that cut for you one of these days, maybe you'll come to the barber with me when I'm not too busy.'

'Where is the other doctor?' I asked nervously.

'Mother of Mercy Ward.'

'Will I have to stay there?'

'That depends on what he says,' he said, adding that he was certain I would be back in his ward sometime.

'Is the other doctor going to be able to make me better?'

'I hope so, after all that's why we are sending you to him, and if he doesn't he will have to deal with me,' he laughed.

I had settled into Saint Patrick's Ward and didn't want to leave, but by now realized that being moved from place to place was an inevitable part of my life. Despite that, every move was a traumatic one. Even though I had witnessed and experienced suffering during my months there and lived with the seemingly endless visits of the priest to administer extreme unction, I had come to like the place, even love it. Nurses and patients were good to me and treated me as someone special. There were lighter moments, like the empty proposals of marriage which always took the form of a question like;

'How would ya like to put yer shoes under the same bed as meself?'

'You're a desperate man,' the nurse would reply, laughing.

'Desperate! Bejasus I am! You can put that to music.'

CHAPTER TWELVE

Mother of Mercy Ward was a small Neurosurgical unit with no more than ten beds. There were two rooms off the corridor reserved for private patients or people recovering from major brain surgery. In contrast to Saint Patrick's, it was very quiet and the patients appeared to be more ill. Many of the beds were screened off, but every patient I could see had a plaster covering part of his head. Some had their heads completely shaved and covered with a heavy cream-coloured sticking plaster. Their faces were stained by disinfectant running like pink tears down their cheeks and along the back of their necks.

The nurses shifted busily around the ward with no real rapport between them and the patients as there had been in St Patrick's. Whenever I made noise I was reprimanded by a nurse. Patients muttered at me, one elderly man shouting at the nurse on duty to 'get that child to hell out of the place'.

I hated Mother of Mercy Ward, hated its drabness and silence. I hated the cranky old men groaning their way out of the world, though by now I had become so used to death that I accepted the ritual of it as just part of each day. I resented having to stay in bed with no-one to play with. Some nurses and visitors would bring in comics which I kept stacked in a neat pile at the end of my bed. I never felt comfortable beneath the bedcovers and so I spent most of the day outside them. Whenever the Matron was expected, I was hastily rushed under the covers which were tucked in tightly to ensure that I remained there. It was the same whenever a doctor, priest or nun was visiting the ward, or during visiting hours on Sunday.

My closest friend during those days was a young nun, a novice of barely nineteen or twenty, freshfaced and good looking despite the unattractive habit she had to wear, which only allowed her face and hands to be exposed. Her friendship towards me and the love I felt for her were in marked contrast to my feelings for the nuns in the School at Cappoquin, who by now were nothing more to me than bad memories. I was so used to calling nuns 'Mother' that I found it difficult to address Sister Catherine as 'Sister' for a while. She spoke softly, even when I irritated her by not bothering to learn spellings she had set me. She often asked me to learn pieces out of an old green covered catechism she had given me and was always pleased when I answered her questions and never angry when I didn't.

One day she gave in to my persistence and had agreed to play a game of draughts with me when the Matron unexpectedly arrived into the ward. She glared icily at the young nun before beckoning to her with her wrinkled finger. Sister Catherine grew visibly distressed as the matron rebuked her for being intimate with a patient. When she reminded the Matron that I had no-one else to play with she responded through her gritted teeth; 'Your job Sister is to look after the patients, not to play with them.'

I felt desperately guilty as Sister Catherine wept openly. I wanted to tell her how sorry I was but couldn't bring myself to. It would have been too embarrassing for both of us. As she walked out of the ward accompanied by the matron I wondered if she would ever talk, never mind play with me again.

The nurses wore white uniforms with white veils that hung from their heads like kites. They were heavily starched and held in position with three white hair clips. They wore badges which gave the initial of their first name. Nurse M. Duffy was giving me my medication one day when I asked her what the 'M' stood for. She refused to answer and, when I persisted, said that the patients were not supposed to know the nurses first names because nurses were not allowed to be familiar with them. Eventually she told me her name was Margaret but warned me never to call her that out loud, or both of us would be in trouble.

'I heard the other nurses calling you Mags,' I said. 'That's what I'm going to call you.'

I teased her and she playfully put her hand across my mouth to stop me. As she did, I bit on the loose skin of her fingers which made her pull her hand away.

'Play a game of Ludo with me Mags and I won't call you Mags.'

'I will not,' she said 'Do you want Drac to catch me?'

'Who's Drac?'

No sooner had I asked the question when I realized she meant the matron. I remembered what happened with Sister Catherine and I understood Margaret Duffy's refusal to play with me.

Not long after I arrived there the consultant neurosurgeon came to see me. Unlike most of the consultants I had come across during my years in hospital, he didn't have a large group of students with him, just one other doctor. He was friendly towards me and adopted the habit of gripping my nose between the joints of his first two fingers and twisting it gently. It was a gesture designed to make me less nervous of him.

Whenever he wanted to discuss something with the staff of the ward or the doctor accompanying him, he stepped back from the bed and stood in the middle of the ward. Though I could always hear what he was saying I didn't always understand it. But I understood when he told the ward sister he wanted to carry out some investigative surgery and would be taking me 'down' the following morning. I trembled at the mention of the word 'down', which could only mean one thing. I was to be operated on. This time under general anesthetic. Using his own head as a model he explained to his house man how he intended to insert plates into my head to be used for various procedures in the future. One would be inserted at the top of my head towards the front and another at the back. He also described the need for 'burr holes' to relieve intracranial pressure. The precise nature of the condition was not clear and the surgery would be purely investigative. Before leaving he twisted my nose and mentioned that he would see me in the morning. I nodded fighting to hold back the tears.

In the afternoon, Sister Catherine came to my bedside, her face strained as she left a covered tray on the bed-table. She asked me softly not to touch anything as she walked across the ward for screens to put around my bed. Her voice trembled as she said she had to get me ready for the theatre. There was silence between us for a minute before she took a small nurse's scissors from a white leather pouch attached to a belt around her waist. She ran her fingers lovingly through my long straight hair before beginning to cut it. As the scissors snipped tufts of hair into her hand I wept silently and though she did her best to comfort me, I couldn't stop. When the scissors could do no more she unveiled the tray and filled a basin with warm water into which she dropped a bar of soap and a shaving brush, similar to those I had seen many men use to lather their faces before shaving. As the brush soaked, she carefully unwrapped a blade from its paper and inserted it into the open jaws of the silver razor. With a circular motion of the brush on the soap she prepared to lather my head for shaving. At first her movements were jerky as the razor jumped over the longer hair, dragging rather than shaving it. Sister Catherine apologised for hurting me, and replaced the original blade. I touched my head and was shocked by how prickly it felt. Other parts had no hair at all.

The Ward Sister came behind the screens and asked how Sister Catherine was getting on. She was satisfied with what had been done and wondered if my head felt cold. When I said it did, she suggested I wear a pixie. She left and returned with a green knitted one. She put it on and I threw it to the floor.

'Don't you like it?' the Ward Sister asked.

'No.' I replied, 'it's stupid looking.'

'Well isn't it better than having nothing at all on your head?'

I kept silent.

'Please yourself,' she said, and left.

Sister Catherine returned to take away the screens. I asked her to leave them.

'Why?' she asked.

'Because I don't want anybody to see me like this,' I sobbed.

'Now be a big man and stop crying, you look fine to me. Nobody is going to laugh at you, I bet they won't even notice.'

She removed the screens. I lay down and wondered if any of the other patients would notice me. They didn't. Later that evening Margaret Duffy woke me and offered me something to eat. I refused at first and only accepted when she reminded me I would have nothing else before surgery.

'Why did she have to cut all my hair off like that?' I asked in desperation. 'And why do I have to have an operation anyway?'

'Your hair will grow again soon, and the operation is only a very minor one. It'll be all over in a matter of minutes and you won't feel a thing.'

I sat up in bed, very self-conscious of my bald head, and wondering if the domestic staff serving the meal would comment. I tapped on the boiled egg, making only a half-hearted effort to break its shell. I pushed the spoon down and the soft yellow yolk ran down along the eggcup and onto the white plastic plate. One of the men was tearing a slice of white bread into strips and dipping them into his egg, I copied him and enjoyed the taste. Once I had finished eating, a 'Fasting' sign was hung at the head of my bed. My locker was searched for food and any that was found removed. I lay motionless wondering what was going to happen to me and thought of other patients I'd seen coming back from the theatre with tubes suspended from their bodies. I could visualize my face covered in pink antiseptic fluid and my head in sticking plaster. I stared at the young man in the next bed who had been admitted just a few days after me. At twenty one, he was the nearest of all the patients to me in age – twelve years my senior. He lay flat on his back, his eyes wide open, never blinking, staring at nothing on the ceiling. His life was sustained by liquid food and glucose from inverted glass bottles hanging from drip stands. His urine passed through a plastic tube into a bottle at the side of his bed. At intervals during the day, a nurse checked it and made notes on his chart. From a hole beneath his chin, a rubber tube protruded which drew off phlegm that accumulated on his chest. The sound made by this tube was the most sickening I have ever heard.

On the evening before my own operation I watched as the parents and friends of this young man gathered at his bed, watching and praying that he would come out of his comatose state. His mother had to be supported physically by his father as she wept and wondered aloud why she had ever allowed her son to become involved in rugby.

Vincent Flynn was in a deep coma as a result of an injury he'd received during a game. A scrum collapsed and he was caught underneath. When play resumed, he was left lying on the ground, motionless. It was his birthday. I watched his mother squeeze her son's hand so hard that her own knuckles went pale. It was as though she was desperately trying to awaken him. She looked at me but I turned away, embarrassed at how I looked and ashamed of myself for being caught prying.

When only Vincent's parents remained at his bedside, they knelt and prayed outloud. His father asked me to join in and I did. They recited decades of the rosary and finally a plea to God to allow their son to be alright 'if it be your holy will'.

Before being given my sleeping tablets, I was checked by a doctor, who listened to my chest and checked my pulse. With a small penlike torch he looked into my eyes and down my throat. I was tempted to say it was sore, because I knew that could prevent surgery. When he finished and was satisfied about my health, he said he would see me in the morning, in the theatre. That night before going to sleep, I was given more tablets than usual.

I was not allowed to wake properly the following morning. I felt a needle puncture my skin but my senses were too numb to react. Even as I was being dressed in a theatre gown, I made no attempt to resist. I couldn't.

My memories of being placed on the trolley and wheeled from the ward are vague. Most of the images are blurs, foggy scenes involving nurses and hospital orderlies. On the way to the theatre I became fully aware of what was happening as the doping effect of the drugs wore off and I became almost fully alert. Whatever potency that remained in the drugs was nullified by the awful sense of terror within me. I tried to sit up but the strong hand of the orderly pressed firmly down on my shoulder making it impossible to move.

I screamed as I was wheeled into the sterile atmosphere of the theatre where doctors and nurses quickly gathered around in an effort to stop me. Within seconds, my arm was strapped to a plastic covered piece of wood and a doctor stood over me with a needle and syringe in his hand. The overhead bright circular light hurt my eyes and as I struggled to break free from the people restraining me I felt my right forearm being pierced. A nurse asked me to count to ten. By three the room was beginning to spin, by five I was losing consciousness. I don't remember reaching six.

When I returned from theatre, I was put into one of the small rooms off the main ward. As I came out of the anesthetic and became more aware I could make out the blurred figure of a nurse sitting beside my bed. I could feel a soreness in my head which I wanted to rub but she prevented me. Every few minutes, her voice reminded me that I was back, and that everything was alright. For the next few hours I drifted from semi-consciousness to unconsciousness, only waking fully when my thirst became unbearable or the pain from the operation overrode the effects of the drugs. I felt the cloth of the sphygmomanometer being wrapped around my upper arm and tightened as my blood pressure was taken, and then the hissing of air as the pressure was slowly released.

'Water,' I said.

'You can't have water just now, it would make you sick,' the nurse said.

'Water,' I pleaded, through cracked, half sealed lips.

'You can have all the water you want in a little while.'

I rolled my tongue around my mouth in search of even the slightest sign of moisture, but there was none. The glycerine applied to my lips was no substitute for the drink I desperately craved.

About two hours after returning from theatre a nurse placed one hand at the back of my head and, raising it gently, held a glass of water to my parched mouth. I wanted to gulp it down but she warned that that would only make me sick. When I snatched at it she whisked it away. The next time I got a drink it was to help me swallow pain killing tablets which were to keep me sedated for the best part of two days.

When I was put back into the main ward I borrowed a small, double-sided shaving mirror from Vincent Flynn's locker. One side gave a normal mirror image, the other side was magnified. It was the magnified side that I chose to look at myself. What I saw horrified me. I was so ugly I wondered how anyone could even look at me. My head seemed to have a big bump on the top where a dressing had been placed after the operation and my face was almost completely pink from surgical antiseptic. I pulled a towel from my locker rail, dipped a corner of it into a glass of water and began to rub my face furiously, trying to remove the pink streaks, but I couldn't make the slightest impression. When I asked a nurse how I could get it off, she said it would fade away itself after a while. Margaret Duffy caught me looking at myself and said that I was being vain.

'I'm not being vain, I just want to see if my hair is growing yet.'

'You hardly expect it to grow two or three days after it has been shaved,' she exclaimed.

'No but I hope I'll have some hair before my birthday.'

'Is that a hint?' she asked, smiling.

'It's my birthday on the nineteenth of May,' I said.

'I thought you didn't know when your birthday was. According to your chart it's not until the nineteenth of June.'

I told her that when I was in Kilkenny I'd said it was in February, thinking it might get me out of the room I was in by myself.

'Did they believe you?' she asked.

'No, I don't think so.'

'Do you know what age you'll be?' she wondered.

'Ten.'

'Ten! I suppose we'll have to have a birthday party for you.'

'I suppose,' I answered, unsure what to say. I had never celebrated a birthday before and wondered if a party would be organised for me.

The ward sister asked if I had been to the toilet and when I said I hadn't, she told me I'd need to drink a lot and eat plenty of fruit or they'd have to give me an enema.

The only liquid I had was water and I looked with envy at the array of soda syphon bottles on the other lockers around the ward.

'Why can't I have something like that to drink?' I asked.

There was a bottle of Lucozade on Vincent Flynn's locker, still wrapped in its orange cellophane paper. She unwrapped it and loosened the black stopper with its rubber band from the bottle, remarking how useless it was to Vincent. I felt guilty, as though I was stealing something from someone who didn't even know.

'Can he hear?' I asked.

'No.'

'Can he see?'

'No.'

'But,' I exclaimed 'his eyes are wide open.'

She told me that Vincent was in a world of his own where everything was dark, just like being in a room where all the curtains were drawn.

'So he's sort of asleep with his eyes open?' I said, and asked her if he would ever wake up. That was in the hands of God she replied. When I asked why he couldn't have an operation to fix him she just said that we would all have to pray and hope for the best.

'Will he die?' I asked finally.

'I think you've had your fair share of questions for one day.'

I asked her why some of the nurses put their finger over the tube sticking out of his throat when they were talking to him. She explained that because of the hole in his wind-pipe he couldn't speak, even if he wanted to. The only chance

170

of hearing anything he might want to say was by closing off that tube.

'Could I put my finger over it,' I asked.

She looked surprised at first, then lifted me the short distance to his bed. She demonstrated how to cover the tube, warning me never to keep it covered for longer than ten seconds. I was frightened as my finger neared the tube and then touched it. I didn't like the feel of the rubber tube or its wetness at the rim, and was frightened too by the vacant stare of Vincent's dark eyes, like two glass discs that gaped from deep caverns in his boney structured face. His arms were down by his sides, completely straight and still. A breathing corpse.

He was extremely good looking and every morning he was given a bed bath, after which he was shaved with a Ronson electric shaver and his jet black hair was combed back from his forehead. During the day, I was allowed to sit on his bed. In my own mind, I had built up a relationship with him, and made every effort to bring him out of his dark, unconscious world. I spent long periods trying to get him to respond to my voice as I repeated his name. Occasionally I would put my finger over the protruding tube, hoping I would be the first to hear him speak. Whenever I spoke to him I kept my mouth as close to his ear as possible, asking him to blink his eyes if he could hear me, but they remained frozen open.

I always protested at being tucked back into my own bed, saying I wasn't comfortable as my foot was hurting me. By now the bending of one toe had spread to the others and my foot used to cramp so badly I was certain the tendons would snap. Instinctively, I knew that something was going desperately wrong. Whenever the ward sister looked at my foot she reminded me that the neurosurgeon was going to put it right, but it would take time and patience. Gradually the amount of medication I was receiving increased and I didn't bother to count the number of pills I took in a day.

'Why can't I get up?' I asked.

'Because . . .' and she hesitated, 'that is what the doctor says. What's the great hurry anyway, won't it be much better for you to be up when you can walk properly?'

'I don't know if I can walk properly any more,' I said. 'Look at the way my foot is twisted.'

She tried to straighten my toes and turn my foot outwards without causing me pain but she couldn't. The level of involuntary movement from me was so great that she was forced to give up. The bones in my ankle were protruding till they threatened to come through my skin and my foot was becoming increasingly deformed looking. When she said she would have to bring the matter to the attention of the surgeon, I asked if it would mean another operation.

'I don't know,' she answered, 'that will be up to the doctor to decide. Anyway you still have the stitches in from the last time, so it's a bit early to be thinking of more operations.'

My stitches were taken out about ten days after the operation. Margaret Duffy, Sister Catherine and the ward sister drew screens around my bed.

Tiny bristles of hair protruded through the heavy white sticking plaster making its removal difficult and very painful. I cried and tried to stop them pulling it but I was restrained and warned not to touch it because of the risk of infection. With the use of ether, the adhesion of the plaster was broken and it was gradually withdrawn exposing the wound to the cold air. Blood stained cotton wool pads from my head were tossed into a steel pedal bin.

With their faces masked and rubber gloves on their hands, they began to remove the stitches, assuring me that I would feel no pain. I felt a tweezers pinch and lift the first stitch then with great caution the cold blade of a scissors barely touched my head as it slid under the loop. A snip and it was gently withdrawn and left in a kidney dish on the trolley. There was an air of tension while the procedure was carried out with hardly a word spoken. When it was finished the sense of relaxation among the staff was almost palpable. A small strip of Elastoplast was put over the area where the stitches had been removed. I asked if I could look at myself in Vincent Flynn's mirror, but Margaret Duffy said I should wait until she had removed all the stains made by the antiseptic from my face. Using a piece of cotton wool soaked in ether, she rubbed gently, taking care to avoid my eyes, nose or mouth. It left my face cold, and its strong smell made me feel drowsy.

When she was finished, she took the mirror from Flynn's locker and held it in front of me.

'Now are you happy?' she asked.

I looked at myself.

'Yeah, I suppose so,' I said.

CHAPTER THIRTEEN

One day when she was not too busy, Margaret Duffy agreed
to play a game of snakes and ladders with me. I set out the
board as she momentarily attended to another patient. During
the game I said I wanted to ask her a question, but that she
had to promise to answer whatever I asked. She protested,
saying she would make no promises. I persisted convincing
her that the question I wanted answered wasn't a hard one.
She agreed to answer.

'Where do babies come from?' I asked suddenly.

She blushed and wondered why I wanted to know.

'I just want to know, that's all.'

'If I tell you, do you promise not to go shouting it around
the ward and get me into trouble.'

I nodded. She shook the dice and scaled a ladder on the
board with her plastic playing counter.

'They come from their mothers' bellies,' she said, 'now will
you throw the dice and stop asking questions.'

'But how do they get in there?'

She reminded me that I'd said 'one question'.

'It doesn't matter anyhow,' I said, 'a boy in the hospital in
Kilkenny told me.'

'You tell me then,' she said.

'I will not,' I replied adamantly.

'Have you a boyfriend?' I asked.

'My God, but you are a nosey little demon. What if I have?
Is it any of your business?' she mocked playfully.

'What's his name?'

'Mind your own business and get on with the game.'

'Will you buy me a money box?' I asked.

'A money box!' she exclaimed. 'What for?'

'I want to save up to buy a watch.'

'And where do you propose to get the money from?'

'I don't know,' I said, 'I'll just leave it on my locker and maybe when the visitors come they might put something in it.'

'Not only are you nosey, but you're as cute as a fox.'

She laughed and I showed her an advertisement I had taken from a newspaper showing the watch I wanted. It was thirty two shillings and sixpence.

'I hope it keeps fine for you!' she said, smiling.

I made her promise to get the box the next time she was in town and she agreed.

By visiting time the next Sunday I had my money box placed strategically on my bedside locker and made a point of rattling it to attract attention. There were six pennies in it, given to me by Margaret with the box. 'That's the sixpence,' she said. 'Now all you need is the thirty two shillings.'

Visitors came over to enquire about what had happened me. The price of an answer was a contribution towards the cost of the watch. It was a well-worked system. First I told them I was saving for a watch, and when their money dropped into my miniature English postbox, I told them I had Polio. If they asked me, as they usually did, if I was getting better I always said no. I would have to have more operations. In most instances this ensured a further donation and a speedy departure of the inquisitor.

It was only a short time before the box was filled and I was confident that I had sufficient money to make my purchase. Getting the money out was a slow, noisy business. I had to insert a knife into the slot and allow the coins to slide out along its blade. The noise irritated the other patients, more than one of whom shouted for a nurse to 'take that blasted box and the child out of here'. The more hatred the men expressed towards me, the more I delighted in annoying them.

When they were reminded that I was only a child they

responded by saying that I shouldn't be in the ward. One man suggested that they 'find a ward full of noisy little bastards and put him in there!'

I was anxious to get the watch and nothing would persuade me to wait until my birthday. After much pressure, Margaret Duffy promised to get it on her next day off. I gave her the money and the advertisement and asked her to bring it to me as soon as she got back from town.

'I can't do that,' she said. 'The nurses are not allowed on to the wards in Civies.'

Her day off was one of the longest of my life. I convinced myself that she would forget or lose the money or there might be no watches left when she got to the shop. When she came on duty Margaret Duffy handed me a neatly wrapped parcel. I tore through the wrapping paper and broke open the cardboard box containing the watch. In sheer delight I looked at the dial, the golden figures, the large second hand that moved jerkily around the face. I listened to the ticking before eventually putting it on my wrist. At first the brown leather strap was too loose and it was only with the aid of the pointed blade of a scissors that additional holes were made to allow the strap to be buckled. I couldn't resist fiddling with the winder, turning it gently to make sure it was wound.

'Once a day is enough to wind the watch,' Margaret said. 'More often than that and you'll wreck it.'

For the first few hours, I kept an almost constant eye on the watch and checked with every nurse that passed by to see if their watches corresponded to my own.

That evening, when the ward was quiet, I took the back off the watch to see what was inside. As I was putting it on again, the second hand fell off. I tried desperately to fix it but couldn't. In exasperation, I left the hand inside the dial and decided to pretend that it fell off while I was asleep.

'Wake up sleepy head. What time is it?' I recognized Margaret Duffy's voice next morning.

I sat up and looked innocently at my watch.

'I don't know what time it is,' I said, 'I forgot to wind it last night and now it's stopped.'

My voice trembled as I handed it to her and I knew I wasn't going to convince her by my story. I started crying.

'Did you open the watch?' she asked.

'I just wanted to have a look inside. I didn't mean to break it.'

When she saw how upset I was she agreed to take the watch back and try to have it changed, provided I promised to say nothing about having opened it. During her break she took it back, carefully wrapped in paper from a present brought to another patient, warning me before leaving not to expect miracles.

Later in the day she returned to the ward smiling broadly. She took a new watch from the large square pocket of her uniform and helped me to put it on, remarking that they wouldn't replace the strap because it had been tampered with.

That night the ward sister examined the wound on my head by gently lifting the sticking plaster that had covered it since my stitches had been removed. There was no need for a replacement plaster and I could touch my head if I wanted to. By now my hair had started to grow and looked just like a tight crew cut. The self-consciousness of being bald was gone and I was looking forward to having a full head of hair again.

But it wouldn't be that way. The ward Sister informed me I would be going to the theatre again. I was shocked and kept repeating that I didn't want to go. It hadn't been long since I was there last.

'Well now,' she said 'if you want to get better . . .'

'I don't,' I said sharply.

'And I suppose you don't want to go to the Zoo either?'

I looked at her.

'Yes,' she said, 'Nurse Duffy and her boyfriend want to take you out for a day soon, but you can only go if you're good and if Matron agrees.'

'When have I to go to the theatre?' I asked nervously.

'In the morning.'

'How could I have to go? The doctor hasn't even been around and the dressing from the last is just gone.'

She said this operation was the second part of the first one and was only a very minor 'job' not to be worried about. The priest would be around later. The routine was familiar. Notification of an operation. Fear of death while undergoing surgery. Then confession. The cleaning of the soul, just in case.

Again, Sister Catherine was given the job of 'prepping' me. She screened off the bed and apologised for having to shave my head again. 'Someday,' she said 'it'll be all over.' She lathered my head and shaved it completely, taking great care not to hurt the previous scar which was still tender. Her hand trembled as the razor removed the freshly grown, downy hair.

'Why do I have to have operations on my head?' I asked.

'I wish I knew,' she said with sadness in her voice. I could feel her concern for me. She was so different. She was kind, laughed a lot and played games with me. Lifting me in her arms she would carry me out of the ward, to a garden at the rear of the hospital where she'd take photographs of me, seated on a blanket, in front of a circular flower bed. Her mother used to buy clothes for me and she took great pride in dressing me and ensuring I looked well. I always received my medication promptly when she was on duty and consequently seldom became distressed or over-anxious. In the times of my greatest stress she made a special effort to alleviate it, always trying to be there as I left the ward for surgery and again when I returned.

Next morning in the operating theatre, the neurosurgeon greeted me by giving my nose a slight twist. When he asked if I was frightened I didn't bother to respond. A needle pierced the most prominent vein in my arm and within seconds I was drowsy and dizzy. Soon I was asleep and he was making further incisions on my scalp in preparation for drilling through my skull.

Later as the trolley was wheeled back into the ward I was partially awake. Drifting in and out of sleep, I heard the sounds I was familiar with. Men coughing. The news being read on Radio Eireann. Through half-open eyes I could see Sister Catherine walking beside the trolley and felt the softness of her hand firmly gripping mine.

I felt well when I woke, not as sick or as thirsty as I had been previously. The thirst I dreaded so much was speedily vanquished by a cup of warm sweetened tea which Sister Catherine held and allowed me to take at my own pace. Within a few hours I was sitting up in bed and having a light meal.

I was ten years of age before I celebrated a birthday. Birthdays didn't happen in the Industrial School and were not bothered about in any of the other hospitals I had been in. In Mother of Mercy Ward, there was a certain amount of excitement when anyone was celebrating a birthday. A request might be played for them on Radio Eireann's, 'Hospital's Requests', and there would be more than the usual amount of visitors. It wasn't unusual to see a relative slip a bottle from a brown paper bag discreetly under the bedcovers of the patient he was visiting. For that day nurses turned a blind eye to what was happening, though next morning the half empty bottle of whiskey would be confiscated after a search of bedside lockers. Wives fussed more than usual and if the opportunity presented itself would draw a screen around the bed, through the folds of which I could see them embrace and kiss their husbands with great passion and urgency.

I woke early on the 19th of May 1961 to a chorus of 'Happy Birthday' from nurses and some patients. Both nightnurses and day-nurses had gathered around Sister Catherine and Margaret Duffy who were carrying a large parcel. A white envelope bearing my name was sellotaped to it. As it was lifted onto my bed, they asked me to guess what it was, but I was too excited to. It felt light and delicate. As they helped to remove the paper, the shining chrome bars of a bird-cage were slowly revealed containing a beautiful, greyish-blue budgie that hopped from perch to perch.

'What are you going to call him?' Margaret asked.

'I don't know,' I answered.

'What about Pedro?' she suggested, pronouncing the 'P' as a 'B'.

'Okay,' I said, repeating the name. I was so delighted and preoccupied with the present that I didn't notice a card pinned on the wall over my bed. It was Margaret Duffy who drew my attention to it.

I looked up at the long unfolded card and read out *PADDY: TEN YEARS OLD.* The words were printed in bright luminous green.

'That was made specially for you,' she said.

'Who made it?' I asked.

'Bernard did.'

'Who is Bernard?'

'He's my boyfriend,' she said, blushing slightly, as she realized she had given his name unintentionally, 'You'll meet him later. You're coming to the Zoo with us.'

I asked to have everything taken off my locker so I could put the cage as close to me as possible. I stared through the tiny rails, my eyes riveted on the bird fluttering around the cage, chirping and occasionally screeching as he hung by his beak from a yellow plastic swing. The noise was annoying some of the patients who were demanding that the ward sister 'take that damned bird to hell out of the place'.

'You should take the bloody child too, and that would solve all the problems,' one shouted.

The Matron arrived as the ward sister was explaining to those objecting that it was my birthday and they should accept the right of a child to have some fun. Matron walked towards me, looking angrily at the budgie. Then the brightly coloured card over the bed caught her eye. She called the ward sister and demanded that the cage be removed from the ward at once.

'We are in a hospital, Sister, not a home for pets,' she said sternly.

The ward sister tried to explain, but the Matron was not interested and said so. I was bitterly disappointed as my present was taken from the ward. Despite my tears the matron warned me that she didn't want to see the bird back in the ward again or the other patients disturbed.

'What is the meaning of this?' she said, pointing to the birthday card over my bed.

'It's a birthday card Matron,' the sister replied. 'One of the nurses got it made specially.'

'It will have to come down immediately. It is more like an advertisement for whiskey and it could be upsetting to the older patients.'

She walked swiftly towards the door, turning to warn that she would be back. As the card was removed, the ward sister told me that I could go to her office anytime I liked to play with the budgie.

Sister Catherine dressed me in new clothes, saying that she 'wanted her little man to be looking lovely when he went out'. She carried me in her arms out to the garden where she took some 'Birthday Photos'. By this time I had great difficulty in keeping still and became very stressed when having a photo taken. The harder I tried to keep steady, the more difficult it became. She looked at the patch on my head where the hair had not grown since my operation, and suggested that I should wear a hat while out. I thought a hat would look silly and when I told her so, she didn't pursue the matter.

As I waited to be brought out, I wondered how I was going to manage to get around the Zoo. I was worried about travelling in the car, remembering how tense and uncomfortable I had been the last time I had travelled in one. I was confused as to whether I wanted to go or not, but I said nothing.

Margaret Duffy arrived into the ward with her boyfriend Bernard and immediately noticed that the cage and budgie were gone along with the card he had made.

'Where's Pedro?' she asked, angrily. 'And what happened the card?'

The ward sister told her what happened. Margaret was furious and referred to her as 'a right bitch'. She laughed at the thought of the card being an advertisement for whiskey.

Bernard looked on, unsure of what was happening. He was a tall thin man with very sharp features and a pale complexion. He had blonde hair and deeply set blue eyes. After we had been introduced to each other the ward sister told Margaret that she had reservations about asking Matron that I be allowed out, in case it would result in a refusal. She suggested that they slip out of the hospital with me as quickly and quietly as possible. Bernard lifted me and carried me down the short corridor to the main hall and out the door into his black Volkswagen. There was a sense of urgency about everything from the time we left the ward until the car was out of sight of the hospital.

When Bernard carried me through the entrance of Dublin Zoo the cashier indicated he would not be taking for me. He suggested that instead of having to carry me around they might like to use one of the buggies lined up just inside the gates. Margaret pulled one out and Bernard put me sitting in it. I was most uncomfortable, my stockinged feet banged relentlessly against the polished steel frame and as my spasms became strong and violent, my feet actually entangled themselves behind the footrests, which could have broken my legs were it not for the swift movements of my companions. Eventually I could no longer endure the pain or discomfort of the buggy. Margaret and Bernard agreed to carry me on a rota basis, and whenever we came to a cage where a lot of people had gathered, she politely asked to be excused. Children asked their parents why I had hardly any hair. Why was I not wearing shoes and why were my feet all crooked? Why did I have to be carried? But the adults and their patronizing smiles were more difficult to cope with than these perfectly understandable questions. Many of them clipped their children around the ear and told them to mind their own business. One child received a tremendous wallop when he said in a loud, musical, Dublin accent 'Hey Ma, that fella looks like a monkey, his ears stick out and he has a furry head'.

I wanted to get away from the crowds and be alone with

Bernard and Margaret. He went to the shop while she carried me to a wooden bench at the edge of a lake. There were just a few people around and I was much more content. The realization that I was being constantly stared at had dampened my interest in the animals, except for a tiger called 'Rama'. Bernard took a photograph of Margaret and me in front of his cage, while in the background the tiger devoured what appeared to me to be a horse's head. The animal's growling was interspersed with the sound of flesh being torn from bone, as the elegant beast held his meal firmly between two enormous front paws.

Bernard returned from the shop and sat to one side of me, sharing crisps, chocolate and lemonade.

'What will you do when Mags leaves?' he said suddenly.

I could feel her jab him furiously in the ribs with her elbow.

I was extremely close to Margaret Duffy and had come to regard her in many ways as a mother figure, someone that I could love, and who would return that love. I had never given a thought to the possibility of her leaving, though deep down I always felt we would be parted by me being moved to another hospital. I was equally attached to Sister Catherine but because she was a nun I felt there was always a barrier between us.

I wanted to be alone with her, to talk. Why was she leaving? Where was she going? Would I ever see her again or would it be just another person I loved and trusted gone forever from my life?

'When are you going?' I asked eventually.

There was a slight agitation in her voice as she answered. 'I don't know.'

'But Bernard said you were.'

'Look,' she said, forcing me to look her straight in the face, 'it's not as if we'll never see each other again.'

The moment she spoke those words I knew that a close friendship was coming to an end. At first I didn't want to know what she intended doing. I made that obvious by remaining silent on the journey back to her boyfriend's flat. My sulking obviously annoyed her and when I was sitting on a bed she caught me by the hand and shook me slightly.

'Listen,' she said, 'I'm very fond of you, you know that. It's not going to be easy for me to leave. Not only do I have to leave you. What about my parents and my brothers and sisters as well as other friends? Do you think I won't miss them?'

I kept silent while we had tea and cakes. While they were washing up I got off the bed and slid across the floor on my backside. Neither of them heard or noticed me. As I touched Margaret's stockinged leg she screamed, frightened by the sudden and unexpected touch of my hand.

'Why don't you tell me where you're going?' I asked.

She squatted down to be as close to me as possible, then with her eyes fixed firmly on mine she said, 'Bernard and I are getting married and are going to live in America.'

I went hysterical and began to scream and throw things around the small bed-sit. I accused her of liking 'that fella' better than me.

'You're the only friend I have in that smelly, stinking ward full of cross old men. You don't care what happens to me. Do you. Do you?' I screamed at her and when she tried to put her arms around me, I pounded my clenched fists into her chest and tried to kick her. As her boyfriend moved to restrain me, she told him she was alright.

'Sister Catherine is very fond of you, and when I'm gone she will take care of you.'

'I hate nuns,' I said.

'That's not true, and you know it.' She was getting angry. 'Sister Catherine is very good to you. Who gets you all the lovely clothes you wear and who goes to the theatre with you. Isn't she always there when you wake up? She takes better care of you than I ever could and it is not fair to say that you don't like her.'

'I wouldn't have to go to the theatre if she didn't shave off my hair,' I shouted.

'Now you're being stupid. You know well she's just doing what she has to.'

I knew she was right and knew also that whether I liked

it or not, I was going to have to let go of her. She had her own life which I could not be a part of.

'Why do you have to leave?' I asked.

'Because I will be finished my training and once I get married I'll have to leave the hospital anyway.'

'Will you ever come to see me?' I asked.

'I'll try, but America is a long way away, and it costs a lot to get home. There's nothing to stop you writing and I will always answer your letters. I'll be dying to know how you're getting on.'

I didn't speak on the journey back to the hospital and as she lifted me from the car, Margaret asked me to say goodbye to Bernard. I grunted something or other and when he pressed money into my hand, saying it was for 'that famous money box' I didn't even thank him. I blamed him for taking Margaret out of my life.

'Are you never going to speak to me again?' she asked as she held my face close to hers, going up the steps of the hospital.

'No,' I growled.

'Not even if I promise to buy you a goldfish and bowl before I leave?'

'That old bitch of a Matron will just take it like she took the budgie.'

She laughed uncontrollably at my outburst. I laughed too. She whispered into my ear that bitch was not a nice word, but that I was right.

That laughter lifted the terrible hatred I felt for her a few hours earlier. When we reached the ward, Sister Catherine and the ward sister brought a sponge cake with ten lighted candles to my bedside. The three of them sang happy birthday and got me to blow out the candles and make a wish. A piece of cake was offered to all the patients, some of whom took it while others refused. While I was eating I stared into Margaret Duffy's eyes and noticed tears in them. She left the cake on a piece of cardboard and rushed from the ward, saying that Bernard was waiting in the car. That was the moment I accepted the inevitability of her leaving for good.

In the days before she left, I made a point of ignoring Margaret Duffy as much as I could and turning my attention and affections to Sister Catherine. I looked to her to play games with me and for praise whenever I did anything.

Sister Catherine was different in every way from the nuns I had grown up with – kind, gentle and not afraid to show affection. She was never cruel to me and when I did require a reprimand, it was usually a playful event, like the day I was being particularly difficult, climbing out of bed and sliding around the ward on my behind. I slid under the patients' beds much to their irritation. She pursued me from bed to bed and suddenly said 'Here's Drac,' with an urgency in her voice.

I came out from under a bed and was sliding across the floor to my own when she swept me up into her arms. I was laughing as she brought me to an upstairs bathroom and put me sitting in the empty bath, telling me to stay there until I decided to behave myself. She hadn't thought I would be able to get out of it, but within minutes I was at the top of the stairs calling her name. From there I could see into the office where she was busy writing the day report into a ledger. She noticed me and rushed up.

'How did you get out of there?' she asked, lifting me into the office. She put me sitting in a chair at the desk beside her while she continued writing. I couldn't resist the temptation to lift the black telephone and hold it to my ear.

'What number do you want?' a male voice said.

There was a board hanging in front of me with a list of numbers on it and I gave him one.

'Are you a patient?' he asked gruffly.

'Yes,' I said.

'Patients are not supposed to use the phone. Where's the sister in charge of that ward, I want to speak to her immediately.'

I slammed down the receiver, shaking with fear and told her what had happened.

'Did anyone see you using the phone?' she asked.

'Just you.'

186

'Me!' she exclaimed 'I didn't see anything.'

If I felt particularly lonely I asked to be put sitting on Vincent Flynn's bed, where I would wave my hands frantically at him in the hope that he would blink. When that did not bring a response I tugged gently at his hair and even twisted his nose in the way the neurosurgeon used to twist mine. I used to read Enid Blyton's 'Famous Five' books for him and tell him silly 'Paddy the Irishman' jokes and laugh loudly into his face. Sometimes I'd hold his mirror in front of him.

For months his parents had been calling to see him every evening, but when it became apparent that he was not getting better the visits became shorter and less frequent. Everytime I saw them I longed for the love and affection of a mother or father. Indeed many times as I watched them hold their son's hand I used to turn my back so they wouldn't see me crying. They always asked to see a doctor about what was being done for their son and sometimes asked about the chances of a particular operation being successful. I had noticed that when Vincent was being taken to the theatre his father was offered a form to sign which I heard a doctor describe as a 'consent form'. I never saw anyone sign a form for me but often wondered who, if anyone, did. The other thought I had constantly was if I had parents, would they have allowed so much to happen to me.

One afternoon while many of the patients slept, I noticed a change in Vincent Flynn's breathing and called the nurse. She was quickly followed into the ward by the sister in charge, who asked that screens be brought to the bed and his parents be contacted.

The chaplain was at his bedside by the time his parents and family arrived. They gathered in a cluster in the middle of the ward as he prayed aloud in Latin. I found myself responding to prayers I had not said since leaving the Industrial School. It seemed appropriate that mine should be the voice most prominent as he died.

I was deeply moved as his body was taken from the ward.

The procession of grieving relations and friends made its way from the ward to the morgue at the rear of the hospital. His death didn't frighten me, though it caused me great sadness. Sister Catherine embraced me, saying that he was better off with God. Her words somehow seemed right.

CHAPTER FOURTEEN

I was starting to lose count of the number of times I had been to the operating theatre. I seem to have the memory of some form of surgery to my head twice in the same week on two occasions. All I can be certain of is that today there are eight scar marks on my skull. Vincent Flynn was dead and Margaret Duffy was gone to live in America. She sent a postcard, saying she had arrived safely, and would write as soon as she settled in. Weeks passed and no letter arrived. Sister Catherine was on duty less and less as she was in 'block', attending lectures in preparation for exams. She was also approaching the time when she would take her final vows which could mean her departure from the hospital.

That summer my head was X-rayed from a number of different angles. A few days later, the neurosurgeon, studied the lunar landscape appearance of my brain on the X-ray viewing frame in the ward and drew imaginary circles around different parts of it. He discussed with his houseman what he proposed doing. He told the ward sister that the procedure was difficult, but if it was successful there should be a marked improvement in my condition. He hoped for a reduction in the amount of spasm and a lessening of my dependence on drugs. Intensive care would be essential in the days following the operation, and a close eye would have to be kept for any emotional or physical changes in me. Before leaving the ward, he twisted my nose and asked me to be brave. He ran his hand over my head, feeling the hair which was just beginning to grow. I could sense that whatever he intended doing it was going to be difficult and though I was only ten I didn't share the apparent optimism of nurses and doctors that the operation would be a success. As I worried about what lay ahead, the ward sister reminded me that even though the operation was going to be longer than the previous one, it would be worth it all. Success would mean that I could walk again and be able to leave the hospital.

'Will this be the last time that I have to go down?' I asked nervously.

'That depends on how successful it is.'

'I don't want to go, please,' I begged.

'Now Paddy,' she said 'if this operation is successful you'll be able to get up and about.'

'But I don't want to have another operation.'

'Wouldn't you like to be finished with tablets and not to be afraid anymore? Wouldn't you like to stop living in wards with old people?'

'I don't mind old people,' I replied.

'Yes, but wouldn't you prefer to be with children of your own age? Your doctor is a good doctor, you have to trust him. All the patients and nurses will be thinking of you and looking forward to seeing you well again.'

I said nothing. I didn't care anymore what they did to me. I hadn't the slightest interest in being able to walk or mix with other children. I didn't pray for the success of the operation and only went to confession out of habit. Not even the prospect of death worried me.

In the late afternoon screens were drawn around my bed and a trolley arrived containing the instruments for giving an enema – a white enamel jug containing saline water, wrapped in towels to keep it warm, a basin of water and a bar of soap. On the lower section of the trolley there was a bedpan covered in a blue check cloth, a funnel, a thin length of reddish rubber hose and a jar containing petroleum jelly.

When the bottoms of my pyjamas had been removed, I was told to turn onto my side and bend my knees up towards my chest. My pyjama top was raised along my back and tucked underneath my arm-pits. I shivered with cold and fear. One nurse held me while a second prepared to administer the enema. I heard the familiar slapping sound of rubber gloves being drawn on and felt a smear of jelly being applied to my anus before my body was penetrated by a rubber tube. As it was being inserted, the nurse told me to shout if it hurt. I managed to look over my shoulder and saw her holding a steel funnel connected to a thin rubber hose, before the first nurse forced my head back towards her. Warm water was poured into the funnel and ran down the tube into me. The feeling was horrible and I wanted to force it back out. I would have only for the constant reminders to 'hold on to it' from the nurses. As more water was poured in the urge to discharge it became unbearable.

'I can't hold it any longer,' I cried.

'Just another minute or two,' they both urged.

I gripped the rubber sheet I was lying on, and clenched my teeth.

'I can't, I can't,' I pleaded.

The tube was withdrawn and before they could get me onto the bedpan, my bowels had emptied onto the rubber sheet. A nurse quickly lifted me off the bed while the other slipped the bedpan beneath me. I was desperately weak and certain I was going to faint. I lay there embarrassed and terrified.

Sister Catherine came to shave my head, a task I'm certain she disliked intensely but had to do. Each time she shaved it there was an extra wound to be careful of where the skin was still delicate and tender.

'Now,' she asked as she finished, 'are you not going to give me a smile?'

'No,' I said.

'Are you still going to marry me?' she asked.

'I don't know,' I replied and asked if she would come to the theatre. Gently, she held my face in her hands and promised to be with me as I was brought down and by my bed when I emerged from the anesthetic.

I was given a higher than usual dose of drugs on the morning of my operation as well as a pre-med injection which sent me into a deep sleep. I have only the vaguest memories of being changed into a green robe and taken from the ward to the operating theatre. One thing I remember vividly though, is the number of people that touched me as the trolley passed down the corridor – a series of blurred images on which I tried to focus but couldn't. I felt their hands touching my cheeks or the light pressure of a palm on my forehead. It seemed as though they were in sympathy with me and aware of how serious the surgery about to be performed was.

The scenes within the operating theatre were familiar, eyes gazing down from the strip of skin between the mask-tops and the green cloth caps, each person indistinguishable from the others. I was less nervous than usual due to heavy sedation. Some medical checks were carried out before the surgeon about to perform the operation spoke to me. I ignored him.

A needle pierced my arm and a male voice asked me to count to ten. Instead of doing so aloud as I usually did, I counted silently. Unconsciously or consciously, I decided to defy the anesthetic, and by the time I reached eight my eyes were still open and fixed firmly on the bright circular light overhead. Then I felt the needle being withdrawn, and the rubber band on my arm tightened. Fingers slapped on the veins in my forearm, to make them more prominent and easier to inject. The needle was re-inserted and, without bothering to count, I passed out.

Years later, one night on BBC radio, I heard an actual recording of a neurological procedure similar to that which I underwent. Naturally I cannot describe the operation I was involved in in 1961 and am not attempting to do so. But it was with an extraordinary sense of terror and fascination that I sat listening to the voice of the surgeon, identifying with the aid of carefully marked X-rays, the area of brain he wanted to deal with. The patient's head was completely daubed and then marked where incisions were to be made before being covered with a sort of artificial skin, a strong, stretchy plastic which clung tightly to his scalp. Cuts were made in it, giving access to the skull and eventually the brain itself. Incisions were held open by surgical clips known as retractors, and dressings were inserted into wounds to absorb any bleeding that occurred before veins could be tied off. The microphones picked up the surgeon and anesthetist in constant conversation, checking pulse rate and blood pressure as well as deciding when the level of anaesthesia needed to be deepened or reduced. Gradually the hard bone of the skull was exposed as the openings became wide and deep.

For the surgeon to reach the brain it was necessary to cut and drill through the skull. It is a manoeuvre requiring great skill and dexterity. As the drill sank deeper, the patient's head vibrated and had to be held steady. The sound of the drill boring its way deep into the skull was shrill and piercing. As one drill bit became less effective it was replaced by another resembling a tiny rose, each petal a small spike. Any bone that could not be removed using a drill was cut out with a fine toothed saw which made a screeching sound as it cut. Bone filings dispersed during the excavation process were collected and mixed with silicone for replacement on completion of the operation. Veins and arteries close to the site where the surgeon wished to extirpate tissue considered responsible for the patient's condition were carefully closed off, and the utmost care taken in the removal of the tissue. There are many complications to this type of surgery, some of which include, anxiety, depression, apathy and bronchial pneumonia.

Listening to the programme brought back the most traumatic event of my own operation, when I woke while apparently still being operated on. Absolute confirmation of this is difficult to obtain, but my memory of the event is sharp and clear. I was conscious of everything that was going on around me. The overhead light hurt my eyes momentarily and I could see the surgeon and other theatre staff looking at me. I was aware of various pieces of equipment close at hand and, most clearly, I remember that awful parched feeling in my mouth. 'Water,' I managed to say before being put back to sleep.

Many hours later I was taken from the operating theatre and put into intensive care. A nurse kept vigilance at my bedside and I remember her being instructed not to leave me alone for a minute and to ensure that I didn't sneeze or become distressed in any way.

I was kept asleep for nearly two days before being moved back to one of the rooms off the ward. I heard Sister Catherine's voice telling me that everything was fine. Slowly and painfully I emerged from the anesthetic to discover my arm tied down while I was given a blood transfusion. I tried to lift my head to take the water being offered me, but it was too painful to do so. Sister Catherine dipped a cloth in the glass and I sucked on it instead.

During the next days I suffered great pain in my head and also developed the severest pain I have ever experienced in my chest. I gasped and screamed, convinced that I was about to die. I begged Sister Catherine not to let me and she promised she wouldn't.

She looked at me with great anxiety as she damped my flushed face with a cloth, suggesting in desperation that I try to think of nice things. She said the doctor would come soon and everything was going to be fine.

'I don't want to die,' I screamed again.

'You're not going to die,' she said, her voice trembling. When the doctor came into the ward, I was still distressed and screaming. He listened to my chest and placed his hand on my forehead before prescribing medication and stressed the need to keep me under constant observation.

I have a very vivid memory of a woman standing in the doorway. I looked at her as she stared pitifully back and, despite the severity of the pain, I clearly remember her walking towards my bed and asking Sister Catherine if it would be alright for her to stay and say a few prayers.

They both knelt and continued to pray even when the neurosurgeon returned briefly to the room. Sister Catherine rose and listened to him as he spoke quietly. The woman moved away and leaning against the wall, prayed continuously, running her fingers along black rosary beads. After the doctor left she handed a brown scapular to Sister Catherine and insisted that she put it around my neck.

I do not know who this woman was, whether she was even real or just the ghost of a fevered imagination, nor do I know the significance of the brown scapular, apart from its reputed curative abilities. I can say with absolute certainty that following this event I went into a deep sleep and when I woke the excruciating pain in my chest was gone.

After about a week, I was taken back into the main ward. It must have been obvious to the doctors and nurses that the operation which they expected so much from was a failure. My toes twitched relentlessly and the degree of spasm in my body had greatly increased. I had no control whatever over the movement of either leg and most of the time they were contracted tightly against my chest. My toes bent so much and the spasms in my feet were so intense that they badly strained the tendons in my ankles which added greatly to my discomfort.

In August 1961, I was taken from Mother of Mercy Ward and returned to St Patrick's from where I had been taken nine months previously. The impact of this move on me was devastating and distressed me more than any previous one.

Sister Catherine's attempts to console and reassure me were futile. I screamed in protest as she carried me from the ward, unable to believe her when she told me I would be back. Under such stress, the ferocity of my spasm was so great that Sister Catherine had to protect herself from being injured by the uncontrollable kicking action of my legs. When I was put to bed in St Patrick's Ward, steel rails were erected on each side of it to prevent me falling out. It was the final indignity.

As she left the ward I shouted after Sister Catherine not to go. She returned to my bed and promised she would do everything possible to ensure I wouldn't have to stay in there.

In March 1962, I was taken back to Mother of Mercy Ward, for what the hospital records describe as 'possible basal ganglion surgery'. The record goes on: 'A small abscess had formed around one of the previous markers

195

and therefore no surgery could be done, but the marker was removed'.

By now Sister Catherine had left to work as a missionary nun in Kenya. I couldn't understand why, though I accepted the inevitability of her departure from my life. There was no nurse in the ward that I recognized and the only familiar face was the neurosurgeon passing through. My biggest worry was that I would have to undergo more surgery and every time I saw him I could feel my entire body tense. He often came to the end of my bed but said very little to me. He had even given up twisting my nose.

I no longer bothered trying to get out of bed and became so withdrawn that I took little notice of anything going on around me. The excitement and fun of Margaret Duffy and Sister Catherine had left an enormous gap in my life. Now the days seemed longer, and though the nurses were kind and caring there was a distance between me and them which I had no desire to remove.

During my final days in that hospital preparations were made for a visit by an East German Cardinal. Every time the nurses tucked me into bed I climbed back out. I couldn't bear the feel of the sheets on my feet and when the prince of the church arrived I was outside the bedcovers.

Perhaps because I was the only child in the ward, he came directly to my bed and extended his hand for me to kiss his ring. Press photographers followed, taking pictures that would be included in the following day's papers.

A photograph from one shows his thumb making the sign of the cross on my forehead. My feet are clearly visible, deformed and obviously in spasm and my newly grown hair is sticking up. What the photographs do not show is the sudden, vivid memory I had, when his ringed hand touched my skin, of the day six years before when my uncle's car halted with a jerk at the door of the school and the hands of Mother Paul, white against the blackness of her habit, beckoned me slowly into her care.

Shortly afterwards, on the 25th April 1962, I was discharged from there. After many inquiries from doctors on my behalf the only medical records I have been able to obtain are three single pages. On the two of them that give details of surgery the column for 'Next-of-kin or Responsible person' has been left blank. The section of the record referring to where I was discharged to reads: '—FD/SH Home'.

I was in fact sent to another hospital.

EPILOGUE

I was moved to St Mary's Hospital Baldoyle also known as 'The Little Willie Hospital'. The first thing I noticed on entering the hospital was a poster of 'Little Willie'; a small boy, his legs in calipers and his body supported on crutches. The image of this child, who was a patient there, was used extensively to raise funds.

I was put into a ward where the other patients were all about the same age as I was. The hospital at Baldoyle was situated near the seafront close to the racecourse and when the weather was fine 'walks' were organised there. Because of my condition and the extent of my involuntary movement I had to be strapped into my wheelchair. I enjoyed these outings, especially when I was allowed to roll around on the grass. It reminded me that the thing I missed most about being unable to walk was the feel of cool grass under my bare feet. I was not used to sandy beaches and disliked the feel of sand, especially when it got anywhere near my toes.

Two things in particular pleased me about St Mary's in Baldoyle; it had no operating theatre and there was an obvious absence of doctors. A consultant did visit the hospital once a month and anyone requiring surgery would be transferred to another hospital. I was taken to the physiotherapy department every day where efforts were made to straighten out my legs. Often my spasms were so violent that the physiotherapist had to enlist the help of other people to help her hold my legs down. The discomfort I endured during this process was great and I often begged them to let me go. 'Just another few seconds, it's all for your own good,' was the inevitable reply. This effort they put into trying to get me walk was the worst aspect of my stay there. My legs had to be forcibly straightened, before iron calipers and heavy black boots could be put on me. I was then brought to the walking bars and made to stand between them and look at myself in a full length mirror. All their efforts were pointless and eventually I was put into a wheelchair and given just the lightest of physiotherapy. Once a week I was allowed into the swimming pool where I was less tense and could feel my muscles relax. However, everytime I was instructed to 'kick' I could not. I desperately wanted to but the more I willed my limbs to respond, the more difficult the task became. The frustration was so great that at times I cried.

While in this hospital, I was prepared for confirmation and brought to the local parish church where Archbishop John Charles McQuaid of Dublin confirmed me a 'Soldier of Jesus Christ'. During the ceremony I paid more attention to the altar boys than to anything else. They were moving silently and elegantly around the altar just as I had done five or six years previously. Now I was seated in a wheelchair outside the altar rails, trying to restrain my legs from banging against its metal frame. I had not been in a church since I was admitted to hospital, now the smell of incense, the sounds of the organ and the Latin prayers I had so often responded to brought me back to Cappoquin. I remembered the day I tripped while carrying the missal and coming to in the sacristy, having fainted during mass. Unbelievably, Sister Paul's voice sounded in my ear as though she was standing beside me. 'You will never set foot inside the rails of an altar again'. Her prophecy had become a reality.

I attended a school in the hospital. It was a fragmented education as I was often taken from the class to the gym. In school I was given the task of teaching the tin whistle to a small class. I had just started learning it before leaving Cappoquin and was able to manage the scale and just one tune, which everyone learned; 'The Dawning of the Day'. The payoff was when the hospital band played this tune on 'The Imco Show' on national radio.

I knew that my stay in Baldoyle would be short – I was there for about nine months – and looked forward to being moved to St Mary's Hospital at Cappagh in Finglas, County Dublin. Reports reached Baldoyle that Cappagh was a better hospital, that the nurses were nicer and the nuns were not as cross. It was also a hospital for big boys.

The move to Cappagh was not in the least traumatic as I had prepared myself for it. It was to be a move of great significance to me and one which would undoubtedly have a massive impact on my future. In the first few weeks I underwent surgery to both legs, the purpose of which was to release the tendons at the back of the knee, allowing them to be straightened with greater ease. The surgery was only marginally successful and the surgeon under whose care I was placed recognized this. He actually told me that I would not have to undergo any more surgery. Instinctively I felt I could trust this man, there was a sincerity in his words I had not noticed before in any of the hospitals I had been in.

As I settled into Cappagh and began to make friends I became a more relaxed person. The days of anxiety and tension were fading and I no longer worried about dying. I was surrounded by lively teenagers instead of old people. Younger boys made plans during the day to raid the convent orchard in the evening, while older lads would try to persuade one of the female patients or a young nurse to meet them at the back of the congress altar, which was used to celebrate Mass every Sunday. This structure had been positioned on O'Connell Bridge in Dublin in 1932 before being moved. It was not unusual for three or four boys with varying degrees of handicap to meet there in the evening for a smoke. Dates with girls were also arranged and it was behind this altar that I got my first kiss. I was now a teenager growing up in an institutional environment but I was happy. I was forging strong relationships with other boys and experiencing the intensity of teenage love. I was enjoying life and being treated as a young adult by nurses and nuns.

One extraordinary event occurred in Cappagh when I began

to answer mass again in Latin, from my wheelchair. The responses to the prayers were still so clear in my mind that I never used a card or missal. I became the hospital altar boy. I was also involved in the Scout Movement and went on regular camping trips to the Dublin Mountains. As my self-confidence continued to grow, my disability somehow seemed irrelevant.

During one of many frequent trips to Lourdes – always paid for by someone hoping I would be cured – I was befriended by a priest. His curiosity about me led to the second meeting between my sister and myself. For her it was to be a traumatic affair. She had last seen me running and walking at seven years of age. Now I was confined to a wheelchair. She still finds it difficult to understand what happened to me in those short years. Many adult years would have to be spent trying, if it was possible, to make up for the lost years of childhood.

I had an interest in music and was tutored in piano by an occupational therapist attached to the hospital. I hated the lessons and tried every ploy to get out of them. I wanted a guitar and finally managed to buy one. I must have banged out the chord of C thousands of times before doing the same with D. The surgeon under whose care I was, listened, unknown to me, as I sang 'What Have They Done To The Rain'. He clapped and said; 'If The Searchers ever get to hear that Doyle, you could end up in jail.' He arranged music lessons for me and paid for them himself.

Nurses were becoming more than just people who looked after patients, they were friends. Two or three played a particular role in my life and one determined its course. She gave me real love, both physical and emotional, and I was able to return it. Sometimes it was difficult for me as a teenager to unscramble love from caring. Could a nurse many years senior to me actually love me, and could I love her? I never wanted to be loved out of a sense of duty or pity, I wanted to be loved for the person I was.

During these years I grew into a strong and confident young man. There were no stresses on me and as a result my physical condition improved considerably, even to the extent that for brief occasions I was able to walk without the aid of crutches or calipers.

I forged a particularly strong relationship with two other boys my own age, and it was not unusual to see the three of us, in the company of three nurses heading for the bus and a day in the city. The nun in charge of our ward was particularly instrumental in ensuring that we went out. Often she called me aside and gave me money, suggesting that I spend it on something other than cigarettes. This nun, now dead, came to my defence when I was caught in the girls' ward, replying, when told by another nun that I was sneaking down to visit a particular girl whenever I got the chance, 'I bet you did a bit of it in your own day Sister'.

I was introduced to a Social Worker and the possibility of my being discharged became a regular topic of conversation. These talks 'primed' me for leaving Cappagh and when the day came I was desperately sad and uncertain about the world I was heading into. I had been in institutional care for most of my life, now I was being discharged from hospital to become part of a family.

I was placed with a most wonderful family. A woman with seven children ranging in age from four to fourteen, was prepared to treat me as one of the family, though I found difficulties in getting used to being part of such a unit. I was actively encouraged to visit Cappagh and to get on with my schooling. I was never made to feel different because I was disabled and I was taken with the family on their annual holidays. There was never a problem about making space for one other person or a wheelchair in the grey Borgward Estate. It was from this family that I gained the confidence necessary to feel I could take my place as an equal in society.

There was an inevitability about my departure from the security of a family. I wanted to challenge life. I wanted society to accept me as I had been accepted by others. I moved into a flat on my own while still at school. The flat was my 'house', there was a sense of ownership about it and I could bring people in when I liked without feeling I was intruding on anyone.

Exactly half the welfare payment I received went in rent for the flat, the rest kept me on a diet of cornflakes, eggs, sausages and bread. There were times when the flat was a lonely place. I wrote a little when I couldn't afford to go out or didn't feel like visiting anyone.

Synge Street Christian Brothers School was nearby and I used to push myself to school each day. I particularly enjoyed those years. I was regarded as 'one of the boys' and loved not only the companionship it brought but, most of all, the respect – not pity – I was given by my fellow pupils. Because I had no basic education I found it difficult to deal with certain subjects in school, particularly mathematics, but one teacher determined that I could get a leaving certificate if I was prepared to work hard in and outside of school. He was right. I passed – though only after a re-check of the maths paper.

By the time I left school I was nearly twenty years old and anxious to get a job. I was involved in a relationship which I hoped would result in marriage and so when the offer of a job in CIE was made to me, I grabbed at it. It was a bad decision, though it took twelve years to realize, by which time I felt my very sanity was being threatened. By the time I had the courage to leave, I was moving towards writing and trying to find out about my past. These ventures, uncertain though they were, have proved stimulating, frightening and rewarding.

In 1974, I got married. Many objected to the idea and voiced their total disagreement to a disabled man marrying an able-bodied woman. People took my wife aside and warned her that she would end up 'looking after' me. What infuriated me most about these interfering busybodies was their blatant disregard for the good sense of either my wife or myself. A half-hysterical matron summoned her student nurse to her office and demanded to know 'what was the meaning of it all?'. People would ask my wife what sort of sex life she could expect. There were times when the pressure almost caused the relationship to collapse. I began to ignore people who interfered, realizing the futility of talking to them about something which ultimately was none of their business.

When all else failed I'd tell them simply to 'fuck off'. This may have been crude but it certainly had the desired effect.

In September 1976 we went to an auction for 'A Victorian House – needing redecoration'. We had looked over the house which had been empty for ten years and, though it was damp and dusty, we decided to try and become the new owners. Our bid was the highest and the auctioneers hammer came down with the words: 'Sold, to the gentleman seated for seven thousand pounds.'

Looking for a house loan and dealing with solicitors delayed us from actually taking possession until six months later. But on a dark, wet Good Friday evening a car and trailer drove up through the overgrown and neglected front garden, carrying all our belongings. My first child ran around the house amazed at its size. My wife, who was pregnant for the second time, stood in the middle of a bare, dusty and damp room. She held the brass halldoor key in her hand and remarked: 'Well, at least it's ours'.

Behind the house a high-speed diesel-engined train hooted as it rushed past, replacing the hissing and panting sound of the steam engines I had been so used to as a child. Looking out the bay window, I fleetingly remembered St Michael's Industrial School. I am typing these words in that same room where trains and granite walls are as close to me now as they were thirty years ago in Cappoquin. I had never been loved there. I am here.

THE END

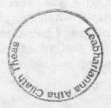

THE HOUSE BY THE DVINA
A RUSSIAN CHILDHOOD
by Eugenie Fraser

'Eugenie Fraser has a wondrous tale to tell and she tells it very
well. There is no other autobiography quite like it'
Molly Tibbs, *Contemporary Review*

A unique and moving account of life in Russia before, during
and immediately after the Revolution, *The House by the Dvina*
is a fascinating story of two families, separated in culture and
geography, but bound together by a Russian-Scottish marriage.
It includes episodes as romantic and dramatic as any in fiction:
the purchase by the author's grandfather of a peasant girl with
whom he had fallen in love; the desperate journey by sledge in
the depths of winter made by her grandmother to intercede
with Tsar Aleksandr II for her husband; the extraordinary
courtship of her parents; and her Scottish granny being caught
up in the abortive revolution of 1905.

Eugenie Fraser herself was brought up in Russia but was taken
on visits to Scotland. She marvellously evokes the reactions of
a child to two totally different environments, sets of customs
and family backgrounds. The characters on both sides are
beautifully drawn and splendidly memorable.

With the events of 1914 to 1920 – the war with Germany, the
Revolution, the murder of the Tsar, the withdrawal of the Allied
Intervention in the north – came the disintegration of the
country and of family life. The stark realities of hunger,
deprivation and fear are sharply contrasted with the day-to-day
experiences, joys, frustrations and adventures of childhood.
The reader shares the family's suspense and concern about the
fates of its members and relives with Eugenie her final escape
to Scotland.

'A wholly delightful account'
Elizabeth Sutherland, *Scots Magazine*

0 552 12833 3

NOBODY NOWHERE
by Donna Williams

'Extraordinarily gripping'
Good Housekeeping

Labelled deaf, abnormal, nut, retard, spastic, mental, moron, 'blonk', crazy, weird, wild and insane, Donna Williams lived in a world of her own. She existed in a state of dreamlike recession, viewing her incomprehensible surroundings from the security of a 'world under glass'. Few people understood her, least of all Donna herself, and she yearned to become 'normal'.

At the age of twenty-five, Donna discovered a word, a new label, which brought with it a handful of answers, a chance for forgiveness and hope for a sense of belonging: that word was autism.

Donna's account of her struggle to come to terms with her condition and to survive the suffering enforced by an unsympathetic, ignorant world is a unique insight into the workings of an autistic mind. She could have been locked up: instead, against the odds, Donna achieved a place at university, lived independently, and has now written this remarkable insider's view of autism. Her book is a landmark in the literature of mental health, a work of outstanding courage, and one of the most extraordinary human stories you are ever likely to read.

'Remarkable autobiography . . . the first ever description by a sufferer of autism of life in the grip of this lonely condition'
Me magazine

'Moving and enlightening'
Woman's Weekly

0 552 99512 6

THE PAST IS MYSELF
by Christabel Bielenberg

'It would be difficult to overpraise this book. Mrs Bielenberg's experience was unique and her honesty, intelligence and compassion makes her account of it moving beyond words'
The Economist

Christabel Bielenberg, a niece of Lord Northcliffe, married a German lawyer in 1934. She lived through the war in Germany, as a German citizen, under the horrors of Nazi rule and Allied bombings. *The Past is Myself* is her story of that experience, an unforgettable portrait of an evil time.

'This autobiography is of exceptional distinction and import-ance. It deserves recognition as a magnificent contribution to international understanding and as a document of how the human sprit can triumph in the midst of evil and persecution'
The Economist

'Marvellously written'
Observer

'Nothing but superlatives will do for this book. It tells its story magnificently and every page of its story is worth telling'
Irish Press

'Intensely moving'
Yorkshire Evening News

0 552 99065 5

A SELECTION OF FINE AUTOBIOGRAPHIES AND BIOGRAPHIES AVAILABLE FROM CORGI BOOKS

THE PRICES SHOWN BELOW WERE CORRECT AT THE TIME OF GOING TO PRESS. HOWEVER TRANSWORLD PUBLISHERS RESERVE THE RIGHT TO SHOW NEW RETAIL PRICES ON COVERS WHICH MAY DIFFER FROM THOSE PREVIOUSLY ADVERTISED IN THE TEXT OR ELSEWHERE.

☐ 99065 5	THE PAST IS MYSELF	*Christabel Bielenberg*	£6.99
☐ 99469 3	THE ROAD AHEAD	*Christabel Bielenberg*	£5.99
☐ 13741 3	LETTER TO LOUISE	*Pauline Collins*	£4.99
☐ 14093 7	OUR KATE	*Catherine Cookson*	£4.99
☐ 13928 9	DAUGHTER OF PERSIA	*Sattareh Farman Farmaian*	£5.99
☐ 99479 0	PERFUME FROM PROVENCE	*Lady Fortescue*	£6.99
☐ 99557 6	SUNSET HOUSE	*Lady Fortescue*	£6.99
☐ 99558 4	THERE'S ROSEMARY, THERE'S RUE	*Lady Fortescue*	£6.99
☐ 12833 3	THE HOUSE BY THE DVINA	*Eugenie Fraser*	£6.99
☐ 14185 2	FINDING PEGGY	*Meg Henderson*	£5.99
☐ 99505 3	TRUTH TO TELL	*Ludovic Kennedy*	£7.99
☐ 99637 8	MISS McKIRDY'S DAUGHTERS WILL NOW DANCE THE HIGHLAND FLING	*Barbara Kingham*	£5.99
☐ 14829 4	FIFTY YEARS IN THE SYSTEM	*Jimmy Laing*	£5.99
☐ 13944 0	DIANA'S STORY	*Deric Longden*	£3.99
☐ 13943 2	LOST FOR WORDS	*Deric Longden*	£4.99
☐ 13822 3	THE CAT WHO CAME IN FROM THE COLD	*Deric Longden*	£4.99
☐ 13953 X	SOME OTHER RAINBOW	*John McCarthy & Jill Morrell*	£5.99
☐ 14127 5	BRAVO TWO ZERO	*Andy McNab*	£5.99
☐ 13356 6	NOT WITHOUT MY DAUGHTER	*Betty Mahmoody*	£4.99
☐ 142883	BRIDGE ACROSS MY SORROWS	*Christina Noble*	£4.99
☐ 13946 7	NICOLA	*Nicola Owen*	£4.99
☐ 13369 8	REVOLUTION FROM WITHIN	*Gloria Steinem*	£5.99
☐ 99512 6	NOBODY NOWHERE	*Donna Williams*	£6.99
☐ 14198 4	SOMEBODY SOMEWHERE	*Donna Williams*	£5.99

NEVADA BARR
BOAR ISLAND

HEADLINE

The right of Nevada Barr to be identified as the Author of
the Work has been asserted by her in accordance with the
Copyright, Designs and Patents Act 1988.

First published in Great Britain in 2016
by HEADLINE PUBLISHING GROUP

First published in paperback in Great Britain in 2017
by HEADLINE PUBLISHING GROUP

1

Cataloguing in Publication Data is available from the British Library

ISBN 978 1 4722 0231 4

Offset in 9.83/14.82 pt Dante MT Std by Jouve (UK), Milton Keynes

Printed and bound in Great Britain by Clays Ltd, St Ives plc

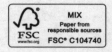

Headline's policy is to use papers that are natural, renewable and recyclable
products and made from wood grown in well-managed forests and other
controlled sources. The logging and manufacturing processes are expected
to conform to the environmental regulations of the country of origin.

HEADLINE PUBLISHING GROUP
An Hachette UK Company
Carmelite House
50 Victoria Embankment
London EC4Y 0DZ

www.headline.co.uk
www.hachette.co.uk

For Julie, a most
excellent friend

ACKNOWLEDGEMENTS

With special thanks to Linda Eddings, Stuart West, Bill "the Rock Nazi" Weidner, June Devisfruto, and all the fine folks at Acadia.

Apologies to the demolition crew that took down the derelict barracks on Schoodic. I rather liked the old heap, so I put it back.

ONE

Fists white-knuckled on the crutches, sweat running into her eyes, Heath grunted like a sumo wrestler. She was walking to the window of her front room. Walking, as in proceeding forward in an upright bipedal manner by putting one foot in front of the other. For some people, toddling around a fifteen-by-twenty-foot room would be as nothing. For Heath it was a miracle, and she was sweating buckets for it.

Eight years before, she had fallen while climbing rotten ice in Rocky Mountain National Park and broken her back: no movement, no sensation below the waist. For an eternity of hopelessness she'd wallowed in self-pity. Finding in Elizabeth a daughter, and in Anna Pigeon a friend, had convinced her to abandon her plan to drink herself to death. It was then she had begun to embrace every nerve's worth of life she could win, earn, fight for, or steal.

During all those years, eye level had been precisely forty-four inches above the floor. One of the first things she noticed when she stood up—stood up out of her wheelchair on her own two feet—was that nobody had dusted any surface more than forty-five inches above the floor in at least five years. Who knew?

She smiled and looked at her reflection standing—*standing*—in the plate-glass window. Dem Bones, Elizabeth called it. Iron Woman in Dem Bones, Heath thought.

Anchored to the outside of each thigh was a long silver-colored piece of contoured metal that linked to a round hinge at knee and hip. Below, another metal lozenge ran down the side of her calf to attach to a horizontal brace that went beneath her shoe. A wide strap, reminiscent of a weight-lifter's belt, circled her waist. A battery pack the size of a hardcover book rode on the belt at the small of her back. On the right hip of her harness was a small control panel with buttons that allowed her to use the electronic exoskeleton to sit down and stand up. The rest was done with body movement. If she leaned slightly forward, wonder of wonders, she *walked* forward. If she leaned back, the walking stopped. The entire assemblage weighed twenty-one pounds three ounces and could be folded into a case slightly smaller than a golf bag.

This was her second day with the skeleton. The first time she had stood up on her own—sort of on her own—she had suffered an attack of acrophobia so sudden and severe she'd nearly fallen. She, who had led precipitous climbs up sheer cliffs for fifteen years, looked down the five feet three inches from her eyeballs to her feet and felt as if she stood on the edge of a chasm a thousand feet deep, a vacuum sucking her into oblivion. She'd managed six steps before she hummed back into her wheelchair, exhausted from movement and terror.

Terror had quickly mellowed into excitement. Still, she felt fifty feet tall, a giantess looking down on a world of dwarves. A rush of power and awe fueled her every time she stood up.

Unfortunately, the machine wasn't hers. There was no way Heath could afford it. She was testing it for her friend Leah Hendricks, the research and development brain of Hendricks & Hendricks. Leah's device had three times the electronics of other models, was smaller and lighter, executed more minute movements, and was able to "learn." Heath had yet to tap into a fraction of what it could do. One of the drawbacks was that Leah had yet to figure out how to get the thing's battery to hold a charge for more than twenty minutes.

In a couple of months Leah would take it back to the lab to tinker with its finer points.

Heath chose not to think about how she would feel, who she would be, when this miracle was taken from her.

For now, she would only think of now, walking now, standing now. Now was good.

Twice she had walked the length of the room. Forty feet. Hooray for the para brigade, she thought. Give us forty feet and we'll take a million miles.

Harsh, repetitive racket shattered her moment of triumph. Rap music, an oxymoron to Heath's way of thinking, rudely pounded down the long hallway from the direction of Elizabeth's room.

Until recently, Heath's adopted daughter had been an aficionado of the lightweight modern version of what Aunt Gwen called bubblegum rock. That and, because children never cease to amaze their elders, anything by James Taylor. Heath had been unaware Elizabeth ever listened to rap. Boulder, Colorado, wasn't much of a Mecca for rappers; too white, too rich, too much spandex. The stuff playing now was ugly and dark, "bitch" and "whore" making up a good percentage of the lyrics.

Why Elizabeth would want to listen to this brand of aural poison was beyond Heath. Why Elizabeth would think Heath would allow it to be broadcast throughout her house, smashing all good karma in its path, was an even greater domestic mystery.

Heath waited a couple of minutes, catching her breath and hoping Elizabeth would come to her senses. The first goal was met with satisfying rapidity. The second was not.

"Wily," she said to the dog laying on the hardwood, watching her workout with narrow, sleepy eyes, "go to Elizabeth's room, boy. Unplug her whatever. Good dog!"

Wily yawned hugely, his mouth wide and crooked like his spiritual guide Wile E. Coyote.

"You're a big help," Heath said.

Pivoting with painstaking slowness, she got herself turned around and centered facing the hallway, the crutch braces biting into her forearms. There was a gizmo built in that gave Dem Bones balance, but she'd not yet come to trust her mechanized lower body, hence the crutches. Leah had tried to explain the engineering to her, but Heath's brain had stalled at the gyroscope analogy.

Fear of falling was an acquired—and necessary—paranoia for paraplegics. Given her fatigue level, it would have made more sense to use her wheelchair for the journey to the back of the house. Still and all, wheeling up, no taller than a hobbit, to lay down the law to a teenager didn't appeal to her.

From behind the crutches, extended like forelegs in front of her, the view down the carpeted hallway—to be replaced with hardwood the moment her bank account caught up with her special needs—looked impossibly long, the doors at the end appearing as distant as the pins in a bowling alley.

Heath sighed and began to hum "Who Were You Thinking Of" as she clasped her crutches through the sweat on her palms and began her robotic version of the Texas two-step. When it came to the two-step, nobody could beat the Texas Tornados.

By the time she'd made it across the living/workout/rehab room to the hall, Wily padding arthritically along behind, she was regretting her impulse to stand high and mighty over her daughter and wishing she'd dropped her rear end, exoskeleton and all, into Robo-butt—Elizabeth's name for the wheelchair.

Having reached the point of no return, equidistant from the rude noise in Elizabeth's room and the security of her wheels, Heath rested a moment before pushing on. Elizabeth had more reasons than an overcrowded psych ward to be moody and rebellious. It was the miracle of the child that she was blessed with a naturally sunny disposition. One of those enviable souls whose brain seems to effortlessly create sufficient serotonin to power a lifetime of optimism in the grimmest of circumstances.

Until a week ago, when sullenness and darkness had replaced the sun.

Or was it two weeks? As much as a month? No. Even a Johnny-comelately mom like Heath wouldn't fail to notice over that length of time.

Heath told herself what she always told herself when she worried that an unmarried, crippled, ex-rock-climber was not the mother a girl as fine as Elizabeth deserved; what she lacked in experience she made up for with love. Also, they had E's godmother—Anna—and Dr. Gwendolyn Littleton. With Anna and Aunt Gwen for backup, Heath figured she could pull off the mother thing.

Leaning against the wall for support, Heath reviewed the past couple of weeks with her daughter. There had been red flags: Elizabeth found in tears and insisting it was "nothing." That was eight or ten days ago. Elizabeth switching screens on her computer, and snapping at Heath for sneaking up on her—as if Heath-cum-apparatus could sneak up on any hearing individual. Had that been a week back? Less. Five days.

The dark, hard rap music started day before yesterday. Elizabeth was listening to it on her iPod so loud Heath could hear the beat. She'd had no idea what the lyrics were, but Elizabeth had looked as if they were driving spikes into her brain.

Then today. The rancid, hate-filled, misogynist rant out in the air, poisoning the hearth fairies that protected the house. Aunt Gwen had made up the fairies when Heath was a little girl and afraid of the dark. This new dark was scarier.

Lots of red flags.

Heath had noticed. She'd mentioned Elizabeth's uncharacteristic behavior to Gwen. As they did with every step in the girl's development, the two of them hashed over Elizabeth's every move.

She was in the midst of the hormonal storms of puberty.

She had a fight with a girlfriend.

She had a secret boy-crush.

She had an embarrassing disappointment.

Heath and Gwen agreed not to interfere.

That was before the rap, Heath thought. This crap was not a red flag, it was a cry for help.

With an effort, Heath pushed away from the wall. White-knuckled, muttering, "Dem bones, dem bones, dem dry bones," she began the final, interminable few yards of hallway, cursing the carpeting with every laborious shuffle of her feet.

Sweat dripping from her nose, breath coming in puffs and gasps, she bumped open her daughter's bedroom door without knocking. Elizabeth was not there.

The bathroom door was ajar, rap blasting out, steam augmenting its hellishness. Forgetting the pain in her shoulders, Heath muscled her way across the room. Using a crutch as a battering ram, she bashed the bathroom door open with so much force it struck the commode.

Tail down, Wily growled.

Steam obscured the mirror and made a wraith of the girl in the tub. Momentarily disoriented, Heath would have fallen if she hadn't been wedged between crutches and doorframe. Vision cleared. What remained was a child—a young woman really, sixteen—in a bath so hot her skin had reddened below the waterline. She was holding a razor blade to her wrist. Tears and sweat poured down her face to fall like rain into the bath. A girl and a razor and an angry voice shouting "fuck that bitch" to the beat of a machine gun in the hands of a madman.

Heath reached over and pulled the iPod out of the speaker. Silence bloomed like a blessing, broken only by the drip, drip, drip of slow tears. Pressing a button on her wrist, she activated the metal bones. With a hum like that of an electric window in an older-model Cadillac, they eased her down onto the seat of the commode. She moved her crutches so they wouldn't be between her and her daughter.

"Honey . . . ," she said gently, and held out her hand. Elizabeth laid the razor carefully in her palm. Heath set it on the sink counter.

Elizabeth had been contemplating suicide with the layered blades of a Lady Schick. At best, she could have given herself what amounted to nasty paper cuts. Though she was in a hot bath, as the media always portrayed suicides for some reason, Elizabeth, being a modest girl by nature and upbringing, was wearing the iridescent blue one-piece bathing suit she wore for swim races.

Much to laugh at.

Nothing funny.

For a minute neither spoke. Elizabeth, flushed with heat, eyes and mouth swollen from crying, long dark hair sleek as a seal's pelt on her shoulders, looked so small and young.

A lump hard and hot as a burning coal formed in Heath's throat. "What can I do?" she managed, her voice burned and choking. "What can I say? Who can I kill? For you, Elizabeth, I will do it. Whatever you need, I will do it."

TWO

Denise sipped her Coke, flat and warm from neglect. Just like me, she thought sourly, then reminded herself not to let the sourness seep into her face. Pleasant expression neutralizing her muscles, she let her eyes casually wander past Peter Barnes and his entourage.

Park picnics had become exercises in self-control. Denise loathed them, but she was damned if she was going to let Peter keep her from attending. Tables were scattered on the grass behind park headquarters. Two, shoved together, were loaded down with hamburger buns and condiments in the oversized squeeze bottles that always struck her as mildly obscene given the flatulent sounds that sputtered out with the ketchup, mustard, and, especially, the pickle relish.

Peter was sitting with his new wife, Lily. *Lily*. Could it get any worse? He couldn't have married a Sheila or a Judy?

Or someone remotely his own age?

Like me, she thought again. Hatred burned like acid in the back of her throat. Peter was forty-six, four years older than she. Pretty little Lily had just turned thirty. Their baby, Olivia, was three months. Married fourteen months and a baby girl. Lucky, lucky Peter. Lucky Lily.

Three years had passed since Denise had been the one sitting next to Peter Barnes at the picnics. More. Thirty-eight months. Yet the wound had not healed. She still felt as if her skin had been peeled from her body, and her flesh, newly flayed, screamed silent and bloody for everyone to see.

For a time—months, maybe as long as a year—Denise had thought things were getting better. Then they started getting worse. Hate would roar like a lion, then tears would sting, but not fall. Thoughts of *them* flooded her mind in muddy rivers, bursting their banks. When the baby came, the flooding grew worse. Some days Denise could not escape endless tape-loops of images of that baby girl.

She hated Peter, hated Lily, though Lily hadn't been the Other Woman, just the next woman. How could she not hate Lily? Lily was young and pretty. Lily had Denise's life, Denise's man, and just to make sure the knife was twisted, the baby Denise could never have.

Could never have because of Peter.

She realized her eyes had been stuck on the happy little family too long, on the baby. Lily was holding the baby, feeding it from a bottle. Lily never nursed. The little cow had no milk.

Lily caught her, smiling, happy, welcoming.

Denise forced a smile that probably didn't work. Peter had undoubtedly told Lily about poor, old, pathetic Denise, the reject who had taken on the role of the ghost at the manor window, always present, never invited in.

Deciding she'd stayed long enough to prove she wasn't broken-hearted, Denise stood and carried her Coke to the nearest trash bin. In an impotent act of defiance, she didn't put the can in the recycle bin. Given that Peter had chosen to trash her life and recycle his own with the lovely, fertile Lily, she was damned if she would support his pet program.

Artie, the gung-ho new district ranger, sat at a table with one of the secretaries. Young and eager, he was trying to make being a park ranger more like being an Army Ranger, itching for black ops. Denise forced herself to smile at him.

After making it a point to saunter slowly from table to table saying her good-byes so it wouldn't look like she was slinking away with her tail between her legs, Denise made it to her Miata. The last few steps she staggered like a drunk. What the hell was that about?

Holding on to the low door to keep from falling, she took deep breaths. Tremors rattled her bones. Almost as if Peter—his eyes, all the eyes—the baby, Lily, everybody knowing, had brought on some kind of seizure, as if around Peter and his postcard-perfect life she could no longer fill her lungs. Bony fingers of a monster hand wrapped around her rib cage, squeezing and squeezing.

Paranoia rampaged through her veins.

No. No monster. No seizures. Hyperventilation is all. Lily doesn't know. They are fooled. I have them all fooled, Denise told herself. For the most part she knew she was right. Certain people had a knack for seeing the ghost behind the eyes. Those people Denise avoided. The rest, when they bothered to think about her at all, believed she had moved on, that she was just as thrilled as they were with the assistant superintendent's spiffy new family.

When she could do so without stumbling, Denise opened the car door and slid into the low bucket seat. A Mazda ragtop in northern Maine was a rich man's summer toy, but a foolish purchase for a woman who could afford only one car. Denise had bought it a week after Peter announced he "needed space," then promptly gave himself that space by throwing her out of the house they'd shared for eleven years.

Two months later he threw her out of his life.

At the time she bought the convertible she hoped it would make her feel free, sexy. For a brief moment it seemed to, then it didn't, and she'd come to hate it. The list of things she was coming to hate lengthened daily, each new loathing attaching to the anchor that was Peter Barnes. The chain of hate had grown so heavy that some days Denise felt she couldn't carry it another foot, that she would collapse under it and lie helpless until all vestiges of life were crushed from her body.

Before—as in before she was ruined and dumped—Denise used to enjoy the short drive on Route 233 to Bar Harbor. August, high summer, hot days and cool nights greened the park. The coast, with its islands like jeweled rock gardens scattering in a sea of whitecaps and blue water, took on a fairy-tale beauty.

Beauty was not yet on the list of things she hated, but she supposed it would come under the pall eventually.

Bar Harbor, draped in schmaltzy cuteness, was a place she'd used to avoid during tourist season. Alcohol, in its myriad forms, was another thing she'd once scorned. This evening, after suffering through another picnic with the royal family, she craved a place as fake as the promise of Happily Ever After, and a beer. Beers. One had ceased being enough long ago.

On the outskirts of town she pulled into the wide circular drive of the Acadian Lodge. In the 1940s and '50s—the heyday of lodges and camps—the almost-wealthy summered at the Acadian, basking in the shadow of the truly moneyed.

There were cottages then. Denise had seen pictures of them—trim, freshly painted, lawns and gardens in careful rustic disarray, and "campers," looking happy and coddled by armies of servants, mostly girls who'd come up from the cities by train to earn a little money and enjoy a summer by the sea.

No more.

The cabins had long since been torn down and the property sold off in half-acre lots. The lodge had grown as sad and tacky as a drunken old woman. Touches of new paint, sporadically and inexpertly applied, soaked like cheap drugstore makeup into the wrinkles and cracks of wood that had weathered too many winters.

In its glory days, the bar had been a fashionable watering hole. Now it was the haunt of locals, lobstermen mostly. It was dark and smelled faintly of the sea and dead fish. Stale cigarette smoke had permeated the walls and carpets so deeply that all these years after indoor smoking had been legislated into a crime, the smell persisted.

Usually Denise drank at home and alone. For reasons she didn't understand—and didn't want to—she was drawn to the Acadian when things in her mind got too ugly. Slipping into a dark wooden booth in a dark corner, she took off her sunglasses. The room was dominated by a once-elegant long bar backed by a mirror easily six feet high and fifteen feet long. Black age spots pocked the silvering around the edges, contributing to the sense that the place was diseased or moldering back into the stone and lichen upon which it was built.

The bartender raised an eyebrow. "Draft, dark," Denise said, and then worked herself into the corner of the booth until the shadows closed around her. Other patrons had no business seeing memories ripping at her flesh, sharp-taloned and as vicious as harpies.

A couple of lobstermen on barstools were talking about the old guy who'd shot another old guy by the name of Will Whitman for robbing his traps and moving in on his territory. Yet another skirmish in the lobster wars that had been waged along these waters for generations and showed no sign of letting up. Law enforcement was worthless for the most part. Whose traps were where, and who ran which lines, was a mystery to everybody but the men who harvested lobsters for a living. They knew the bottom of the ocean around Maine as well as landlubbers knew the streets of their own neighborhoods.

Denise had heard that the dead man's son, Walter, had been excommunicated from the fishing community because everybody figured his dad was guilty of robbing traps—sins of the father, acorns falling near trees, chips off the old block. She smiled to herself. The bozos knew nothing.

Lobsters disappeared, lobsters were never there in the first place, lobsters were poached. These jokers in their little boats on top of the water could only guess who or what happened right underneath them.

A young couple—tourists, lost or slumming—slid into a booth on the end wall. Both on the same side. The old Denise would have thought it romantic. This new Denise wanted to bite their heads off and spit them into their imported beers.

At the near end of the bar, where the wood curved gracefully toward the mirrored wall, a lone woman sat hunched over a glass. Bleached-blond hair formed a curtain between her and the lobstermen. Denise's booth was on the opposite side of the ersatz veil, so she could see the blonde's face. She was sporting a black eye and a split lip.

Revulsion swept through Denise in a sick-making wave. She couldn't stand that the woman's outside was a public image of her own insides: battered, abused, ashamed, and drinking alone.

Despite that, every few minutes, Denise's gaze found its way back to the blonde on the barstool. Denise had been in law enforcement all of her adult life. A national park ranger, she'd seldom dealt with city-cop stuff. Parks were peaceful places for the most part, even in Acadia, where park and town and resort and sea came together in a patchwork of populations, each with its own agenda. Not once had she pulled her gun, used her baton or her pepper spray. What minimal compliance and self-defense training she'd gotten at the Federal Law Enforcement Training Center in Georgia had long since been forgotten.

Black eyes and split lips, though, were a form of violence she was familiar with. Family troubles don't go away on vacation; they get worse. The damaged face wasn't enough of a novelty to hold Denise's interest, but something was. As she sneaked peeks over the rim of her first beer glass, her second, and then her third, she tried to figure out what was so fascinating.

It became evident that the battered blonde was known to the bartender. Maybe a regular. Denise hadn't seen her here before, but then she never came to the Acadian this early in the evening. The lobstermen came here a lot. Usually, by the time Denise slunk in, they were three sheets to the wind. They might know the woman. Either the acquaintance was slight or they didn't like her. Both pointedly refused to look in her direction. This suited Denise. If they didn't look at the blond barfly, they couldn't look at her.

There was something bizarrely familiar about the woman. Had she arrested her? No. that process was long and, in many ways, intimate. Denise would have remembered.

Acadia, for all it had a large and fluid population in the summer months, was a small town for year-round inhabitants. Had she seen the blonde in a grocery store or, given the face, a hospital emergency room? In her capacity as an EMT she had been to the ER at Mount Desert Island Hospital enough times with injured people.

The woman looked to be in her late thirties or early forties. The barstool made guessing her height tricky, but Denise figured she was about the same height as she was—five foot six—and probably weighed about the same, one hundred thirty pounds. Her face—without the obvious damage—was the kind that can be dressed up or down. Makeup and a good haircut and she'd be pretty. Without it, she was fairly ordinary. Still, there was something . . .

After a while the blonde began looking back. Their eyes met, and Denise stopped her furtive surveillance. The last thing she wanted was to get into a "what're you lookin' at?" bitchfest with a stranger.

Another beer, a trip to the ladies' room.

The lobstermen got up and left. As they passed the blonde, working on her third drink since Denise arrived, one ducked his head and said, "Miz Duffy." The other nodded politely.

Miz Duffy. No lobsterman Denise had run across would call a woman "Miss" unless she was their kid's schoolteacher. Miz Duffy must be Mrs. Duffy. As Denise made her way unsteadily back to her booth, she wondered if they'd made a point of ignoring Mrs. Duffy because they didn't think a married woman should be alone in a bar, or because they were acquainted with Mr. Duffy, and the fact that he'd beaten on his wife made social intercourse awkward.

Mrs. Duffy watched them go, a tired look on her face, and something more energetic in the curl of her upper lip, disgust possibly.

The blonde shifted on the stool. Again their eyes met, this time in the long mirror backing the bar. Realization hit Denise with the force of near-sobriety. Not disgust. Hatred was what burned in the blonde's eyes. She knew. Denise had seen it. It greeted her in the bathroom mirror every morning. For a long time they sat, eyes locked, watching a slurry of emotions, memories and shocks flickering across the faces in the glass at dizzying speed. Never breaking eye contact, the blonde stood, picked up her drink, and carried it over to Denise's booth. She slid into the shadows on the opposite side.

"I was beginning to think I'd made you up out of whole cloth," she said, and laughed.

The laugh made the hairs on the back of Denise's neck prickle.

THREE

Elizabeth wouldn't tell Heath why she'd been contemplating slitting her wrists. When pressed, she cried and looked so desperate it scared Heath into silence.

Dem Bones hung like a Space Age suit of armor on its stand in the corner; Heath, collapsed in the familiar embrace of Robo-butt, was putting water on for tea. While the water heated, she rolled onto the back porch to call Gwen in her persona of doctor and great-aunt. She also called Anna Pigeon in her persona of law enforcement ranger at Rocky Mountain National Park and Elizabeth's godmother. Surely, between medicine, the law, and Heath's blind determination, they could find out what had driven Elizabeth to despair and put the child back together again.

Curled up on the oversized leather sofa, and in her pajamas though it was not yet sundown, Elizabeth accepted the tea without comment. Elizabeth couldn't care less about tea, but it was all Heath could think to offer, and she was grateful her daughter took it.

Heath had not seen E this hopelessly totaled since, at nine years old, she had wandered out of the night woods weeping and nearly naked.

A year earlier, during a nightmare canoe trip on Minnesota's Fox River, Elizabeth had been as strong and canny as any battle veteran. Heath had almost forgotten she wasn't Rambo; she was a sixteen-year-old girl. Evidently, whatever this evil was, it was of a variety that struck at the heart of where that wonderful, vulnerable girl lived.

Anna arrived first. Soundless in moccasins without socks, she appeared in the doorway between the kitchen and living room. She must have dropped everything and left work as soon as Heath called. Heath probably sounded as panicked on the phone as she was. She refused to feel guilty. They were talking about Elizabeth's life.

Anna had changed out of her uniform. She was wearing Levi's so worn the knees were white and stringy with age, not artifice, and an oversized, man's white shirt, probably her husband Paul's, rolled up to the elbows.

A while back Anna had turned fifty. More gray twined through her braid now than when Heath had first met her. Decades in the sun had freckled and creased her skin in a way that suited her skull and her soul. Anna had grown to look like a person you would want to tell your darkest secrets, all the while harboring an uneasy sense she already knew what they were.

"Hey," Heath greeted her. She didn't expect a hug. Anna was not a touchy-feely kind of woman. Both in greeting and departing, Anna nodded. A modified bow of respect, Heath guessed. Or dismissal.

Perhaps because Elizabeth was so young and damaged when she'd met Anna, she had crept through those boundaries. Leaping off the sofa, the girl threw herself into the ranger's arms. As tall as Anna, and a few pounds heavier, Heath expected Elizabeth's onslaught to knock Anna back into the kitchen, but Ranger Pigeon stood staunch as an oak and wrapped her arms around the clinging girl.

Relief only slightly tainted with jealousy washed over Heath. Chest muscles loosened. She drew her first deep breath since she'd found Elizabeth in the bath. It saddened her that, physically, she could not be Elizabeth's rock. Without bitterness, Heath knew she'd gotten the harder job, to anchor and support her emotionally.

Anna folded down onto the floor, her back against the sofa, legs crossed Indian fashion. Elizabeth curled up on the seat behind her and played with Anna's pigtail the way she'd done when she was a little wreck of a girl, still in shock from the multiple ordeals that brought her into Heath's life. Holding on to the braid, Elizabeth whisked the tail over her eyes and cheekbones as if sweeping away cobwebs.

"I wish you hadn't changed out of uniform," Heath said to Anna. "I was kind of looking forward to having a gun close to hand."

Before Anna could respond, Gwen blew in through the outside door. Gwen was in her late seventies, small-boned, fragile-looking, with wildly curly hair that she ignored with the exception of taking time every three weeks to keep it as resolutely red as it had always been. Dr. Gwen Littleton was the antithesis of a little old lady. Heath thought of her aunt as a whirlwind, a dust devil, a genie in a tiny bottle, a force that, though small in size, was most definitely to be reckoned with.

She gusted into the living room, dropping the black leather doctor's bag she'd been given when she graduated from medical school—and still carried every day—on the floor. The air that came in with her was the kind that can only be found during dry high-mountain summers, a draft so light and crisp, so warm and full of optimism, you feel that if only you could spread your wings wide enough you could fly.

"I left the door open," Gwen announced. "Fresh air. My unbottled, un-patented, priceless, free cure-all." Dumping her purse, Heath's mail, and a long turquoise-and-gold scarf she'd been carrying for some reason, she put her hands on her hips, surveyed the three of them, and said, "Okay, now, what's this all about?"

Elizabeth started to cry again, mopping at the tears with the tail of Anna's braid. Though it had to be absorbing a bit of snot on the side, Anna didn't look like she had any intention of rescuing it.

Gwen swooped down onto the sofa and folded her great-niece in her thin arms. Anna took one of Elizabeth's narrrow feet between her roughened hands and began to massage it gently. Heath rolled nearer, closing Elizabeth into a circle of love. An impenetrable circle? Probably not. Love did not conquer all, but sometimes it made it bearable.

"Baby, what is it? You have to tell us," Gwen crooned.

"Or we'll never go away," Anna added.

"Not even to go to the bathroom," Heath said. "How disgusting would that be?"

"I am so ashamed," Elizabeth mumbled through her tears and the soggy end of Anna's braid. "I swear I'm going to die of embarrassment. Just die! I want to die," she said with bone-chilling sincerity. "I'm so ashamed." Tears clogged her throat then, and she sobbed into Gwen's boney bird-shoulder.

"I accidentally fell on a friend of mine and killed her," Anna said. "That was pretty embarrassing."

Heath almost blurted out, "What the fuck?" Leading technical climbs for much of her adult life, Heath was fluent in the modern vernacular, and "fuck" was such a jolly good bad word. But when Elizabeth came into her world, Heath had determined to clean up her language. Saying the F-word was one thing; hearing it on the lips of a fairylike little girl was obscene. Worse, it was tacky, low rent.

Anyway, it had been ruined. On the Fox River one of the thugs had, quite simply, used it up. He had used all possible, probable, and improbable applications of the word, finally rendering it absurd. Now, when E and Anna and Heath heard someone say "fuck," they'd lift an eyebrow, exchange a smile.

Left without it, Heath fell back on the classics. Twelve apostles and forty thousand cowboys couldn't be wrong. God damn it to hell, bastard, SOB. All were workable.

"The hell you say," she amended. From the corner of her eye she noted Elizabeth was listening. The sobbing had quieted.

"No kidding," Anna said somberly. "Squashed her throat. Now that's something to be ashamed of."

"I once told a woman her fetus was going to be stillborn," Gwen admitted. "She mourned and wailed through seventeen hours of labor. The baby never moved, its heart never beat, I swear it! The moment she was born, that baby girl was wiggling and giggling. The wretched little thing had been lying doggo, or hiding behind Mom's liver or some darn thing. I thought I was going to die of humiliation before the mother killed me for scaring her to death. Thank God that was back before mothers sued for every little birthmark. I was so ashamed I didn't show my face at the hospital for nearly a week. When I did, doctors, and even some nurses, started calling me Dr. Lazarus."

"I never killed anybody or scared anybody half to death," Heath said. "But in college I got drunk and made a bet with this guy that I could free-climb the front of the administration building, no lines, no belays, no shoes, no gloves, no nothing. Bet him a hundred bucks. He upped it to a hundred and fifty if I did it totally naked. I was halfway up and doing great when the cops showed up with the spotlights. I was charged with drunk and disorderly, disturbing the peace, and—this hurt worst—defacing university property, apparently by plastering my bare-naked ass on it."

"You did not!" Gwen exclaimed.

"Spent the night and half the next day in jail. I was too ashamed to call you. The only reason I wasn't expelled was that the boy who made the bet with me was the president of the university's son. Cross my heart and hope to die."

Elizabeth stared at her wide-eyed, completely engaged now. "Oh gosh, Mom, how did you stand it?" she cried.

Absurdly pleased that her tale had trumped accidental death by falling on, and nearly terrifying to death by misdiagnosis, Heath said, "This was before everybody had iPhones. I was only totally humiliated in front of twenty or thirty people, not millions on the Web."

Elizabeth's face went deathly pale. Heath had read the phrase "deathly pale" many times, but this was the first time she'd ever witnessed the phenomenon. It was as if she watched the blood drain from beneath her daughter's skin, leaving a gray pallor in its wake. For a moment she thought E was going to faint or scream or vomit. What she did was far more frightening. She began striking herself in the face with her balled fists.

Heath ached to hold her. She knew that the best she could manage was to lurch upon the pile like Frankenstein's monster. Cursing the ice that had bested her, she turned her wheelchair sharply and sped from the room, left the hardwood and hit the carpet without slowing down. Robo-butt had never moved so fast. In an instant she was down the hall and in Elizabeth's room. The pink iPhone, a gift from Gwen, was on the bedside table. Elizabeth's laptop was on her desk, holding pride of place in the midst of a landfill's worth of cosmetics, tissues, magazines, earrings, and whatever else had been dropped there over the past two years.

Heath took both electronic gadgets and dropped them into the saddle-bags on her chair. Another twenty seconds and she was back in the living room parked beside the couch. "Elizabeth," she said in a tone that cut through the soft fuzzy outpourings of Gwen and the somber attentions of Anna. Elizabeth looked up, eyes and cheeks wet, lips red and swollen.

Heath held up the pink cell phone.

"Noooooo," Elizabeth begged. She covered her ears and squeezed her eyes shut as if waiting for the fuse to burn down to the dynamite.

"Yes," Heath said. "Rotten ice." Rotten ice was their code for *This will try to kill you. Face it or run away fast.*

Gwen glared at Heath. Anna nodded slightly. In the minute or less Heath had been gone, Anna must have figured it out. Heath pushed the message button. Seventeen new messages in the in-box. "I've never had seventeen messages in my entire life," Heath said. A small whimper from

Elizabeth. Not funny. Heath opened the first message and read it. Then she read it aloud in a flat voice. " 'Have you been on the page? Dweeb said you did the basketball team. TNT?' "

"Kimmy?" Heath asked as she noted who it was from.

"She's in my geometry class," E said miserably.

"TNT? Explosive?" Anna asked.

"Totally Not True," Elizabeth said. "How could she have to ask?" Tears started. She knocked them from her eyes with the backs of her hands.

E was going to be brave. Heath hoped she was. She opened the second. " 'Check The Page.' Tiffany sent this one," Heath noted. "The Page?" She raised an interrogative eyebrow.

"It's a blog the kids all read." E hid her eyes with the tail of Anna's braid. "Somebody posted that I did things I didn't do."

"Like the basketball team?" Anna said dryly.

"Like that," E said.

Heath opened the third message: " 'Who hasn't screwed you yet?' My God, this stuff is insane. Somebody is going to get their skull bashed in if I have any say in the matter."

The fifth had a picture attached, an image of a woman being mounted by a Great Dane. Heath didn't read it aloud. She passed the phone to Gwen.

" 'I guess you like being done to by dogs.' "

"Holy Mary Mother of God," Gwen whispered.

Anna had taken the laptop from the saddlebag and had it open on her thighs. "What's the address of the blog?"

E told her. Anna typed it in.

Heath rolled her chair over to read it. " 'EJ pulled a train—you hear that? After the game.' "

" 'True. I was the caboose.' That one's signed Spike," Anna said.

"It's this creep everybody calls Dweeb. He signs himself Spike,"

Elizabeth said. "God, the *Dweeb*!" E cried. "Nobody could think I'd have anything to do with the Dweeb!"

"'No sloppy seconds for me.' This one is signed IceBlow."

"A slime bag Dweeb hangs with. You should have let me kill myself," E whispered.

"'Sloppy twenty-seconds more like,'" Anna read on relentlessly. Heath considered stopping her, saving Elizabeth the pain, but she believed Anna was right in what she was doing. Elizabeth already knew what they said. Aloud, in Anna's flat, almost bored tone, they lost some of their snickers-in-the-dark malice and sounded as stupid as they were. Almost.

"'Not in all orifices.'" Anna looked around. "Orifices?" she asked no one in particular. "Big word for this moron." She returned her attention to the computer and read the last two quickly, as if the whole thing were too foolish for words.

"'No shit?' asks bozo," Anna said.

"'Meat sandwich with a blow job topper.' This from thug number two. Who started this ball rolling?" she asked Elizabeth in cold even tones.

"I don't know," E sobbed. "The only names I recognize are Dweeby Spike and his creep pal, IceBrain. If cooties weren't extinct, they'd have them big-time."

Of course, Heath thought. Once the story was out, the dweebs and the creeps wanted to be part of the action. If a girl was having sex with the other boys, why not them? "This is good," Heath said. "Nobody cares what they say. They're creeps." That sounded good and might even be true.

"Your Facebook password?" Anna asked.

"WilyCoyote2015," Elizabeth said softly. "Capital W, capital C." At the sound of his name, Wily thumped his tail on the floor. Pushing to his feet, the old dog ambled over and stuck his head under Heath's hand. It was as comforting as it always had been.

Anna looked up from the laptop. "More of the same," she said. "Where else?"

"Everywhere," Elizabeth said hollowly. "There's a website the kids go to, like a Mean Girls thing. That blog. I've found three others. Things are forwarded to my whole class sometimes."

Cyberbullying: vicious, anonymous, all-pervasive. Heath forced her voice to calmness, then asked, "Who started sending these first?"

"I don't know," Elizabeth whispered. "Honest, I don't know. Don't tell anyone," she begged. "Anna, promise me, no cops. No cops, Heath, nobody. Gwen, no doctors, and please, please, please don't talk to any of my friends' parents. Pleeeeease!"

For a second, Heath suspected Elizabeth knew, not only why she was being targeted, but by whom, and her sixteen-year-old mind was telling her that if she ratted out the culprit, it would dump her into a hell worse than the one she was already in. The one that could only be escaped by razors to the wrist.

Heath changed the subject. "When did"—and she waved the cell phone rather than speak the evil words—"this stuff begin?"

"I don't know," Elizabeth said automatically. Then, "About a week after school let out for the summer." Elizabeth was a rising senior at Boulder High. Not in with the in crowd or the jocks, but at the moderately comfortable level of acceptable anonymity that allows a majority of kids to survive high school without permanent scarring.

"Who?" Anna demanded.

Shocked into honesty by Anna's tone, Elizabeth said uncertainly, "Tiffany?"

"Tiffany? Tiffany's your best friend," Heath said. Not a friend of Heath's choosing. The girl's parents were Christian fundamentalists, or at least her mother was. Heath figured Elizabeth had suffered enough at the hands of religious fanatics for several lifetimes, but Tiffany seemed like a nice girl.

In Heath's opinion the friendship was more one of opportunity than genuine attraction. Tiffany, her folks, and her two-year-old brother, Brady, moved into the house next door; she and Elizabeth were the same age and starting their freshman year together; both settled at the same level in the high school pecking order. Admittedly, Elizabeth seemed to enjoy Tiffany's company. Most days either she was at Tiffany's or Tiff was over here. It suddenly occurred to Heath she'd not seen the girls together for a while, a week or more.

Rotten mother, she scolded herself. Blind as a bat.

"I don't think we're friends anymore," Elizabeth said.

"Did you guys get in a fight?" Heath asked. She should have asked this a week ago. She should have been paying better attention.

"Not exactly. Momma, could I have some more tea? It really helps." When Elizabeth called Heath "Momma," either they were having a moment or Heath was being conned. Obviously Elizabeth really, really did not want to talk about this. All three adults homed in on the vibe like hounds on a scent.

The only thing missing was the baying.

FOUR

Bad idea to be doing this drunk, Denise thought, but continued dragging the straps of her scuba tank up over her wetsuit. Cold water would sober her up quick enough, she rationalized. If it didn't, and she drowned, that was all right, too. Since all of her children had been murdered, and Peter had thrown her away like so much damaged goods, death didn't seem like such a bad option.

Except that Peter would be glad she was dead.

Except that the son of a bitch would go right on living his spiffy little life. With his precious Lily and the baby. They would watch the baby that should have been hers grow up without caring that Denise was fish food.

Mouthpiece adjusted, gear hooked to her harness, she made a final check of the gauges with her flashlight. How drunk could she be if she remembered to check gauges? It wasn't as if she was planning on going deep or staying down long, half an hour max. Hell, I dive drunk better than I do sober, she thought. *Drunk diver.* The phrase amused her, and as she went over backwards into the ocean, she forgot to hold on to her mask. Cursing and sputtering, she managed to catch it before it sank and get it back on. So much for the "better drunk" theory of diving.

Mask adjusted, she got her bearings. The night was perfect. Warm, overcast, and as dark as the inside of Jonah's whale. Her navy blue runabout on a midnight sea in a great big ocean was as close to invisible as a corporeal body was likely to get.

She upended.

Following the anchor line toward the bottom, she thought about Will Whitman, the lobsterman who got shot for robbing that old guy's traps. Whitman might have been rustling lobsters, but the traps he got shot over were in her territory. The murder had renewed hostilities in the long-running feud.

Not that she cared. People shot people. People did a lot of awful things to other people. Nobody gave a damn. Her own mother had dumped her. She'd been adopted by borderline assholes. Cry me a river; nobody cares about anybody other than themselves.

Enough! she told herself and quieted her mind. Stopping thoughts from spinning was hard. It was like her mind had developed a mind of its own, and maybe neither one was her friend.

No! she shouted silently. The dueling minds couldn't have this place. Clenching her jaw, she forced herself to look outward.

She loved that only the circle of her lamp and the anchor line existed. Under the Atlantic at night was the only time she felt anywhere near free or whole anymore. Contained in apparatus and silence, held in weightlessness and peace, she savored the balm to her soul. Above, in the light, in the world of men, she devoured herself, ripped the flesh from her bones with her teeth, like a coyote chewing off its own leg to free itself from the jaws of the trap.

Watching the line play through her gloved hand as she descended, she let herself think about the woman she'd just met in the bar of the old Acadian Lodge.

Neither one of them had said anything for the longest time after the blonde slid into the booth and made her cryptic announcement. "I'd begun to think I'd made you up."

They sat and stared at each other in the dim light of the bar. Denise was struck dumb. She'd never quite known what was meant when people said that. She did now. There were no more words in her head at that moment. Had there been, she wouldn't have been able to move her tongue or push out the breath to say them. Words had become futile pathetic little things, not fit to bring into the immensity of the idea that had slipped in with the blonde.

"Takes some getting used to, doesn't it? I've been thinking on it for months now, so I'll talk while you get your mind around it, how's that?" the woman said. Her voice sounded creepy, the way Denise's always did when she heard herself on a tape recorder, familiar but alien. Not right.

"My name is Paulette Duffy. I'm forty-one." She smiled. Denise drank down the last of her beer, then waved at the bartender for another. Paulette's teeth weren't the same. Denise had gotten her front incisors busted in a schoolyard fight and had neat straight caps. Paulette's leaned in as if they needed each other for support.

"I think I'm forty-two," Denise managed. "But that could be off a year either way."

"Forty-two on March sixth of next year," Paulette Duffy said. Her hand shot out for no reason Denise could see and banged the metal napkin holder. "Sorry," she laughed. "I guess I'm turning into a klutz in my old age."

"Nerves," Denise said to be saying something. "Happens to me more and more." Her head was swimming. Too much beer. Too much everything. Sitting back, she let her head fall against the cracked leather of the booth. "Forty-one," she whispered. "Forty-two on the sixth of March. That kind of makes a person real, doesn't it? Knowing when you were born, knowing somebody cared enough to write it down."

"You never knew?" Paulette asked softly. Denise hated being pitied for her rotten childhood, hated talking about it, wouldn't talk about it. Peter was the only one to whom she'd told all the grit and grime, and now, every time he looked at her through the scrim of his new clean wife and spotless baby, she could see every bit of shit she'd ever been through clinging to her in his eyes.

Now she wanted to spew it all out like vomited beer here in this booth for Paulette Duffy. "Never knew," she said. "I'm not ready for any of this." She pulled the man's wallet she favored out of the hip pocket of her pants, then dumped the contents on the table. It was probably enough to pay for her drinks three times over. She didn't care. "I'll never be ready for any of this." Standing unsteadily, she waited a second for the room to stop spinning.

"Here," Paulette said. She scribbled on a bar napkin. When Denise didn't hold out her hand to take it, Paulette shoved it in Denise's pants pocket. "This is my address and the number of my cell phone. I got one of those prepaid ones at Walmart. I have lots of minutes left. Call me. Promise. Promise you'll call me."

Denise didn't promise. She made it to the Miata. Then to the runabout. Then to the sanctity of lobster rustling under the sea.

The ocean floor coalesced out of the gray-green circle of gloom at the farthest reach of Denise's light. Turning herself so her feet pointed earthward, she came to a gentle landing on the sand. Froglike, iridescent green in the glow of the lamp, her swim fins squeezed small swirls of liquid dust puffed from beneath her.

The depth gauge read twenty-six feet. Habit was all that made her check it. This stretch of Davy Jones's locker was, metaphorically speaking, the back of her hand.

Moving with the slow grace of a hippopotamus on the bed of the Nile she turned, letting her light drift in a circle until she saw the yellow line snaking down from the buoy she'd anchored near, the marker of a line of lobster traps. With a lazy kick she rotated to the horizontal and swam toward it.

Traps were on the end of lines connected to Styrofoam buoys on the surface. Lobstermen checked their traps every day, putting fresh bait in if they needed it. The buoys were marked with the license number of whichever fisherman owned the trap.

The traps on the ocean floor out from Somes were the old variety, wooden crates covered in rope mesh, with a circular opening just big enough for a lobster to crawl in. Occasionally, Denise mused, surely a lobster, smarter than her fellows, after having consumed the bait, would crawl back out to live and reproduce. Maybe man had created the ultimate evolution facility, and one day the giant spiders would take over Silicon Valley.

The first trap had two lobsters in it, but they were small. She passed them by. The next had one enormous old fellow. Lobsters could live a hundred years, though most didn't make it more than ten or fifteen. This guy looked to weigh close to two pounds. He had been around a while.

Careful to avoid the claws, Denise reached in and dragged him out. Her hand twitched as if she'd been hit by an electric shock, much the way Paulette Duffy's had. Her knuckles rapped on the side of the trap, and her fingers opened. With a flick of his tail, the lobster shot into the darkness.

Nerves.

Over forty and falling apart, Denise thought. The big spider would have been a good addition to the canvas sack trailing from a tether attached to her dive harness, but, in a way, she was glad it had escaped. Sad to end one's life in a tourist's stomach.

When she had ten good-sized lobsters, she switched off her light. Her bag could easily hold as many as fifteen, but she made it a rule never to take every one she found. If a trap had a couple of lobsters in it, she'd take only one. Those she emptied, if there was any bait left inside, might lure in another crustacean before the licensee came to check his catch. This way she figured the lobsterman would be pretty sure his traps had been poached, but not a hundred percent sure.

Denise rotated her lobster rustling through four different patches. All they had in common was that they were shallow and easily accessible from Somes Sound, where she moored her little boat. Other than running into somebody night diving—and probably up to no good either—while she was in the act of robbing the traps, there was no way she could get caught.

Denise liked that the lobstermen knew they'd been had, liked that she was thumbing her nose at the holier-than-thous in the park service, the Peter Barneses. Liked the feeling that, at least in this, she was the one in control. It was she, Denise Castle, who was making fools of them all. That was as important as the money she got for her catch with the less than honest owner of the Big Fat Lobster Trap, a seafood restaurant on the outskirts of Bar Harbor.

Lobster rustling was petty payback for what had been done to her since she was old enough to remember. Pathetic, if she thought about it, but it was the best she could do.

Until now.

Paulette Duffy.

There were possibilities opening to her that hadn't existed before.

Kicking off the bottom, she let herself rise gently to the surface. She had not been deep enough, nor down long enough, to make any decompression stops necessary. At the surface, she bobbed, a black sea creature in a black sea. Finding her boat was the most challenging aspect of her midnight forays into the seafood aisle of the Atlantic.

Under the gunwale, on either side of the bow, she had mounted three small LED lights. They were green. She'd been careful not to put them in a line or evenly spaced—the telltale marks of a work of man, not nature. Glimpsed by anyone, they'd be taken for a reflection, a bit of phosphorescent sea vegetation, or a trick of the light. For her they were homing beacons.

After a minute or two she saw them winking as the boat rose and fell on a gentle swell. She swam toward it. Having tied her sack of squirming arachnids to the starboard cleat, Denise heaved herself over the gunwale. As always, her first action was to remove and stow her dive gear, then pull on Levi's, a sweatshirt, and a ball cap to cover her wet hair. She'd established her reputation as a woman who enjoyed night diving. Still, diving at night, alone, was considered dangerous enough to raise questions she'd rather not answer on the off chance she ran into anyone. The lobsters she could always cut loose back into the ocean if need be.

An innocent, if nocturnal, ranger once again, enjoying the resource and preserving it for blah, blah, blah, she started her motor and headed back toward Somes Sound. Bear Island loomed to her port side, dark and forbidding, its mysterious, reclusive owners seldom in evidence, then Boar Island, smaller and virtually treeless. Boar had a jagged silhouette that reminded Denise of a ruined castle, the turrets half crumbling. The lady who owned it had a bad heart and was currently in a convalescent home in Bangor.

That's what happens to women who have no children to care for them, Denise thought. In old age they become orphans and are thrown on the state for their keep. Denise did not want to end her life the way it had begun, an unwanted orphan beholden to the state of Maine for a meal and a roof over her head.

That brought her back to the battered blonde, Paulette Duffy.

And all the new possibilities.

FIVE

Elizabeth knew she'd stepped in it, Heath could tell. As three adult stares bored into her, she groaned and rolled her eyes toward the ceiling. This show of sass did more to cheer up Heath than a thousand clowns in a barrel full of monkeys. "You said you 'didn't exactly' have a fight. What is 'not exactly' having a fight?" Heath asked.

Regardless of the incidents that should have aged Elizabeth before her time, she retained that magnificent innocence of face one seldom sees in anyone over the age of ten. When she was with people she trusted, or too tired to keep her guard up, her emotions could be as easily read as those of a two-year-old. Heath watched in loving fascination as Elizabeth decided to lie, thought better of it, decided to cry, changed her mind, and, finally, began.

"You know Mr. and Mrs. Edleson, Tiff's mom and dad?" Elizabeth asked. The question was meant for Gwen and Anna. Of course Heath knew them. Sam was around forty, thick sandy hair, nice build. If he hadn't been cursed with a seriously weak chin he would have been a handsome man. A chin implant probably would have changed his life. As it was,

Heath noticed, Sam vacillated between arrogance and obsequiousness. Terry, his wife, said he worked as an apartment and condo manager for a company that rented real estate to vacationers by the week or month. Ostensibly this job was what brought the family from Coeur d'Alene, Idaho, to Boulder, Colorado. Terry was a part-time bookkeeper for an auto-body company. In her mid-to-late thirties, she ran to fat, twenty pounds or so overweight, no longer particularly obese by American standards. Her hair was the same color as Sam's, but hers was from a bottle. Overall she seemed pleasant: pleasant face, pleasant voice. Heath couldn't think of any serious drawbacks to her as a neighbor—or even as the mother of Elizabeth's best friend—except that Terry talked too much in general, and too much about her God and her husband in particular.

The moment she'd spot Heath outside, words would begin to flow, a river with no end in sight. Heath wasn't as quick at escaping as she'd been in her salad days. There was a long trek from the mailbox to the ramp beside the kitchen steps with nothing but a low hedge between her property and the Edlesons'. During these rolling social events, Heath had been informed in far more detail than she cared for that Sam was cut out for bigger things, Sam was unhappy in his job, Sam had always thought . . . God had a plan for Sam, but . . .

"I vaguely remember the Edlesons," Anna said, cutting into Heath's thoughts. "You had Paul and me over as backup when you invited them for dinner last summer."

Last summer. Heath was surprised. She'd thought she'd made it a point to socialize with her neighbors, and especially the parents of her daughter's best friend, at least two or three times in the past year. Evidently not. There'd always been an excuse not to set herself up for an evening of Sam's seesaw personality and Terry's mouth.

"I say hi whenever I see them," Gwen said. "Though if it's Mrs. Edleson, 'hi' can take a chunk out of one's day."

Elizabeth laughed. If the sound had been a dead fish, both Heath and Wily would have rolled in it. A child's laughter, particularly after tears, wasn't something Heath had ever fancied getting dewy-eyed over, but she was, and not for the first time, either.

"Well, me and Tiff—"

"Tiff and I," Gwen corrected, then looked abashed that she'd interrupted at such a time.

"You and Tiff," Heath said to get Elizabeth going again. She didn't want to give her time to reconsider that lie she'd seen sneaking across her face earlier.

"We were supposed to be looking after Brady, Tiff's little brother," she explained to Anna and Gwen, in case they'd forgotten about him. "He's a monster. A real monster—he bites and spits; he just never lets his mom see him doing it, so she thinks he's like this little angel and Tiff and I are the evil stepsisters or something. Anyway, we were supposed to be watching him because it was Wednesday night—remember, Mom? I wanted to go over even though we'd be babysitting so Tiff and I could decide what to wear on the last day of school? Not like it matters, but there's always stuff on the last day and, well, you know."

Heath nodded, though she didn't know, and didn't remember that particular Wednesday.

"Wednesday nights are big church nights. Usually Tiff and her brother both go, and sometimes her dad, but Brady had been pretending to have the flu all day, so Mrs. Edleson let him stay home if Tiff would watch him. Mr. Edleson stayed home, too, though I got the feeling Mrs. Edleson wasn't happy about that. Then, around eight or so, Brady disappeared to pull the wings off of flies or whatever—"

"Does the kid torture animals?" Anna asked darkly.

Elizabeth was untouched by the ice in her voice. "No," she said. "He's not like a little Hannibal Lecter in the making or anything. At least not that I've seen. He's mostly into torturing high school girls, as in Tiff and me.

"So Tiff went out to the backyard—you know what a big yard they have, part of it borders on the creek—because that's where the little monster likes to hide out in the dark and leap out and scare the bejesus out of us. I didn't want to deal, so I stayed in the living room, where we'd been watching boring kid movies to keep Brady happy.

"Turns out Tiff wasn't in the yard looking for Brady." Elizabeth faltered to a stop.

Heath, Anna, and Gwen waited in respectful silence. Heath wondered if they worked as hard as she did not to demand answers.

Elizabeth sighed deeply and resumed. "Her dad had intercepted her coming in and sent her and Brady out for something at the drugstore. So, anyway, I was sitting on this big couch they have in the living room playing solitaire on my phone, and Mr. Edleson comes down from upstairs and sits on the couch and starts asking me the usual lame questions. How do I like school and what do I want to be when I grow up. Then he asks if I have a boyfriend, and I say don't I wish, and he starts in this long thing about some tribe in darkest wherever, and how fabulous it is that the old guys, uncles even—gross—introduce the virgins into womanhood. Way gross."

She looked up from where her hands were picking at the edge of a fray on the hem of her pajama top, swept an inclusive glance over Heath and the others, then returned to her hands. "It reminded me of something Father Sheppard would say."

Father Sheppard—Dwayne Sheppard—was the leader of the pseudo-Mormon cult Heath and Anna had rescued Elizabeth from when she was nine years old. Sheppard believed in multiple wives, the younger the better. Heath could feel her blood pressure rising. Anna and Gwen were as stone.

"Then what happened?" Gwen asked softly.

"He like put his hand on my thigh and leaned in and kissed me. A wet sloppy kiss that Wily would be disgusted by. I was, you know, so totally freaked, for a second I didn't do anything. I mean, I didn't kiss him back, but I just froze. I guess he thought I was saying what he was doing was okay." Elizabeth's eyes filled again, and her hands came up to hide her face.

Gwen took hold of Elizabeth's wrists, prying her hands from her cheeks. "You didn't do anything wrong. Nothing. Nada. Zip," she said firmly.

"And he didn't think what he was doing was okay," Anna said. "He's nearly forty, he is your best friend's father, and he's married. He knew it was not okay. You did not bring this on yourself. Mr. Edleson is a scumbag."

Anna rose to her feet. Heath, tuned in to the finer details of human locomotion, noticed she didn't move with the effortless grace she once had; still, she rose fluidly. Only the faintest of grunts and the crack of a knee or ankle attested to the effort.

"What are you doing, Anna?" Heath asked warily.

"I'm going to pay a call on the neighbors," she replied.

"Noooo," Elizabeth wailed.

"I'll take care of that end of things," Heath said, a hint of territorial challenge in her tone.

For a moment Anna swayed like grass in a gentle breeze. Heath waited to see if she would respect the role of mother or if she would go tear Sam Edleson's house down. Heath wasn't sure which outcome she was hoping for. Anna settled, folded down, and took up her position on the floor beside the sofa.

"Was that the whole of it?" Heath asked, sensing it wasn't and dreading the rest of the story.

"No," Elizabeth admitted. "While he was slobbering on me, and grabbing, Tiff came in. She hadn't gotten all the way to the drugstore. He'd given her the keys and told her to take Brady with her in the car! Tiff has a learner's permit, but it's not a good idea for her to be driving at night, even if it's only to the Walgreens. And not with Brady screaming and bouncing around."

Maybe because of what she'd been through in Sheppard's house of wives, Elizabeth seemed to censure Sam Edleson more for endangering his children than for making a sexual assault on her. At that moment, Heath loved her daughter so fiercely she thought she might explode.

"How long was she gone?" Anna asked. Heath moved rapidly from angry and proud of Elizabeth to shaking inside and terribly cold. Had the cretin stopped at a slimy kiss and a grope?

"If she'd've gone to the store, it would have been maybe half an hour. I don't know exactly. We've kind of quit speaking to each other. I guess she came back for something, and she came into the room while her dad was grabbing at me. I'd got over myself and was shoving and hitting to get him off me, and he was sort of flopping around. I don't know if he was trying to stay on me or get off me without getting kneed in the balls, because that was what I was trying to do.

"Tiff started screaming, and Mr. Edleson fell onto the floor. Right then Mrs. Edleson walked in, back way early from her church thing. It usually goes till nine."

"My guess is both Tiff and Terry felt there was something fishy going on," Anna said. "It probably wasn't the first time good old Sam had tried to get time alone with the girl next door. He may have been run out of Idaho for all we know. I'll check it out."

Elizabeth went on, "I managed to get up. Mr. Edleson had torn my blouse—not torn it, really, three of the buttons just popped off—and I was holding it shut, not knowing what else to do. Mrs. Edleson starts yelling, and Tiff stops screaming and starts yelling. Mr. Edleson is a creep, but I didn't want to hang around to watch him get chewed out. TMI big-time." Elizabeth stopped again and fell into what looked almost like a trance.

Staring at her hands, she turned them back and forth as if she'd never seen them before. After a few seconds Heath saw a tear fall like a raindrop on her left palm.

"Momma, they weren't yelling at *him*," she whispered. "They were yelling at *me*."

SIX

It was late when Denise parked her Miata a few houses down from the address Paulette had given her when they were at the Acadian. Several days had passed, full days for Denise. Acadia was at the peak of its busy season. That wasn't the reason she'd put off visiting, however. Twice Paulette Duffy had called her cell. Denise hadn't picked up.

There was a lot to think about before she could distill even part of it into words. Paulette Duffy—Paulette—had had years to grow used to the idea. Until they'd met in the old lodge, Paulette had no proof, but she'd long had suspicions. Not Denise, not the trained law enforcement officer, taught to seek out disparities and make sense of them. Denise hadn't had a clue.

She had always been at pains to give as little thought as possible to her so-called family. Home wasn't "the place where, when you have to go there, they have to take you in," as Frost had written. Home was where, if you had to go there, you might as well put a gun in your mouth and blow your brains out. You'd be doing yourself a favor. The Denise who had suspicions was a deep-secret Denise, a Denise that Ranger Denise Castle had thought long dead.

Three days and two phone calls passed, and finally, at quarter past ten in the evening, Denise was parked on the outskirts of the small village of Otter Creek on a two-lane road that cut through a dollop of public land still extant in the midst of Acadia National Park.

When she'd first bought the Miata, the only concession to good sense she'd made was disabling the interior light, a practice customary in police vehicles. No sense in lighting oneself up for whatever miscreant might be waiting in the dark to take a potshot at the local constabulary.

Denise was grateful for that moment of sanity. Tonight she didn't want to be seen entering or leaving Paulette's place, wasn't sure she wanted the two of them to be associated with one another. Not sure she wanted any of it to be real. Not that she loved the devil she knew, but she was used to him. Paulette would change everything.

Moving quietly and casually, she sauntered the hundred yards between her car and Paulette's cottage. Should one of the scattered residents happen to look out a window, she would appear to be an innocent out on a stroll enjoying the sweet-smelling night.

Paulette's home was what Denise's high school art teacher used to call a two-bit picture in a thousand-dollar frame. Because of its location, the smallish plot of land had to be worth a fortune. The tiny but picturesque shack squatting on it was hardly worth the match it would take to burn it down. It had to be family land. Paulette's husband's, Denise guessed. Had it belonged to Paulette, surely she would have sold it and run away on the proceeds.

Paulette's husband, Kurt Duffy, wasn't home. Paulette had said that in the text that finally brought Denise to Otter Creek.

She stepped into the deeper shadow of the dilapidated porch. Through the four frosted panes in the front door shone the bluish wavering light from a television. Either the volume was off or the old house had better soundproofing than its gaping weathered siding suggested.

Denise rapped lightly on the frame of the screen door.

The door opened so suddenly it startled her. Paulette must have been waiting and watching for her. "Come in," she whispered, as if she shared Denise's desire for secrecy.

The house's interior was as sorry as its exterior. A battered, stained sofa, cigarette burns on the arms and one of the cushions, slumped against the left-hand wall, facing off with a huge television. The TV was the old-fashioned kind with a rounded glass front and three feet of tubes forming an ugly black hump on its back.

A scarred coffee table filled the space between, cup rings overlapping on the ruined finish, the surface littered with orange crumbs from a single-serving bag of Doritos. Blinds with broken slats, dents in the plaster walls, dirty finger marks on the woodwork, and the cracking linoleum floor attested to the misery Denise had sensed in the battered blonde on the barstool.

Nausea tinged with panic rose quivering and cold in Denise's midsection. Like Paulette's bruised face, the room was an outward manifestation of the ruin Denise carried inside herself. Scrupulous attention to her outsides kept it hidden. She hoped. Her apartment was spotless, neither cluttered nor Spartan; the art was tasteful, the dishes carefully selected. The same could be said for Denise—sharply pressed clothes, well-cut hair, clean unbitten nails, painstakingly maintained so no one would suspect that her life was no better than if she were living it out in this sad room.

Anger at the tawdriness of Paulette's house flared up, hot and bitter. This place was a slap in the face, insulting.

Paulette read her expression, or maybe her mind.

"It's not me," Paulette said hurriedly. "This room, it's not mine. What I mean is . . ." Shoving the ruin of bleached hair back from an eye now haloed in the faint yellows and greens of a fading bruise, she let her eyes wander over the desolate interior landscape. A sigh of such exhaustion Denise's anger was blown away on it emptied Paulette Duffy's lungs.

"I made it nice, not rich, but orderly and clean, and, believe it or not, it had charm. I'm good with my hands."

Denise was good with her hands. For Peter's house she'd sewn curtains and created flower beds, stenciled bathrooms, and carved tiny animals on each kitchen drawer pull. For Peter's house. For Lily's house. For the baby's house.

"Kurt liked it once. Then, I guess, he knew how much it meant to me . . . I don't know. Things changed. Things got broken," Paulette finished with a resigned smile.

For Denise, too, things had changed. Things had gotten broken.

"Please, please, come," Paulette begged, and to Denise's surprise, Paulette took her hand and tugged her farther into the house. More to Denise's surprise, she didn't jerk her hand free. It was okay. It was good. It was right that her hand was in Paulette's hand. Nothing had ever been so right before. It was like she and Paulette were alone, alone together.

Paulette led her to the pathetic couch, where they sat side by side, knees almost touching. Paulette began to talk of the little girl she'd been. The joy she'd found in the tide pools, each a tiny universe of beings so incredible it was hard to believe they were real and alive.

Denise had felt the same.

Paulette spoke of a puppy she'd had in fourth grade. Rex, she'd called him. Rex was a mixed breed with dark mottled fur and a depth of intelligence in his canny brown eyes.

Denise, who hadn't been allowed pets—or much else in the way of comfort—had found solace in a stuffed dog, his fur mottled beige and brown. She'd named him Rex.

Paulette remembered winning the fifty- and hundred-yard dash in track meets all through grade school.

Speed was one of Denise's strengths. Every morning until the snow got too deep, she ran five miles before breakfast. In a strange intoxicating way, Paulette was telling the story of Denise's life, not factually, of course, but perhaps the life another Denise Castle had lived in a parallel universe. Which, in a way, was the case.

At some point they moved to the kitchen, and Paulette made tea—not coffee, tea; not fancy, Lipton. Both women drank it unsweetened with a dash of lemon juice.

Seamlessly the conversation shifted to Denise, and she found herself telling not of the wretchedness of her bouncing around the foster system but of a pair of sunglasses, the lenses shaped like hearts, the plastic frames canary yellow, that she'd had in the second grade, her prize possession, then basking in the warmth of Paulette's throaty laugh of understanding.

Paulette's had been shaped like the eyes of a cat, the frames fire-engine red.

Paulette had grown up on Isle au Haut, the only child of a lobsterman and his wife. Her mother "did" for the summer people who kept houses there. Much of Isle au Haut was part of Acadia National Park, the southernmost patch in the patchwork quilt of federal lands.

In her work as a ranger, Denise had been by the tiny one-room school where the island kids went dozens of times. She'd been by Paulette's house. There had to have been times she had missed Paulette by hours, or even minutes.

At sixteen Paulette married Kurt Duffy, the son of a lobsterman who ran lines out of Frenchman Bay, and moved to the mainland, then to a tiny house on Otter Creek Road—a thin slice of public land cutting through the main bulk of the park on Mount Desert.

At sixteen Denise had planned to elope with a boy named Chuck Miles. He had been killed when a logging truck hit his Honda as he was coming to pick her up.

Paulette worked at Mount Desert Hospital.

Emergency medical work was Denise's favorite thing about being a ranger.

Paulette worked mostly nights. She loved the night.

Denise loved the night; she volunteered for the latest shifts.

Twice Paulette had gotten pregnant, and twice Kurt Duffy had beaten her so bad she lost the baby. After the second time she could never get pregnant again; there were complications.

Denise had gotten pregnant with Peter's child. He'd slaughtered it. Slaughtered all her children.

Kurt told Paulette that if she ever left him he would track her down and kill her.

Peter had made a family that Denise was not part of. A family with a baby.

Sometime after midnight they found themselves in the cramped bedroom Paulette shared with her husband when he chose to come home. Shoulder to shoulder, hip to hip, they sat on the edge of the queen-sized bed and stared at their reflections in the wide mirror over what had once been a fine dressing table. Denise's dark hair was pulled back from her face into a low-maintenance ponytail at the nape of her neck.

Paulette pulled her desiccated blond mop back and secured it with a scrunchie. Then they stared. Smoking had roughened the skin around Paulette's mouth, and the blow to her face had discolored the flesh around her left eye. Other than this, they were the same. The ears were identical; their noses were the same, a little long with a squared tip and thin nostrils. Their eyes were the same shade of blue. Each had a brown fleck in the iris of her left eye, dead center below the pupil. Paulette's eyebrows had been plucked, but the arch and the long winged taper matched Denise's.

"I always felt you out there," Paulette said, her voice soft with wonder. "When I was little, you were my playmate. Mom said you were my imaginary playmate. I knew better."

Denise said nothing. She was afraid if she spoke she would cry or, worse, the woman beside her would vanish.

"Did you sense that I was here?" Paulette asked timidly.

Denise shook her head, fascinated at watching her sister's—her identical twin sister's—lips move on precisely the same mouth as her own. "I felt you as not here." Denise tapped her chest over her heart. "Like I wasn't all here. I felt part of me had gone missing. I thought maybe the doctors had accidentally cut off some part of me when I was born. It confused me because I couldn't see any part the other kids had that I didn't. No extra toes or arms or anything. When I got a little older, maybe eight or nine, I lived with a fairly decent family that attended a Presbyterian church. For the eight months I was with them, I went to Sunday school every week along with their kids. The teacher taught us that people had souls. After that, I assumed that I had accidentally been born without a soul. That that was the part that was missing.

"After that I put it out of my mind."

For another few minutes they sat in silence marveling at the faces in the mirror. Denise realized she must have known from the beginning that the battered blonde on the barstool was the part of her that had gone missing.

She had recovered her lost soul.

SEVEN

The specter of Sam Edleson filled the room with the stench of sulfur. Heath caught herself grinding her teeth and made herself stop.

"I'm going to make a few calls," Anna said, and slipped from the room as soft-footed as the apocryphal Indian.

Elizabeth excused herself to go to the bathroom.

Heath and Gwen waited in terror, neither saying anything, both afraid Elizabeth had gone to harm herself, both afraid they would never again feel safe when the girl was out of their sight.

"Should I go check on her?" Heath asked.

"No," Gwen said. Then, after a minute, "Do you think I should?"

"No."

Gwen began feverishly tidying the room. Heath pored over her daughter's cell phone, rereading the sordid texts, wanting to delete them but knowing she shouldn't. They were evidence. Elizabeth was adamant; she didn't want the police involved. Elizabeth was also sixteen. Heath wasn't sure police could do anything about the cyberattacks anyway. To ease the pressure, she finally allowed herself to delete one message. It was from herself to Elizabeth reminding her to put the wash in the dryer.

After what seemed a cruelly long time, Elizabeth returned. Relief flooded Heath when she saw she'd washed her face and combed her hair, signs of hope.

Then the three of them waited, Heath spinning her mental wheels. Gwen, having straightened every cushion, and aligned every book and magazine, sat on the sofa watching her great-niece with such intensity Elizabeth finally pelted her with a pillow.

Irritation, another sign the girl was beginning to engage in the world outside her misery.

Anna returned. "Edleson left his job in Idaho for making improper advances to a seventeen-year-old high school intern. In Idaho it's only a felony if the girl is sixteen or under. Nobody wanted to press charges, for all the usual reasons. The company didn't want to fire Edleson because of the adverse publicity and/or unemployment compensation. He was told to quit, and did. Shortly thereafter the family moved to Boulder." Having delivered the message in as few words as possible, Anna waited, her weight on the balls of her feet. Heath guessed she was hoping to be shot toward Sam Edleson as an arrow is shot from a bow.

"You called the cops!" Elizabeth cried.

"I did," Anna said. "The Coeur d'Alene, Idaho, police. They have no jurisdiction over you."

Reassured, Elizabeth's attention jumped to the next awful conclusion. "He's done it before?" she demanded, sounding shocked.

"Probably more than once," Anna said. "That's how these guys are."

"Then why were they yelling at *me*?" The indignation in her voice went far to soothe Heath. Because she was female, it was inevitable Elizabeth would be thinking she had done something wrong, brought this upon herself.

"Elizabeth, would you get my boots, please?" Heath asked.

"Which boots?" Elizabeth asked warily. "Your old climbing boots?" This last was asked with a small note of hope.

"Nope," replied Heath, dashing it. "The turquoise and silver." Elizabeth groaned. Almost said something, thought better of it, and levered herself up off the sofa cushions to vanish down the hall.

"What's with that?" Anna asked.

"Now we're going to pay that nice neighborly call," Heath said. Her voice came out flat and dark. Even if his wife and daughter lied to themselves and the world about Sam, Heath wanted him to know in no uncertain terms that she knew what he had done.

"No time like the present," Anna said.

"Good cop, bad cop?" Heath asked. She felt silly saying it, but it worked on television, and was the only plan that came to mind.

"Only if I can be the bad cop," Anna said without a trace of humor. "Are you going to wear your carapace?"

Heath thought she detected a note of excitement in Anna's voice. The electronic exoskeleton fascinated the ranger. Leah, whom Anna had gotten to know on their ill-fated trip down the Fox River, had strapped Anna into the prototype. Though she'd fought the machine as if it were trying to take over her body, she'd come to respect and admire it. Whenever Heath used it, Anna would whistle through her teeth or shake her head and mutter, "I'll be damned."

"Not tonight," Heath said. "I've used up my quota of energy on that scale. Robo-butt will have to do the heavy lifting."

"Let me get my—" Gwen began.

Heath cut her off. It was best not to let the juggernaut pick up any speed. Gwen lacked self-control around people who harmed children. Though Heath wanted to rend the Edlesons limb from limb, burn their house down, and sow the land with salt so nothing would grow there for a thousand years, she suspected she would gather a lot more workable leverage and information by using subtle threats and blackmail.

"I don't think this is a good time to leave Elizabeth home alone," Heath said.

"Of course not," Gwen agreed immediately. "I'll make a fresh pot of tea." She smiled wearily. "It's good to have something to hate that can easily be dumped down the drain."

As if he understood every word that passed, Wily heaved himself to his paws with a sigh and made ready to follow them. "Protect the children and old people," Heath said fondly as she rubbed his head. There was a time she would have taken him. He was courageous and as wily as his namesake, but the years were creeping up on him.

Elizabeth returned carrying a pair of worn but beautiful turquoise cowboy boots with silver threading. "What's wrong with your sneakers?" Elizabeth asked forlornly. "Or even your hiking boots?"

"Tonight I intend to kick some ass," Heath replied. Elizabeth flopped down, her body awkward, her resentment obviously at war with what Heath suspected was the joy of having a champion, regardless of whether she rides out on a white horse or in a gray wheelchair.

Gentle, as she always was when touching her adoptive mother, Elizabeth waved away Heath's hands and put the boots on her feet for her.

"Aren't those a bit dressy for an unannounced call?" Gwen remarked, coming in from the kitchen with the threatened pot of tea.

"Power suit," Elizabeth said.

Anna said nothing, following as Heath rolled toward the front door.

The sun was behind the mountains, and though it wasn't dark, shadows pooled and the sky had grown soft and infinite. The day's warmth was drifting away from the skin of the mountains on a gentle down-canyon breeze carrying the scent of pine.

Lights were beginning to come on in the neighborhood, people home from work and cooking supper. Sam's truck was in the drive, an outsized

Dodge Ram that one should not keep if one doesn't own a ranch where it can run and play. Expertly, Heath wheeled around it. Fortunately, the Edlesons' house had a wide brick walk and a front door without a step, a rarity Heath hadn't noticed before her disability. Given this was to be a confrontation, she was glad she didn't have to be dragged up a front stoop, then wait while Robo was hauled clanking up behind like an albatross.

When they arrived at the door, Anna reached over Heath's head and banged the frame of the screen door. There was a doorbell, but Heath was happier with the "Open up. Police!" sound of Anna's knuckles and left it alone. Disquiet murmured from inside, muttering, then silence, as if a television set had been switched off.

More silence.

"Curtains twitched at two o'clock," Anna murmured. Heath had caught the tiny movement from the corner of her eye—Sam or Terry or Tiffany peeking out the front-room windows to see who was at the door. The phrase "at two o'clock" threatened to make her giggle hysterically, and she wondered when her anger had turned to fear. Heath had no fear that Sam would do them physical damage. Bizarrely enough, given she would probably come out on the wrong end of a physical encounter with a well-muscled man, she would have welcomed that. A compulsion to feel his flesh under her fists—or between her teeth—coursed through her so fiercely that, for a second, she felt she could rise from her chair and kick the door down. Her fear was that something she or Anna might say or do would make it worse for Elizabeth.

Anna banged again, louder and longer this time. Heath didn't allow herself to wince.

She was beginning to think the Edlesons weren't going to answer the door when she heard the bolt thunk back. The door opened halfway. No lights were on in the front room. The one in the kitchen, a light Heath had noticed when they crossed the drive, had been turned off. Dim behind the screen door, Terry stared out at them, her eyes like black holes in a dead-gray face.

"Hi, Terry," Heath said pleasantly. "This is Anna Pigeon, a friend of the family and, for the moment, chief chair wrangler." She smiled crookedly. Poor little paraplegic couldn't hurt a fly. It wasn't one of Heath's favorite strategies, but she wasn't above using it now and then if she thought it would give her the upper hand. Maybe she heard a faint snort from Anna; she wasn't sure. "Could we come in for a minute?"

Terry didn't want to let them in. She was breathing hard through pinched nostrils. Heath could hear each sniff. Terry's lips, usually full and soft-looking, were pressed into a tight little frown.

"I'm afraid I don't handle the chill of evening as well as I did before . . ." Smiling again, Heath waved a hand over her lap to indicate just how very sad and debilitated she was. Terry still didn't want to let them in, but, like a lot of people, she was intimidated by the wheelchair. How could she say no? Heath was a *cripple*, for Christ's sake. The door opened a bit more, and Heath got a wheel in, then, with a push from Anna, she was over the sill and into the house. All Terry could do was get out of the way so Heath wouldn't run over her feet.

Before the fall from Keystone, Heath had been brash and ballsy. After, she had been angry and self-destructive. When she finally realized that, though she couldn't walk, she was still a whole person, she found she'd changed. From the bastion of Robo-butt, the world was different, more layered and complex. Heath learned patience. She learned to watch people, to really listen, to genuinely *see* them. Something she'd not done much of when she was superwoman climbing tall mountains. Another skill she'd picked up was canniness, an ability to manipulate situations to her advantage, to manipulate people when she had to. Cunning wasn't a strength much lauded in literature or the media, but it was a strength all the same, and Heath respected it.

Once they had breached the walls, as it were, Terry's mood didn't warm. She did, however, assume the role of hostess, offering them coffee. Anna didn't accept. Heath did. Hard to toss somebody out before they've finished their drink. She parked herself advantageously, blocking the big, leather, man-of-the-house chair so the only remaining seating was on a couch that was too soft or a straight-backed chair that was too hard. She didn't want Goldilocks getting too comfortable.

Anna leaned against a dark wood highboy, her ankles crossed, her arms crossed, looking deceptively relaxed.

In the minute it took for this arrangement, Terry was back with two cups of coffee on a tray along with a bowl of powdered creamer and half a dozen packets of Sweet'N Low. "Sure you won't have anything?" she asked Anna politely. Being the hostess, probably along with the fact that neither Heath nor Anna had lit into her, seemed to have dialed her hostility down a notch. Coffee served, Terry perched on the edge of the couch, her mug hands as plump and white as the Pillsbury Doughboy's. Where there should have been knuckles there were babyish dimples. The rest of her was as amorphous; her bland oval face just missed being pretty due to a lack of definition in her features.

"The girls haven't been seeing much of one another lately," Heath opened conversationally.

"That's so," Terry said, then took a careful sip of her coffee. "I think it will be good for them to have a little time just with family." She was recovering her equilibrium. Heath wanted none of that.

"So do I," she said flatly.

Terry looked up, annoyed or startled. Sam appeared behind her, backlit in the kitchen doorway, shoulder against one side of the frame. His hair was tousled, that nice gold-shot Robert Redford hair, and he wore a plaid shirt half unbuttoned. Heath suspected he'd been in the bathroom primping until this entrance.

"I know you sexually assaulted Elizabeth," Heath said to Sam. "Elizabeth's sixteen. In Colorado that makes your behavior child molestation. A felony."

Sam stopped leaning. He, at least, was scared. Not so Mrs. Edleson. Clacking her mug down on the tray, she tried to nail Heath to the wall with a malevolent glare. "Now see here, Heath, Sam didn't do anything! Do you hear me? You daughter, your *adopted* daughter, is no better than she should be, and you don't know the half of it."

Heath looked over Terry's head. "Sam, I know you arranged to be alone with Elizabeth, then assaulted her. I'm thinking the only reason it wasn't rape was that your wife and daughter got wind of it and came home before they were supposed to."

Terry was on her feet. "Your daughter made advances to my husband!" she shrieked, looking like she might fly at Heath and claw her eyes out.

Anna's voice cut cold from where she still leaned against the sideboard, ankles crossed. "Elizabeth's sixteen. Sam's forty—"

"Thirty-eight," he interrupted, his first words since entering the fray.

"She's a minor. He touched her. Either way it's a felony. Either way Sam goes to jail," Anna finished.

Terry quivered, fumed, sat, took up her coffee cup, breathed, sipped. "There's no need for that kind of talk," she said softly. "There's no need to embarrass yourself—or your daughter—by calling the police. I don't blame Elizabeth. Girls like Sam. He's a very handsome man."

A snort from the sideboard, and a murmured "Chinless wonder."

Heath suppressed a smile. Terry pretended not to hear. Sam's hand flew to hide the lower half of his face.

"Elizabeth made a pass at Sam," Terry said. The threat of jail hadn't silenced her, but it had toned her down.

"Just like the girl in Idaho made a pass at Sam?" Anna asked. She pushed out from the table she'd been tucked against and stepped into the light from the kitchen. Menace radiated from her. Heath could never figure out how she did it. It was just there, palpable, a sense of imminent threat that could be felt against the skin of the mind.

"That girl . . . that girl was . . . she . . ." Terry, her righteous anger temporarily damped, was flailing for words to fan it back to life. Heath took this moment of vulnerability to unlock Elizabeth's cell phone and open a text. Wheeling close enough that she bumped Terry's knees, she thrust the cell phone into the other woman's hands, where she couldn't miss the photo of a woman and a dog fornicating.

"Is that why you sent this to my daughter?" Heath demanded. Terry dropped the pink cell phone as if it were a used tissue.

"This is sick," Terry hissed at Heath. "Your daughter is disgusting and sick. This proves it."

Sam pushed his wife aside, then reached down to retrieve the phone. Heath watched him narrowly as he turned the phone right side up on his palm and pushed the button to unlock it. "Shit!" he said in what sounded like genuine shock. Terry tried to slap it from her husband's hand, but he dodged her blow. Anna moved from the shadows to stand behind Heath's chair. Making plans for a quick retreat, no doubt.

Before the Edlesons could stop their squabble to launch a counterattack, Heath broke into their concentration.

"Sorry to introduce that into your world so suddenly," she said acidly. "Someone has been using the Internet and cell phones—Twitter, texting, you name it—to cyberstalk Elizabeth. I need to find out who is behind it. Since the girls were at odds, I thought Tiff might be able to help me."

"Tiff had nothing to do with that!" Terry snarled. "Nothing. I kept her away from your . . . *daughter*." She made the word sound like an epithet. "Because Tiff is a good girl." Terry's doughy round face hardened and took on a sly look. "Since there is no problem, but you are troublemakers, what about I help you, and you promise not to try and get my Sam in trouble with the police?" she asked shrewdly.

"I promise," Heath said solemnly.

"What about you?" Terry glared at Anna.

"Elizabeth doesn't want the police involved," Anna said.

"We don't know anything about these . . . these filthy things," Terry said. "We don't know people who even know where to get filth like that. Nobody we know would ever *get* anything like on your daughter's phone. There. Now we're out of it. That's all the help I can give you."

The bitch was throwing it back on Elizabeth. Heath said nothing, and that nothing burned in her throat like fire on gasoline.

Sam, still staring at the phone, as if loath to take his eyes from the image of the woman and the dog for fear it would vanish, sat down on the sofa with a thump. "I've never seen anything like this stuff." He was thumbing forward on the touch screen, no doubt hoping for more.

Terry snatched the phone from her husband's hands. Heath was willing to bet she knew what Sam was, knew the lies she told herself so she could stay in the marriage.

"Is Tiff home?"

"You are not going to show this to Tiffany!" Terry exclaimed in horror. Marching over, she dropped the phone in Heath's lap with an exaggerated moue of distaste.

"The girls are estranged," Heath said. "Maybe Tiffany is doing this because she's angry, because you told her Elizabeth tried to seduce her dad."

"Tiff wouldn't do this," Sam said. "Tiff wouldn't even know what this is."

Heath could feel Anna hovering behind her like a brewing storm cloud. She shot her a warning glance; they needed to talk to Tiff. "I don't need to show her the photograph," Heath said with as much patience as she could muster. "But I would like to talk to her. The girls are close; Tiffany might know who wants to hurt Elizabeth."

Terry's eyes narrowed. "We're done here," she said. "Take your daughter's filth and get out."

"We need to talk to Tiffany," Heath insisted. "If you want to be around when we do, go and get her."

Sam stood, trying to pull his manhood up around him despite the missing chin. "You heard my wife," he said, and took a threatening step toward Heath.

Anna moved from the shadows behind Robo-butt. Her right arm shot out, stiff and sudden, the heel of her hand catching him in the solar plexus. With an *oof* he sat again, his moment of macho a thing of the past.

"The girls are not close," Terry hissed. She stomped past Anna and jerked open the front door. "Elizabeth brought this on herself. She probably gets stuff like that all the time. She probably likes it."

Anna had turned the wheelchair so Heath was facing the harridan at the door. Throughout this adventure in futility Heath had remained relatively calm. Terry's smugness and accusations blasted her self-control. The old Heath rose from the ashes of the one born of the ice fall. Heath never moved, but she saw, actually saw, an image of herself rise from her chair like a zombie from the grave, arms outstretched, fingers curled into claws the better to tear out and devour the flesh of Terry Edleson's throat. Maybe Terry saw the projection. Heath didn't know. All she knew was that a look of abject, pants-wetting terror deformed the other woman's face.

Heath bared her teeth and braced her hands on the arms of her chair. Murder could be done in a state such as this. Had her legs been viable, she would have probably left the Edlesons in a squad car, never to see the outside of a prison cell again. As it was, blind rage could not be sustained more than a moment. Anna swept up behind her. Heath leaned back into the loving embrace of Robo-butt to be rolled unceremoniously over the sill and onto the brick walk. "You assaulted Sam," Terry shouted. "I helped

you! So you can't call the police. They won't believe you. You promised!"
She glared at Heath.

"I did," Heath said.

"You are a witness," she yelled at Anna.

"I am," Anna said.

The door slammed. The dead bolt thudded into place.

For a moment Heath and Anna stared at the door.

"Now we call the police?" Anna asked.

"Now we call the police," Heath agreed.

Empty and exhausted, she slumped back in the seat and said nothing
more, letting Anna push her down the walk. The long summer dusk had
settled into true night. A streetlight made shadows stark and colorless on
the concrete sidewalk beside the asphalt. Black and white, Heath thought,
and missed a time when she saw right and wrong that clearly delineated.

"Ms. Jarrod?" came a whisper.

Anna stopped pushing. Heath came out of her slump into full alert.

"Ms. Jarrod, it's me, Tiffany." The girl, her blond hair gray in the cold
light, separated herself from the side of her dad's truck and crouched
down by Robo-butt. At first, Heath thought it a sign of unusual sensitivity in a teenager, but realized it wasn't. Tiffany didn't want her parents to
see her consorting with the enemy.

"I gotta get back," Tiff said. "Tell Elizabeth it's not me; my folks
won't let me call. They took my phone and my laptop and I'm like in
a black hole. I can't call anybody or get on Facebook or anything! I hope
she's okay. Tell her I'll write her and put the note under the hedge where
we used to crawl through when we were little kids. Nobody'd ever
think of that."

"Elizabeth's being cyberstalked," Anna said curtly. "Do you know
who's behind it?"

"I know about the stalking—everybody at school does. I don't
know—"

"Tiffany!"

"Gotta go. I know what Dad . . . I . . . gotta go." She stood and ran, probably hoping to get back inside the house before Mom and Dad figured out she'd defected.

Anna pushed. Robo-butt rolled. Heath rode. Only the crunch of the chair's rubber tires on bits of escaped gravel accompanied them back to the kitchen door. Gwen, Elizabeth, and Wily were waiting for them on the couch, tense and wide-eyed.

Anna parked the chair, then sank down in her former place. Heath set the brakes.

"Well, open the envelope, for heaven's sake!" Gwen exclaimed.

"No winner," Heath said wearily. "It probably isn't Tiff, which is good news. She couldn't, her folks confiscated her cell phone and her laptop."

"Gosh," Elizabeth breathed, evidently shocked at the draconian nature of the punishment. "What did she do?"

"She saw," Anna said.

"Tiff said she would write you about it and leave the note under the hedge where you kids used to crawl back and forth to each other's yards," Heath said.

"On paper?" Elizabeth asked.

"No. She's going to scratch it on a piece of slate with a stylus," Heath retorted.

"That Tiffany wasn't doing it, that's good, isn't it?" Gwen asked.

"Not really," Heath said.

"We haven't a clue as to who is behind it," Anna said. "So we have no way to make it stop. Nobody to come down on. We don't have a motive. We don't, do we, Elizabeth?" The adults again stared at the teenager in her pj's like hawks at a baby duckling.

"No," Elizabeth said sadly. "At school everybody likes me, or I don't even know them. You know how it is. There's a bunch of boys who make a game of getting girls to have sex with them, and they keep score.

They're creeps, and they've done some creepy things—you know, post-ing about the girls who put out, and even meaner posts about the ones that didn't. Both Tiff and I got asked sort of out by one of their bottom feeders—not like a date or anything, just stupid stuff by a guy who wants to be in on the game but is a total loser. Maybe the creep boys could be doing it. I don't think so, though. I mean, at school, I'm not all that *impor-tant*. Why take the trouble to stalk me? I'd probably be worth, like, half a point."

"Half a point?" Anna asked.

"You know, a cheerleader's worth five points, a girl on the student council two points. Like that."

"Time to cull the gene pool," Anna murmured.

"God, I'm glad you're here, Anna," Heath burst out as a boil of anxiety burst inside her. "For all we know this could turn to physical stalking."

Anna said after a moment: "Starting next week, I've got a twenty-one-day detail in Acadia National Park. Acting chief ranger. Their chief is fighting that big fire in Southern California."

This last was said without affect, but Heath knew it rankled with her friend. Like many rangers, Anna neighed and fretted like an old war horse when fire season came around. Heath couldn't understand this love of fighting wildfire. For some it was about overtime and hazard pay.

For others it was an addiction. Anna belonged to the latter group. She'd taken a bullet during the Fox River adventure, and her left arm never fully recovered. Though Anna'd never admit it, she probably hadn't the strength to swing a Pulaski for long.

To be acting chief in a park as important as Acadia would be welcomed by most rangers, a nice step up the ladder to being permanent chief somewhere else. Anna had dithered about the promotion to district ranger. Money meant little to her. Being out of doors and away from human beings meant a lot.

"You're leaving?" Elizabeth wailed.

Heath flinched, not because her daughter cried out like an abandoned five-year-old but because, for an instant, she thought she'd done it herself and was mortified.

"They don't need you!" Heath said, then stooped to threats. "They're liable to give you a promotion."

"I'll be sure and offend the higher-ups," Anna said with a dry smile.

"Send someone else," Heath said, hating the whine in her words.

"Wildfires in California. Everybody is short-handed," Anna said.

Heath said no more. She'd already said too much.

Gwen, whose usual upbeat enthusiasm seemed to have been squelched by the points game and creeps and stalkers, perked up. "Acadia National Park? In Maine? Of course in Maine! For heaven's sake, I'm getting dotty. My first job out of med school was near there. I have to make some calls. Heath, Elizabeth, pack. We are going to Maine with Anna!"

Gwen kissed the air around everybody's cheeks, snatched up her black medical bag, and blew out on the wind the way she had blown in.

"Mary Poppins," Heath laughed.

"Who does Aunt Gwen know in Maine?" Elizabeth asked.

"Dez Hammond and Chris Zuckerberg. A couple of old hippies from the day," Heath said. Heath had met them on two occasions when they'd visited Boulder. She remembered liking them. "Chris comes from money. She inherited an island off Acadia. They spend most of their time rehabbing an old mansion and hosting artists."

"Where's Arcadia?" E asked.

"Acadia," Anna corrected. "Northern Maine, lobsters and nor'easters."

"I'm going to be marooned on an island with four old ladies," Elizabeth cried.

"In a crumbling old mansion," Heath said.

"You'll be there, won't you?" Elizabeth begged Anna.

Heath was annoyed that, though she had more years under her belt than Heath, Anna was not among the designated Old Ladies.

"Not me," Anna said. "A desert isle in the vast Atlantic? Too boring for this child."

Elizabeth groaned.

EIGHT

"D o you want to see where I really live?" Paulette asked. The question should have seemed sudden or peculiar, but it wasn't. In her core—her soul if the metaphor held—Denise knew her twin, her other self, could not truly live in this tragic wreck of a place with paper peeling from the walls and ancient linoleum curling at the corners and buckling along the seams.

They stood at the same instant, laughing at themselves and one another simultaneously. Denise felt as if scales, dirt, fragments of rotting lumber, cracking mortar, and broken roof slates were sliding off her. In the dim light of the bedroom's single shaded lamp, Denise imagined she could see dust rising from the cascade of debris as her old, worn-out, worthless, piece-of-shit life crumbled. When the dust settled, a new, clean, sun-filled life would be built around her and her sister. Denise communicated none of this. Paulette, she was positive, was feeling the same sense of sloughing off a diseased and decrepit skin.

Wordlessly, Paulette led the way through a dilapidated kitchen—appliances right out of Sears circa 1970—and through the back door of the cottage. As they crossed the small weedy yard, a children's swing set, one chain broken, a rotted seat dangling like a broken limb, formed the yard's epitaph.

Paulette reached out. Hesitantly, Denise took her hand and was led into the black night forest.

"I don't go home much, and I always go a different way," Paulette whispered as they made their way through the darkness beneath the trees. "If Kurt found out, he'd spoil it just to be mean; just because he likes to hurt me by ruining my things. He thinks it's funny. Hitting isn't enough. He can't hurt me bad enough with his fists short of putting me in the hospital, which costs a lot, or killing me."

Holding tightly to Paulette's hand, Denise followed blindly, her story—her sister's story, their story—surging through her veins and arteries, down the capillaries until each and every cell in her body was caught up. Waves of fury crashed over deep valleys of sorrow; seas of compassion rose and receded. It had been a while since Denise had felt anything for anyone but herself. The hatred she harbored for Peter had hardened into bitterness. Wormwood and gall had been all she could taste, smell, see, touch.

Dead; she'd been dead to herself in every way that counted. Coming alive in this womb of pine-scented darkness, her hand warm and safe in her twin's, was so overwhelming she staggered like a drunk and fell to her knees, dragging Paulette with her.

Denise felt her sister patting her hand. "Shh, shh," Paulette murmured softly. "It's okay. We're together." Those words were the first and only lullaby Denise had ever heard. She began to cry.

Usually sick helplessness came on the heels of Denise's crying jags. This time, when the tears finally stopped, she felt renewed, as if the tears were poisons her body had expelled.

"We're almost there." Paulette's voice came from the darkness. Denise allowed the gentle tugging to bring her to her feet. "This land belonged to Kurt's mom," Paulette whispered as they crept along. "His grandma lived here. When she died we moved in. It's not like a city lot. It's only about forty feet wide where the house is, but it runs way way back, getting skinnier and skinnier like the tail of a comet. Kurt doesn't care anything about it except that it's his. I wanted him to sell at least part of it because he could get a lot of money for it and we wouldn't have to live in a shack. 'Shack's good enough for the likes of you' was his big-deal answer. If he ever found this, he'd kill me.

"We're here." Paulette let go of Denise's hand. The connection broken, for a second Denise felt as though she were falling, falling and freezing. It was only a dream: the twin, her soul, the Acadian blond barfly. All of it. A dream. A wail rose in her throat, as lonely as the howl of the last wolf on earth. The sound of fumbling, the scratch of a match being lit, then a flame that, born into such a lightless universe, hit Denise's eyes with the force of a supernova, aborted the cry.

Her sister was there. No dream. Tears began to flow again. No paroxysms of grief or wrenching sobs, only warmth and joy in liquid form. Fleetingly, Denise remembered a self that was not given to emotion, a self made stoic by life. No more. In the past months emotions came in sudden overwhelming waves. These were the first that didn't threaten to tear her apart.

Paulette lit an old kerosene lamp she took from beneath a rusted over-turned bucket, adjusted the wick, then handed the lamp to Denise to hold. They were standing at the door of a small shed. The eaves cleared Paulette's head by less than six inches. They would have to stoop to pass through the door without banging their skulls.

By the light of the lamp, Paulette found a short piece of dirty frayed string caught in a crack between two pieces of weathered siding. She pulled it out to reveal the key tied to the end.

"There are so many park visitors, folks would be wandering in all the time," she explained as she turned the key in the padlock that secured the door. "Visitors don't seem to know what's public land and what's private."

"Or care," Denise said.

Paulette pushed open the door, stepped inside, took the lamp, and held it up so Denise could see the room. Bitterness vanished. Delight took its place. The room—the entire house—wasn't more than a hundred and fifty square feet, roughly twelve by twelve, and the ceiling closer to seven feet than eight. On each of the four walls was a large many-paned window, the mullions, frames, and sills clean and painted white, the glass old, from back when glass had ripples and imperfections in it. The walls were painted soft gray, the color of a dove's breast, and hung with pieced fabric stretched over wooden frames, the bright bits of cloth making flowers and mountains, trees and ponds.

On the worn planks of the floor was a simple rag rug. A white crib with a small stuffed bear looking through the bars, a three-drawer chest painted China red, a round table with a lamp of the same color, and a rocking chair completed the nursery. Nothing fussy, nothing out of place, everything clean and necessary and beautiful.

As Paulette closed the door behind them, Denise walked around the room. The windows weren't windows at all. Frames with glass, sills, and half-pulled shades had been mounted on the wall. Behind them were paintings of a forest, much as it might look were the windows real and she was looking through them in the early morning. Shafts of sunlight slanted through dark trunks. The shadows of leaves dappled a small green clearing. Wildflowers surrounded a granite boulder. A bunny grazed fearlessly on new grass.

"I didn't dare make any changes to the outside," Paulette said. "Kurt doesn't come back here, but when people can look in, they can break in, and will. And if Kurt did come this way for some reason, I didn't want to call attention to this old shed."

"He'd ruin it," Denise said. It wasn't a question. She knew he would as if she'd been with Paulette each time he'd made a wreck of what little beauty she'd managed.

Denise reached over the bars of the crib and laid a finger between the stuffed bear's ears. Though she'd never had much in the way of toys—at least not new ones—this one felt familiar to her.

"Kurt's a monster. A big fucking monster," Paulette blurted out.

At the outburst of obscenity, Denise turned to her sister.

Paulette laughed and covered her mouth the way Denise had done until Peter told her it made her look childish. Child*like*, she thought as she watched her twin. Childlike and charming. Another thing Peter had taken from her.

"I've never said that out loud before. Awful as it is, it felt good to say it. Isn't that weird?"

Denise didn't know what to say. It wasn't weird. Not at all. None of this was weird. All of it was exactly how it should be. That was what was weird.

Paulette sat in the rocking chair and let Denise explore the small ornamental boxes, the few books, the fabric art. "When I got pregnant the first time, I bought all these wonderful things for the baby's room. Then, you know, I lost the baby. Kurt said I had to take them back if I'd bought them, or sell them on eBay or whatever if they'd been gifts from my mom and dad—they were still alive then. But I couldn't. I just couldn't. I dragged them all back to this shed and told Kurt I'd given them to Goodwill. He half beat me to death for not getting any money for them. The second time I got pregnant, we got a few more things. Not as many. Mom and Daddy had passed. They were pretty old when they adopted me and died within three months of each other.

"I did the same thing with the new stuff; told Kurt I'd given it away. After that, I used to come out here and kind of fix things up, thinking it would be a nice place for the new baby. I got my nursing degree and started working at Mount Desert Hospital with newborns and infants."

"A nurse!" Denise was pleased. Another thing they had in common: nurse/ranger. Both were jobs helping people.

"When I found out there weren't going to be any more babies," Denise said with a shrug, "I just sort of kept on coming out here to get out of Kurt's sty for a while and remember who I am."

It was easy to forget who you were, Denise thought. She'd forgotten. No, she and Paulette had not forgotten who they were; who they were had been taken from them and thrown into the garbage. Forever, Denise had thought. Now here it was, her true *self*, with her sister's *self*, in an empty nursery in the woods.

"Peter's baby's name is Olivia," she said without thinking. "Olivia Barnes. The name I got was Castle. Now you're Duffy. What was your name before that?"

"Mallory, Paulette Mallory. The Mallorys adopted me. They were good people."

"Then when we're together, I won't be Denise Castle. I will be Denise Mallory," Denise said, and they both smiled.

Paulette stood, the chair still rocking as if her ghost remained behind, and walked over to a small painted table between windows half open on an imaginary forest. "I had time to get used to the idea of us, remember me saying that?" She didn't wait for Denise to answer, as if knowing that, of course, Denise remembered. Miracles tend to stick in memory, and everything about finding a twin sister was miraculous. "I felt you, but then these started appearing in the newspapers in the personal ads. I've only found three. They could be in papers in Bangor and Portland and other places. We only get the local stuff. I've never bothered to try and do a search. I wouldn't know where to begin. Here." She handed Denise a clipping from a newspaper. It wasn't much bigger than the slip of paper found in a fortune cookie. "That one I came across four years ago and for some reason just cut it out and kept it."

Denise turned the bit of newsprint toward the lamp and made out the blurred message. *Seeking identical twins, female, born on the sixth of March and separated at birth. They would now be thirty-seven years of age. Ur-*

*gent they contact me. Family legacy. If you believe you may be such a person send
a postcard to P.O. Box 1597, Post Office, Bar Harbor, ME.*

"March sixth, our birthday," Paulette said.

"No name or zip code," Denise said.

"This one was from year before last." Paulette handed her another
scrap. The message was the same but, this time, included a zip code. Still
no name. "And this is from January this year."

"The legacy," Denise said. Her brain, unable to absorb so much so
quickly, had slowed to a crawl for the moment. "It would be money,
wouldn't it?"

"Or maybe a house or land, like that," Paulette said.

"Our birth parents, do you think?" Denise asked, not sure whether
she would be overjoyed or furious if she were ever to lay her eyes on her
birth mother or biological father.

"Maybe," Paulette said. "Or another relative."

"A lawyer," Denise said, unwilling to have any more relatives at the
moment, wanting to be just sisters alone in a magical cabin in the woods.
"We're the right age, aren't we?"

"And female and twins and separated at birth. How many can
there be?"

"You'd be surprised," Denise said, remembering all the studies done
on identical twins separated at birth.

"Born on the sixth of March? Girls who would be forty-one years old
now, thirty-seven when I found the ad," Paulette said. "The babies must
have been from around here, or who would run the ad in a tiny town like
Bar Harbor?"

Before Denise could think of another reason the ad wasn't for them,
the sound of sleigh bells or wind chimes leaked into the room, tinny and
cheap.

Paulette pulled a cell phone out of her pocket and looked at the face of
it, then up at Denise.

"It's him!" she whispered with all the terror of a trapped bird. Denise could hear her sister's frantically beating wings inside her own skull.

"I have to answer," Paulette said pleadingly.

Denise nodded. Of course she had to answer. If she didn't, Kurt would kill her.

Denise sat on a tiny chair with a rattan seat and a cavalry trumpet carved into the top slat on the back, a perfect, plain, lovely chair for a child, and listened as her sister made excuses for not being in the house when her husband called the home phone; listened to her lie about where she was and who she was with; watched tears roll over Paulette's cheeks, and the way her lips curved down as she rocked herself, begging him not to be mad, promising to be at the house next time.

When she was finally able to hang up, she let the hand with the phone in it fall as if lifeless beside the rocking chair.

"Kurt really is going to kill you," Denise realized suddenly.

Paulette nodded. "I've felt it for a while. He hasn't said anything, and hasn't hit me much, and not real hard. But I know he's planning on killing me and burying my body under the house. When he looks at me I can see it in his eyes as clear as anything. I can see him thinking about how he's going to get the shovel and hide it under the house so it will be ready."

Denise had spent her life in law enforcement. There was no evidence Kurt was plotting murder. He hadn't said he was. He'd laid no concrete plan. Yet Paulette felt it, saw it in his eyes, and believed her husband was planning to murder her.

Denise did, too. She, too, could see it.

This seeing of things hidden wasn't new. It had been growing for months. Change had crept into Denise around the time the park was informed Lily was pregnant with Peter's child. Though subtle, creeping, the change was in both mind and body. Her body responded with small betrayals of the kind that had let the lobster escape. Her mind responded by focusing ever more sharply, by knowing—sometimes—what was in the minds of those around her, just as she now knew her sister believed Kurt would kill her, and knew that Kurt, her *brother-in-law,* did, in fact, plan to murder his wife.

Paulette was her identical twin. Denise knew without asking that she, too, had come to see things that others had hidden in their hearts.

"Kill him first," Denise said, and was mildly surprised that the idea was not shocking. Killing Kurt Duffy was no more than a simple act of self-defense.

"They'd know it was me. Everybody knows he beats me. Not that they care. They'd know it was me. I'd go to jail forever."

"Not if you had a solid alibi," Denise said.

NINE

"Everything is so green and blue," Aunt Gwen said for perhaps the third time. Her red curls as wild as Medusa's snakes in the wind, she was yelling over her shoulder to Heath. Robo-butt, with Heath in it, and Wily grinning on her lap, was firmly lashed in the aft of a small outboard motorboat piloted by a gruff cliché of a New Englander. At least seventy, maybe older, he smelled strongly of tobacco and bay rum, had a couple of days' worth of beard, squinted from a leathery face, and clenched an unlit pipe in his teeth. Central Casting couldn't have done it better, Heath thought.

Aunt Gwen sat in the seat next to him, no doubt charming the pants off Matthew. Luke? Something biblical and manly. Elizabeth, her back toward the rest of them, perched on a gunwale to Heath's right, her mouth set in a rigid line that added years to her face. The rest of the boat's limited deck space was piled with the women's luggage.

Anna had been sent to Acadia several days earlier. Left in Boulder, Heath felt childishly helpless and exposed without her friend. It was embarrassing. A big chunk of the eleven days since Heath found E in the bath with the Lady Schick had been spent getting ready for this trip. The other chunks had been spent watching Elizabeth turn from the compassionate, resilient girl she'd watched grow up to an angry, whining teenager, whom she felt like she didn't know.

Who she sometimes felt hated her.

The change depressed and confounded Heath. E wanted to escape the bullying, yet seemed angry and afraid to leave it behind, as if, unattended, it would metastasize until the cancer destroyed her life. The promised solitude had gone from a reprieve to a prison sentence in the girl's mind. In Heath's as well, on bad days. Like this one. Only Gwen had maintained her optimism. It had been temporarily damped by the news of her old friend Chris's heart attacks, and finally a stroke. The sadness was touched, Heath guessed, by a fear of her own mortality; Chris was sixteen years Gwen's junior.

No one was equipped to fight invisible monsters, Heath realized. Monsters of the Id or the Internet. The kind that worked in the dark, unknowable, motives as twisted and murky as eddies in a polluted river. Creeping poisonous fog that insinuated itself through the cracks of the mind.

The kind Anna couldn't shoot and E couldn't run from.

"That be Boar," the pilot said. He lifted an arm and pointed with a hand that looked to be carved from an old oak tree. Arthritis bent his little finger at the second joint, poking it out to the side at an odd angle.

"You've got to be kidding," Elizabeth said.

"It'll be fun," Heath insisted with more determination than faith. The island was right out of *The Count of Monte Cristo,* or some other nineteenth-century romance. It looked like a broken molar thrust a hundred feet up from the ocean's surface. In the cavity of the jagged tooth, protected by a rugged cliff to the northeast, was the house they would be staying in for the foreseeable future. As luck—bad for Gwen's friend, the island's owner—would have it, it was unoccupied for the present. Chris was recuperating—or dying—in a medical facility in Bangor.

Heath hoped the house would prove less forbidding than the land it rested atop, and their sojourn there more salubrious than that of the former occupant.

The boat pulled neatly up to a stone jetty. The pilot turned off the engine, then, line in hand, jumped nimbly onto the jetty to tie the boat off. Wind keened around the granite base of the island. None of them spoke; Heath, Gwen, and E were staring up a fifty-foot cliff, steps carved into the stone.

"John, are you sure this is the right island?" Gwen asked the pilot. John Whitman, Heath remembered.

"Yup."

"This is not happening," E said.

"Why didn't you tell us?" Heath asked.

"Didn't ask," John said.

"Anybody mind if I shoot your pal Chris?" Heath asked.

"Ms. Zuckerberg is ailing." John said with mild rebuke. He tied a second line to secure the stern of the boat. Wily hopped from the boat to the jetty. Not hopped—his hopping days were behind him; scrambled was more like it.

John scratched Wily behind the ears.

"I think I might be able to do the stairs on my butt," Heath said. "Might" was the operative word. Leah had grudgingly given her permission to bring Dem Bones, but she was not to use it anywhere there was salt or damp. Not all that useful under the circumstances.

"Slippery as eel snot if there's any wind. And there's always wind," John said around the stem of his pipe, which he was lighting.

"That's insane," Elizabeth said. "This whole thing is insane."

"You could lose your balance and be killed," Gwen said.

"That would take the fun out of it," Heath admitted. She didn't have the kind of money it would take to stay in a hotel. The airfare had just about cleaned her out.

"Does this mean we get to go back to Boulder?" Elizabeth asked.

"Can you spell 'stalker'?" Heath wasn't going to let E anywhere near anywhere until she found out who was stalking her. The police didn't much care about cyberstalking—or, more probably, hadn't a clue what to do about it. Private detectives charged a fortune, and Heath doubted they could do anything she couldn't do if she put her mind—and Gwen's and Anna's—to it.

All she needed was three things: to know E was safe, a Wi-Fi connection, and time.

"This place has everything we need. I'll just carry my butt up those stairs, and we'll be moving in," she said firmly.

John puffed on his pipe and said nothing.

Wily watched with the somber attention of a fan at a tennis match.

"It's too dangerous, Heath," Aunt Gwen said.

"Could we just not do this?" Elizabeth whined.

"Can't be as hard as it looks," Heath said with the desperate good cheer she'd taken to injecting into the platitudes she seemed incapable of avoiding.

Elizabeth snorted. She sounded like Anna, Heath realized, and was careful not to smile, not to notice at all.

A metal ramp borrowed for the occasion was laid from the boat to the jetty. Heath and Robo-butt debarked in a maneuver as complex and intricate as the landing on Omaha Beach. Gritting her teeth against what she knew was going to be an event fit for the Special Olympics, she rolled to the first of the stone steps soaring in zigzags up the face of the cliff.

That she wouldn't make it, that she would slip off and tumble into the Atlantic, or worse, the rocks, that she'd get halfway and give out, and there'd be the huge humiliation of a ranger rescue: These thoughts she shoved deep into the well of hopeless thoughts in the back of her brain.

She wasn't taking Elizabeth back to Boulder. She was taking Boar Island. The temptation to yell, "Charge!" was tempered by the fact she'd be advancing butt first.

"I'm not climbing that," Elizabeth said. "No wonder Ms. Zuckerberg had heart failure."

"Elizabeth!" Gwen admonished, then said to Heath, "Let's wait and call Anna."

"For what?" Heath responded irritably. "Her to carry me up on her scrawny back?"

"Maybe she could drag you like a sack of laundry," E suggested.

"That I'd like to see," John said. "Still and all, if it was me, I'd take the lift."

Heath and Gwen glared at him. He squinted into the wind and puffed his pipe complacently.

Heath's hope of a Batcave-like super-elevator bored into the living rock was quickly dashed. The lift was a wooden platform with rails made of old pipes. Steel cables were attached to the four corners, then tied off ten feet up on a ring at the end of another cable that snaked to the top of the cliff, where it disappeared into a rusted iron wheel.

"Electric winch," John said as he led them to where the conveyance sat, graying wood and dull pewter-colored metal rendering it almost invisible against the granite. "When Ms. Zuckerberg had her first heart attack, and Mrs. Hammond came to look after her, she got this put in. Steps too hard for carrying groceries and what-all."

"First heart attack?" Aunt Gwen asked.

"This was the third."

"She didn't tell me that. Neither did Dez," Gwen said, her voice sharp with concern.

The boatman swung open a hinged section of the welded railing. "Who's first?"

"Don't look at me," Elizabeth said.

"I'll do it," Gwen said tentatively.

"No," Heath decided. "It has to be me."

"Right," Elizabeth said scornfully. "Who's going to hold it while you roll off? Could we please go back to the real world now?"

"The real world sucks at the moment," Heath said.

"Will it haul us all at the same time?" Gwen asked.

"Might could," John said.

"Forget it. I'm not getting on that thing," Elizabeth said, and got back into the boat.

Gwen and Heath would go first, leaving John to unload and get the luggage on the lift. Heath harbored no expectations that this new Elizabeth would help him. Wily whined and yipped and showed no inclination whatsoever to get on the thing, with or without people.

"Come here, Wily," E said. She lifted the dog back into the boat with her.

Once Heath, with chair, was rolled onto the lift, she locked her wheels. John handed her a small metal box hooked to a cable. The box had two buttons on it, one red, one green.

"After you're off, just push the button. That'll send the lift back down," John said.

"I take it green is up," Heath said with a look at John.

"We'll see," he said.

"Tally ho," Heath said idiotically, and punched the green button. Had she not been half blind with terror, the trip up would have been stunning. Through the waves of panic that crested each time the lift lurched, or Aunt Gwen squeaked, she barely managed to register the glittering expanse of unbelievably blue sea and sky, the dense green of the hardwood forest above the cliffs, breaking waves painting white lace around their feet. These were the good things. Heath kept her eyes resolutely on them. The one time she looked down, her daughter, her dog, and John were growing ever tinier, looking more and more like specks of chewed food caught in the sharp teeth of the rocks.

She wished controlling what she heard was as simple. Fear honed her ears to batlike sensitivity. Each creak of the winch wheel or groan of the platform signaled failed machinery and a splatty death before the eyes of her only child. In the end, she gave up, stared skyward at the wheel reeling in the cable, and prayed that God would not let a nice lady in a wheelchair die on such a sunny day.

"We're here," Aunt Gwen said as the last terrifying clank announced the end of the line. Heath was pleased to hear the quaver in her aunt's voice. It was not good to be the lone coward in a group. Moving from platform to clifftop wasn't as formidable as Heath had feared. The lift rose through a square hole in a larger platform, where it could be secured in place by four sliding metal plates about the size of a magazine. Ms. Zuckerberg had clearly envisioned a day when she might be commuting by wheelchair.

When the plates were set, the lift was as stable as the platform. Heath wheeled easily out onto solid ground. High, certainly, but solid, and worthy of a quick word of gratitude to the almighty.

The luggage followed, with John to unload it. He sent the lift back down. Heath refused to roll near the edge and holler at E to come up. Not yet.

"Used to be only a lighthouse here until city folk began piddling around in 1922," John said. "Waste of a good rock, if you ask me." He left them to get a cart for the luggage.

High on an island in the ocean, Heath could feel the elements in a way she usually didn't. The sun was a force against her skin, the wind a living thing twining in her hair; the light refractions from the sea were as sharp as the salt smell. Suddenly she felt very alive. Leaning her head back, she looked up a hundred and fifty feet to the top of the old lighthouse. The base had to be at least forty feet in diameter, and the walls fourteen feet thick, at least at the bottom.

The lighthouse was the single bit of architectural grace. The rest reminded Heath of the Winchester House in California, as if each owner had been driven to keep on building regardless of how haphazard the design. Forming an awkward V, with the lighthouse at the point, two wings—one of them two stories, the other three—blew back from the original tower, then petered out in drunken angles to finally die in piles of stone and timber. A century of winds had piled the debris along the skirt of the high granite wall on the northeast side of the island.

"If this place isn't haunted, I want my money back," Gwen said.

"I'm afraid we'll turn out to be the evil spirits," Heath said, thinking of the sudden—and to her, inexplicable—changes in her daughter. "Elizabeth has gone from Junior Jekyll to Rising Senior Hyde. It's like she's turned into a different person in a matter of days. Did I ever act like that?"

"For a year or two. You went through a bad patch when your dad remarried."

"Everything I do is wrong." Tears of self-pity and frustration flooded Heath's eyes. "Wind," she said, wiping them away. "I haven't a clue how to respond to her this way."

"Do what she asked you to do about a million times," Gwen said.

Her aunt's sharp tone offended Heath. It was as if Gwen thought she was a fool, or worse. "And what is that?" Heath snapped.

"Give her electronics back," Gwen said.

"You're joking," Heath said, aghast. The night of Lady Schick and the tub, Heath had taken everything of E's that needed a charge to run.

"That's what she wants. I think she's made that clear enough," Gwen said.

E had complained bitterly for a few days, then quit speaking of it. Why? Heath asked herself. Because she accepted that Mom was right? Decided her cyberlife sucked and she was glad to be out of it?

"Give her back her iPad, iPod, iPhone—whatever-all teens carry these days. Life as she perceives it is in the toilet, and now you're forcing her to go through withdrawal. Electronic media is an addiction of E's generation," Gwen said with exasperating patience.

"Addiction my ass!" Heath grumbled. Cocaine was an addiction. Heroin was an addiction. A telephone was not an addiction. It was an affectation.

"You saw the crap she's getting on her phone and laptop," Heath said.

"So did she. She knows what is there; is it any worse imagining what's there? Not being able to communicate with friends because *it* is there? Because we don't understand being addicted to social media doesn't mean it doesn't exist. Addicted isn't even the right word. It is the new normal. She feels like you're punishing her for something she has no control over," Gwen said.

Heath resented the intrusion into her maternal bailiwick as much as she wanted her aunt's advice. Lose-lose situation. "The last time I checked, there was one of a threesome with her face Photoshopped over the woman's. I can't bear the thought of her looking at that stuff," Heath said.

"How do you think she feels having you see it? Or me? Though I've delivered hundreds of babies, she sees me as a little old lady who doesn't know where babies come from."

"She doesn't see you that way, you know," Heath said.

"Elizabeth is drowning in shame."

"She's been through worse, real threats, and she was so strong," Heath almost wailed, and cursed herself for being a weakling. For respectable mothers, children are Achilles' heels.

"But she can't fight this one. You can't fight this one. The enemy has no face. The enemy might be her friends. Her friends might be sniggering at the pictures and talking behind her back. It's anonymous, horribly personal, and public all at the same time."

"We should have stayed in Boulder. I should have gotten her a psychiatrist," Heath said. A second mortgage on the house and it would have been feasible. Cheap if it helped E.

"Maybe. Since you didn't, you have to let her be an adult with you.

She survived the Fox fiasco because she fought back. This is her fight, and you've confiscated the field of battle. You two have to come to terms about how you're going to deal with this as a team."

"So sayeth the goddess of youth," Heath said with a wry smile.

"So sayeth the goddess," Gwen affirmed.

The winch groaned to life and began spinning up steel cable.

"Give her back her electronics," Gwen said. "I'm going to help John."

TEN

Anna sat across the kitchen table from Lily, sipping extremely good coffee and watching Peter Barnes make goofy faces at Olivia.

"Nice being your boss," he said. "We don't have much crime here, so I may order you to babysit." He grinned.

"Sure," Anna said. "I met a baby once."

"This may be Gris's last fire. He's been muttering about retiring for ten years. I wouldn't be surprised if he up and does it. Your duty station here might end up being for more than three weeks. Maybe for years."

"That's a lot of babysitting," Anna said somberly.

Anna had known Peter nearly twenty years, since law enforcement training at FLETC, the Federal Law Enforcement Training Center in Brunswick, Georgia. In the day, he'd been the epitome of "tall, dark, and handsome": black hair, brown eyes, a few inches over six feet, with thick thighs and upper arms. In a test of endurance, Anna could best him. When it came to sheer physical power, she was as a spider monkey to a bull ape.

In his forties, Pete was still tall and handsome, but the dark at his temples had been painted gray—enough to suggest he was experienced, not enough to suggest he was getting old. Fatherhood was the big change. The Pete Anna knew always referred to children as ankle-biters and rug rats, harped on overpopulation, and eschewed the institution of marriage as nothing but a piece of paper.

Yet here he was, married and dangling a wee daughter on his knee, familial bliss oozing from every pore.

"They're pretty doggone cute, aren't they?" his wife, Lily, said with a smile and a wink at Anna. "I think Peter wanted progeny because a big man with a tiny baby is a megawatt chick magnet."

Anna laughed because it was true. Even she, happily married to the finest man on earth, was finding Peter positively adorable.

"I told Anna she could be chief babysitter as well as chief ranger," Peter said, never taking his eyes off baby Olivia's face.

"I could keep her alive," Anna said seriously. She was mildly offended when they laughed. "In Texas, I kept a younger baby alive under seriously adverse circumstances."

"They don't all make it," Peter said, gooey-eyed over Olivia.

"Culling the gene pool," Anna said.

"You don't mean that!" Lily said in the warm tones of a good person.

Actually, Anna did mean it, but had learned not to flaunt her darker side. Much as she liked Peter, her personal jury was still out on his new wife. So far she'd seen nothing not to like about Lily. Still, it was good to wait a few years before rushing into these sorts of decisions.

"I'd best go make myself presentable," Lily said. Having stopped to kiss first Olivia, then Peter on the head, Lily escaped upstairs.

"Sorry about the quarters. The fancy digs are getting repainted. Are you settled in on Schoodic?" Peter asked.

"I am," Anna replied. She liked the Schoodic Peninsula. Situated across Frenchman Bay from Bar Harbor, an hour by car, less than half that by boat, it was part of the patchwork of public lands that made up Acadia.

The forested peninsula was mostly owned by an absentee landlord. The NPS had only the stony tip where it thrust into the sea.

With fewer tourist amenities, the peninsula received only a fraction of the park's visitors. On Schoodic, Anna could occasionally feel a hint of how it must have been when it was wilderness.

Peter was humming "Twinkle, Twinkle, Little Star" as he fed the child from a bottle.

He looked up and saw Anna watching. "Formula's not the best, I know, but sometimes, well, the magic doesn't work. Lily has no milk," he said as if Anna had asked, as if she cared, which she hadn't and didn't.

"You're the most beautiful girl in the world, yes you are, yes you are," Pete crooned, bobbing his big square head back and forth.

"You do know you look like an idiot," Anna said kindly.

"I *feel* like an idiot! I'm a prisoner of love," he said with an exaggerated sigh and a hand to his heart. "Who knew? Your own kid is different."

Anna would have to take his word on that. She'd never wanted kids, never had kids, and never regretted the choice. Kids were great; watching them was fun, talking to them edifying, and working with them occasionally revelatory. Anna liked kids. Then, too, she liked Irish wolfhounds. She just never much wanted one in the house.

The first few notes of Alice Cooper's "School's Out" sounded from the other room. Peter groaned. "Here, you hold her."

"I can," Anna said defensively as she took Olivia into her arms. Peter went to answer his phone.

"Hello, little citizen," Anna said. Round blue-gray eyes stared unblinkingly into hers. The infant interrogation technique. Anna always felt she was being asked, "Are you worthy? Can you keep me safe?"

"No," she said, and, "I'll give it my best shot."

Olivia stared at her in the unfathomable way of infants. Then her eyes squeezed shut. Her pretty little mouth formed an ugly square. She started to cry. Anna sighed. Babies almost always cried when she held them. It hurt her feelings. Was it that she smelled funny? Or was it that she was so paranoid about dropping the squirmy little beggars that her muscles tensed up until the creatures felt more as if they'd been nailed into a peach crate than enfolded in loving arms?

Peter appeared in the kitchen doorway, cell phone in hand. "That was Artie, the district ranger for Mount Desert. Courtesy call. They got an e-mail tip that your pal on Boar is receiving contraband." The look he gave her reminded Anna of how long it had been since they'd spent any time together, as if he was thinking that if he could turn into Father of the Year, maybe she could have turned into a person who consorted with underworld types.

"I told him we'd meet them at the jetty on Boar," Peter said. "Lily!" he roared, sounding like the old Peter. "We've got to go."

Anna's cell phone buzzed. She pulled it from its case. A text from Heath: *Weird shit getting weirder. Come when you can.*

"Ready when you are," she said to Peter. He led the way to the white Crown Vic, an older model. The NPS was a frugal organization. Anna slid into the passenger side, buckled her seat belt, and prepared to enjoy the view.

Visitors often asked her which park was her favorite. She'd never come up with a satisfactory answer. Today, a body of water encompassing a universe of light and life, a thousand blues in waves that rose and broke in sun-silver celebrations, the surf whispering secrets just out of hearing, it was Acadia.

The fancy houses infesting the multitude of islands scattered in the ocean should have made the coast feel cozier, more inviting of human habitation. Instead, on the rugged coast of the Atlantic, the grandest homes man could devise seemed mere shacks. They hugged the rocky shore as if afraid to venture from sight of land. Those on the tiny islands were like orphans lost at sea.

Anna loved it when nature made humanity seemed trivial. It was a comfort to pretend that she was of a relatively harmless race; she felt safer when she could delude herself that in the battle of Man against Nature, Nature had a chance. For the short duration of the boat ride out of Somes Sound to Boar Island, she could almost believe Internet bullies and weird shit getting weirder did not matter.

The ride up the lift, accompanied by the towering form of Peter Barnes and the hulky muscle-bound district ranger, Artie Lange, was a tad more exhilarating than Anna liked. Not for the first time, she wished more of her compadres were small-boned women, less inclined to strain machinery. Still, she appreciated the view.

The bedrooms in the lighthouse, accessed one through the other by the original circular iron stairs, and the rooms around the lighthouse's base had been renovated. The rest of the place, two wings, blew northeast and west like a tattered cape in a gale. Damp, winds, and harsh winters had had their way. The remains were more ruin than mansion.

"That was quick," Heath said as the lift creaked the last few inches to its mooring fifty feet above the rocks. "And with reinforcements," she said, not sounding particularly pleased. Heath, in Robo-butt, was sitting in the shade, an iPad on her lap. Wily lounged beside her, his chin on his paws. With a deep groan he forced himself to his feet and ambled over to greet Anna. Anna and Wily were old friends; they were pack. She was glad of the sun on his old bones, and the new interesting scents for his nose.

Scratching behind Wily's ears, Anna introduced Heath to Peter and Artie. The young district ranger was looking at Heath keenly, undoubtedly hungering for a perp worth his ambitions. Anna had never worked with Artie, never met him before coming to Acadia, but she suspected he would have been happier on a SWAT team than a bucolic island getaway. She also suspected he thought—hoped—Heath might be a major drug dealer and Anna a co-conspirator.

Suppressing a sigh, she asked, "Where are Elizabeth and Gwen?"

If Artie was going to get all Long Strong Arm of the Law, she didn't want Heath accused of drug crimes—or, gods forbid, arrested—in front of her daughter.

"John took E and Gwen into Bar Harbor for mail and groceries," Heath said.

Peter shot Anna a look. Clearly he knew his district ranger and wanted Anna to take the lead. Anna folded down with her legs crossed Indian-style, the better to commune with Wily. Peter and Artie remained standing.

"You're looming," Anna said.

Peter sat down on the waist-high stone wall separating the patio from the drop to the sea.

Artie, continuing to loom, said, "I've never been on Boar. I'm not classy enough for Ms. Hammond and Ms. Zuckerberg. Mind if I poke around a bit?"

"Poke to your heart's content," Heath said easily.

Anna wished she hadn't. It was always a bad idea to let law enforcement— especially guys like Artie—"poke around." But then, Heath thought they were here to help her with weird shit, not investigate an anonymous tip. Before Artie could go more than a step or two, Anna said, "Artie got a tip. An e-mail that said you were receiving contraband goods. Drugs. That you and Elizabeth were dealing to the kids in Boulder."

"You're kidding," Heath said, obviously—at least to Anna—stunned. Heath laughed. "You are kidding?"

"Nope," Anna said.

"You've stolen my thunder for weird shit today. This is what I got." Seeming completely unconcerned with the accusation, Heath rolled over to where Anna and Wily sat shoulder to shoulder and handed her the iPad. "Hit REFRESH," she said.

Anna did as she was told. Reading the screen was almost impossible in the direct light of the sun. Shielding it as best as she could, she squinted at the line of comments scrolling down the right-hand side.

"That's usually where the comments of people Elizabeth follows on Twitter show up," Heath said. "This guy—or girl—has been tweeting like a damned canary since last night."

The expected obscenities were in evidence, but the thrust of the argument had changed. Anna read aloud, "'Kill yourself. The world will be better off when you're dead. Slit your wrists. Your Mother tried to abort you. When that didn't work, she dumped you. Put a bullet in your brain. You alive will make Heath kill herself. Die, bitch, die.'"

Peter rose to his feet. Artie decided this was more interesting than poking around.

"I kind of like that last one," Heath said. "It has a certain simplicity the others lack."

"Has E seen these?" Anna asked.

"All but the last few. They came in after John took them in the boat. She may have seen them by now. She has her phone with her."

"I thought you were keeping her away from electronics," Anna said, her voice flat to keep the censure from leaking through. Anna had not rushed headlong into the twenty-first century. People scarcely noticed as life was remade by cell phones, GPS, Amazon, YouTube, Google, and Facebook. Big Brother was a mere piker compared to Amazon and its fellows. Clicking "accept, accept, accept" to unread contracts, whole countries and their children became citizens of this sudden and stunning world of bread and fabulous circuses without a thought or a backward look.

Anna knew there would be a reckoning. Even in the twenty-first century she doubted there was anything like a free lunch.

"Aunt Gwen made a good argument against it," Heath replied a bit defensively.

"Like E needs to see this stuff?" Anna growled.

"Like E needs to have a sense of control. That and addiction," Heath said with the exaggerated patience Anna knew she'd inherited from her aunt.

"Addiction?" Artie asked. Had he been a dog, his ears would have been pricked.

"Evidently," Heath said. "Aunt Gwen said it's common, almost epidemic."

"Gwen Littleton is a pediatrician," Anna explained to Artie and Peter. To Heath, she said, "Elizabeth is not an addict," and then, "Addicted to what?"

"Electronic media," Heath said.

Anna snorted. Peter wore a neutral ranger mask, the kind put on when taking reports of flying saucers and sightings of Kokopelli.

"Be that way," Heath said to no one in particular. Shaking a cigarette from a pack kept in Robo-butt's saddlebag, she went on. "For all the reasons we had talked about, I did take E's iPhone, iPad, laptop, everything but her Kindle." Cigarette in her teeth, Heath cupped her hands to protect the lighter's flame from the onshore wind and lit it. "E grew sullen, irritable, had trouble sleeping, had little appetite, trouble focusing, exhibited obsessive behaviors, paranoia, hypersensitivity—all the things she would have if she'd been a cocaine addict and I'd cut her off cold turkey."

"Or heroin," Artie said.

Heath glanced at him, mild confusion in her eyes, then went on. "The only thing missing was hallucinations." Taking a deep drag of the smoke, she glared around at the three of them.

Wily, Anna noted, was not included in the malevolence.

"She's been under a lot of stress," Anna said.

"That, too. But after Gwen convinced me, I Googled it."

"That's asking the dealer about the junkie," Anna said.

"As Ripley said, believe it or not," Heath retorted.

"So you just handed her back everything? Fornicating threesomes, goats, pederasts, and donkeys—the whole filthy business?" Anna asked.

"We talked. I told her she had to show me everything. If it was so shaming she just couldn't bring herself to let me see it, she had to forward it to you."

"Thanks a heap," Anna said, but was honored.

"I gave her electronics back and the symptoms cleared up almost immediately," Heath said.

"Freaky," Anna said, shaking her head. To her, social media was about as entertaining as mosquitoes whining around her ears.

"Yup. Strange but true," Heath said, the wind whipping the cigarette smoke from her lips.

The bell on the pole by the lift clanged; then, with a piteous groan, the machinery began paying out steel cable.

"That will be my little addict now," Heath said.

The love in her voice made Anna smile.

Minutes later the platform appeared filled with bags, Gwen, Elizabeth, and John. When the retired lobsterman saw the field of green and gray, his eyes narrowed and his teeth clamped harder on his pipestem. Acadia was one of many parks that had frequent interface with previous residents, inholdings, shared or debated boundaries, and clashing cultures. Locals often eyed park rangers askance, figuring they were only around to make up rules about things that were traditionally none of their damn business. Conserving resources for the next generation was of little interest to those of the present generation who were just trying to get by.

Anna didn't blame them, but it was of greater importance that the native plants and animals survive and thrive. Humans had much in common with kudzu, Russian thistle, and other invasive species. They needn't be wiped out entirely, only uprooted where they threatened the natural balance.

Gwen, her hair made wild with salt wind, looked fifteen years younger than she had in Boulder. The sea air? The change of scenery? No, Anna decided; it was John. Gwen was enamored. The boat pilot had the same sort of sex appeal as Spencer Tracy, Humphrey Bogart, and Robert Mitchum. The kind that doesn't depend on youth or good looks.

Even E appeared happy enough. When she saw Anna studying Gwen, she rolled her eyes and made a face. At sixteen, geriatric romance was grossing her out. A wonderful problem, given the other things that had been grossing all of them out for the last weeks.

"John, get the cart so we can get the perishables in the fridge," Gwen bossed him happily. From the look on the man's face, he was teetering between enchanted and terrified.

"Got a present," Gwen said as she dumped envelopes and a shoe-box-sized package on Heath's lap.

"Do you want me to come help put groceries away?" E asked, batting her eyes innocently.

"That won't be necessary," Gwen said.

E flopped down beside Wily and Anna. "I just offered to annoy her. For a while there in Bar Harbor I thought she was going to ask him to carry her books or give her a ride home on his bicycle. That or get a motel room. Yuck."

"*Amore*," Anna said, and sighed deeply.

"Somebody to sit next to at the old age home more like," Elizabeth said. Then, "Sorry, Mom. I know she'll want to park her wheelchair next to yours."

"Not if I take my medicine," Heath said, waving her unfiltered Camel. "The cure for old age."

E was not amused.

Nor was Anna.

"What's in the box, Ms. Jarrod?" Artie, the district ranger, cut in. Anna had totally forgotten why they'd been called to Boar, the anonymous tip that Heath and E were drug dealers come to the East Coast to corrupt the youth.

Now a box appears right on cue.

"Haven't a clue," Heath said and began ripping at the paper.

"Don't open it," Anna said suddenly.

"Think it's a bomb?" Heath asked, laughing as she smashed the paper beneath the box so the wind wouldn't snatch it away. She was as gleeful as a child on her birthday. Relief from stress, Anna guessed.

"It's not ticking," Heath said as torn paper revealed a shoe box.

"Bombs don't tick anymore," Anna said as she leapt to her feet.

Heath lifted the lid off. "What in the hell . . . ," she said.

The District Danger Ranger was beside Heath's chair in an instant. "I'll need that box, ma'am." Before Anna could snatch the box or slap Heath upside the head, Artie had it in his big, long-fingered hands.

Wide-eyed, curious, Heath waited like a sitting duck.

"Looks like heroin to me," Artie said with barely suppressed glee. He bounced the box in his hand as if weighing it. "An eight-ball or there-abouts."

"Like *heroin* heroin?" Elizabeth asked.

"This could be serious," Heath said. Now that it was too late, she was finally catching on, Anna thought, but Heath wasn't paying any attention to the drugs in the ranger's hand; she was staring at the wrapping paper spread across her knees.

"This wasn't forwarded from Boulder," she said. "This was sent to the PO box we rented in Bar Harbor."

"The e-mail was sent to Acadia," Anna said.

Unconsciously, Elizabeth raised her hands to her throat. "Whoever it is knows where we are," she said softly.

ELEVEN

Denise and her sister had neither seen nor spoken to one another since they'd decided something had to be done to keep Kurt Duffy from beating—or killing—Paulette. Not that Denise wanted to be alone; she never wanted to be alone again. Space to think was what she needed. After three days of thinking, of no contact with Paulette, she went to her sister's house during the day when she knew Kurt would be at sea. She moored her runabout in Otter Cove, a tiny inlet with little to lure visitors. From there she hiked overland to Otter Creek and her sister's back door. This way no one would see her car parked anywhere near Paulette's. The car was one of the things she had thought of while she was in her lonely thinking space.

Not phoning Paulette was another thing. Cell phones were wired to record every call, every text, and, with GPS, where the phone was at any given time. Denise didn't know how many of these invasive pieces of technology dwelt in her phone—it was four years old—but if they were going to do something serious about Kurt, she didn't dare take chances.

The previous night she had taken her phone apart, cooked the SIM card in the microwave for a few minutes, then cut the nuked card into pieces with tin snips. That done, she smashed all the parts of the phone that could be smashed with a three-pound sledge hammer. Over the remaining rubble, she poured lighter fluid and burned what would burn, melted what would melt. The resulting black mess she tossed overboard where the channel was deepest.

It never made sense to her that criminals couldn't destroy evidence properly. She had to suppose they never really put their minds to it. Paulette's prepaid cell from Walmart would have to be destroyed as well.

The way her sister's face lit up when she saw who was tapping on her kitchen door made Denise's heart fill her throat. Along with her soul, she'd thought unconditional love went missing when she was born. The open trust and joy she saw in her twin's eyes she'd only ever expected to see in the eyes of her newborn child.

Paulette came out onto the porch. She was wearing a calf-length skirt in lime green and pink. The pink was in geometric patterns and the green in paisley swirls. The waistband and the bottom third of the skirt were green, the rest bold pink. On her feet were mules of tan-colored canvas with green ankle ribbons and wedge heels. Over the skirt she wore a white tunic, belted with a narrow lime green ribbon.

Denise wore trousers. Always: for work, for home, for fancy dress. The palette of her wardrobe ran the gamut from dull Park Service green and gray to totally grim. Seeing "herself" in a bright skirt, she was startled at how pretty she was, they were.

Without any need for discussion, Paulette headed toward the trees. Again she led Denise in a circuitous path to the nursery so there would be no obvious trail worn in the duff. Neither spoke until they were closed behind the wooden door, lamp lit against the artificial night inside the windowless shed. This time Denise sat in the rocking chair and Paulette on the child-sized chair with the trumpet carved on the back.

"That's a nursing rocker," Paulette said of the chair Denise had taken.

"That's why the arms are so low and curved; so you can hold the baby and rest your forearm on the wood."

Unconsciously rounding her arms as if she held an infant, Denise rocked gently. "It feels right, good," she marveled. For a long moment, both she and her sister gazed out at the never-changing forest painted behind the window frames, a world no one but they could inhabit, no one but they could alter.

Paulette began as if telling a story that would be important to Denise, one that Denise had been asking for in her head. "I first brought the baby things out here fourteen years, two months, and nine days ago; you don't forget the day you lose a child. I was just storing them, you know, for the next baby. Hiding them from Kurt so he wouldn't sell them or break them. He wasn't too bad back then."

"He beat you so hard you miscarried," Denise said.

"I guess. Yes, I mean, I know he did," said Paulette with a wan smile, her head shaking slowly from side to side. She looked as if she were fighting clear of a fog she'd been lost in for a long time. "I guess what I was thinking was that back then, when he hurt me, he didn't mean it like he does now. He'd get stirred up over money, or he'd get jealous of the way I supposedly looked at some guy, or he'd get mad because I wanted to go visit Mom and Dad or whatever. He'd get mad for some reason, lose his temper, and take it out on me.

"At the hospital we've got this old man who comes in every few months. He's got this awful abscess on the side of his calf that fills up with yuck and bursts. We clean it up, the doctors prescribe salves and antibiotics, and it seems to heal. Then, in a month or two, he's back in. Kurt used to be like that, this abscess that filled with yuck. Then he'd get drunk and beat up on me, and he'd be okay for a while. Even sorry in the beginning. Shoot, by the time I was twenty-six we'd been married nearly ten years. What else did I know? I guess I figured most men slapped their wives around. I didn't have much in the way of girlfriends to compare lives with." She smiled at Denise. "I didn't have a sister."

Denise smiled back without thinking, and realized she had been so strung out, weirded out, on guard, and paranoid for the last few months that she'd reacted in the same way Paulette had to Kurt's abuse. It had become the norm, the real, the way life was. This sudden relaxing of vigilance was a revelation. Abuse was not the way life was. It was the way men made it. Women could subject it to change without notice.

"After I lost the first baby, I never forgave Kurt. Him beating me, I could forgive that. But not beating the baby to death inside me."

That was why Denise couldn't forgive Peter. Dumping her? Sure. Marrying a younger woman? That, too. The loss of her baby? Never. Maybe Peter was another person who needed to be dead. He hadn't beaten her, but he had certainly browbeaten her into getting an abortion. Murder twice removed was still murder. Even in a species gorging on death every day, killing babies was genuinely despised. Nobody cheered baby killers. They didn't get medals. People paid more than lip service to wanting to stamp them out.

"Then, three years, three months, three weeks, and five days later, I lost a little girl, my daughter. She was fairly well along. Tiny hands and fingers, a nub of a nose, ears, all perfect. I saw her in the the bathroom overhead light. That's where I miscarried. Kurt looked sick seeing us there on the floor. I thought he was going to pick us up, but he sort of shook all over like a goose walked on his grave and said, 'Clean up the mess.' He didn't come back for a couple of days, and when he did it was like nothing happened. Nothing. He comes through the door, turns on the TV, and says, 'What do you have for supper?' That was it. After that he didn't hit me for a long time. A year or more.

"That's when I fell into a kind of sleep, I think. I gave up on the house, except for keeping it clean enough to be sanitary, and I'd come back here and tidy up. Bit by bit, this room became what it is. While I was walking in my sleep all those years, this was the dream I was dreaming. Does that sound crazy?"

"No," Denise answered. "It's a beautiful dream. A wise dream. I must have fallen asleep, too. I dreamed of dark places and rotten people. Walking around this park we so loved when we were little, I would see nothing but my pain. Finally, my world was made of pain, and that world got smaller every day."

Denise knew she hadn't been a child in Acadia National Park. While her twin was being raised by kindly old folks on Isle au Haut, Denise was being kicked around trailer parks in Brewer and Bangor and Winterport. Still, she wasn't lying; she knew that their childhood playing in tide pools was more real than hers playing on train tracks and around warehouses. Paulette would know this, too.

For an instant she was outside herself, looking at the two of them sitting in the painted room. Panic surged up her throat; she was going crazy, had gone crazy, Paulette did sound crazy.

Then she was back in her body. The terror abated. She looked around the space her sister had created, calming herself with the fabric art pieces, the windows that showed the world as it should be rather than as it was, the crib with the stuffed bear, bright-eyed, head tilted inquisitively. The true insanity was not what she and her sister dreamed. It was the actions of those who had made their lives so miserable they needed to dream it.

"Then I woke up," Paulette said simply, cutting into Denise's thoughts. Still on the little chair, her skirt flowing to the floor in a bright blossom, she spread her hands with a shrug. "About a year ago . . . six months . . . I don't know. Around that time I started feeling again, then I started feeling everything was odd, off somehow. At first Kurt didn't notice I'd woken up. When he did, he didn't like it. He knocked me around some—not a lot, but I could feel he meant it this time. Meant to kill me."

"*The Burning Bed*," Denise said.

"I loved that movie."

"Self -defense. There's no way around it."

They were quiet for a moment, the only sound the soft beat as the rocker rocked back and forth on the wooden floor.

"Do you know how to kill people?" Paulette asked. "Rangers have guns and all. Do you teach you that?"

"Not in so many words," Denise said. "They use the word 'stop.' A gun has to have 'stopping' power. We shoot at targets shaped like people, and we learn to aim for center body mass—bigger and easier to hit than the pinhead of the usual criminal. We learn to hit people with batons in places that will disable them."

Paulette thought that over for a couple of minutes. Denise rocked and thought about killing. Death was standard operating procedure: Cows died for hamburgers, grass died for cows. Little lambkins were slaughtered for Easter dinners. Turkeys died by the millions for Christmas and Thanksgiving. Animals were different, the people who ate them always insisted. People pretended that killing people wasn't the same as killing animals, that killing people was horrific. Then they voted to fight in Iran, Iraq, Afghanistan, Vietnam, Korea, Libya—always somewhere, and mostly not because anybody wanted or needed soldiers marching around their backyards shooting. Humans liked killing humans. They were good at it. They celebrated it with medals and movies and songs. Then they pretended to themselves that a woman killing a violent bastard like Kurt Duffy was so horrible she had to go to prison forever. It made no sense. Either it was okay to kill people deemed bad or it wasn't. It was pretty obvious to Denise that in America, as well as the rest of the world, the consensus was in: Killing was fine and dandy, good even. Admirable.

The only thing bad about killing was *saying* it was okay. Like the "family values" politicians: They could fornicate, whoremonger, go with same-sex hookers, commit adultery, and still get reelected by the Evangelicals as long as they *said* those things were wrong.

So nobody was going to care that Kurt Duffy was killed. Not a bit. They only paid lip service to the idea that killing a Kurt Duffy was wrong. Really, most people didn't care at all; they just wanted to curl up on the sofa and watch *Saw III* or *Dexter*. What she and Paulette needed to do was find a story that would help people explain the murder of Kurt Duffy to themselves so they could stop thinking about it, stop pretending it was bad, and get back to their own rat killing, as one of her old high school teachers was fond of saying.

"I don't want to disable Kurt," Paulette said. "I think he needs to be dead for a long, long time."

"For the rest of his life," Denise said, and they both laughed at the absurdity.

"My gosh!" Paulette gasped, covering her mouth. "Are we awful? I mean, we're laughing about killing people. Killing *Kurt*! I don't feel awful, but I know I should."

"Don't feel awful," Denise said when they'd stopped giggling. "He does need to be dead."

"Poison?" Paulette ventured.

"Do you know anything about poison? I don't," Denise replied.

"We'd have to buy it somewhere. That would make a trail," Paulette said. "I could burn him in bed, like Farrah Fawcett did in the movie. She got off on a self-defense plea."

"It wouldn't work a second time. Too obvious," Denise decided. "Besides, you can't be anywhere around when it happens. You have to have an iron-clad alibi. We could screw with the brakes on his truck. I know how to do that."

Paulette shook her head. "He only drives from here to Bar Harbor and back. Nothing bad would happen, not bad enough anyway."

"Yeah. Bad idea. Even if it worked, we wouldn't know the exact time it would happen, so maybe no alibi. How about the lobster boat?" Denise asked.

"I don't know how to sink one even if we could get near it, and his crew would go down, too. Probably they'd all drown and Kurt would swim to shore and come kill us both. If he knew there was a both. Me for sure."

"Push him off a high place?" Denise mused.

"No. He's too big and too lazy. When he's not on the boat he doesn't exert himself at all. If you managed to get him to go up on some rock, somebody could see. You can't be seen to be with us, with me."

Denise sighed. "Okay. We shoot him."

"We shoot him three times," Paulette said firmly.

TWELVE

Heath lay in the ground-floor bedroom of the tower, exhausted from the sheer effort it took to go to bed. Before she'd been hospitalized, this had been Gwen's friend Chris Zuckerberg's bedroom. Other than a few pieces of truly stunning artwork, the decor was not what Heath had expected from a woman who owned an entire island. Though the mattress and the bedding—down comforter over fine cotton sheets—were excellent, the bed was narrow, an old-fashioned kid's bed. The armoire, obviously made for this lighthouse or another round dwelling, was an antique but in bad condition. The single wooden chair and writing desk were scuffed with use.

Gwen said Chris was land- and house-poor. The place was a money pit on a grand scale. Probably most of it went to fixing leaks in roofs and buying better mousetraps. There had to be mice. The decaying wings of the house looked like prime rodent habitat.

The room still held Ms. Zuckerberg's scent, faintly spicy; her clothes still hung in the armoire, and papers were strewn across the desk as if she'd expected to return. Something Gwen thought was unlikely. In the days since they'd arrived, and Dez Hammond had phoned to welcome them to the abandoned house, Ms. Zuckerberg had suffered several more transient ischemic attacks.

Heath found the Spartan utility of Chris's room pleasing. Simplicity had always suited her. The world presented enough treats and turns for her eyeballs that she didn't feel the need to spread too many of them around indoors.

The room above Heath had been used by Dez Hammond. Dez was a childhood friend of Ms. Zuckerberg's. Aunt Gwen said Ms. Hammond moved in pretty much full-time after her husband died and Chris's health began to fail.

This second-story room was claimed by Elizabeth of the young strong legs. It boasted two wide windows. The view, so Elizabeth said, was spectacular.

The topmost room, where the lighthouse's lantern had been housed, had a three-hundred-sixty-degree view. It had been Chris's before the first heart attack had driven her to ground level. The penthouse suite was where Gwen had chosen to bunk.

Heath's ground-floor room had only two windows, slits that medieval bowmen would have found claustrophobic. Despite the lack of a view, she liked the space. There were times when only a fortress on a crag surrounded by a cold, deep moat could make one feel safe.

Pulling the comforter up under her chin, she stared at the electronic suit Leah had so generously allowed her to bring. In this historic environment it looked at home on its hanger, more like a suit of armor than an exoskeleton. Though she had yet to try it on Boar, Heath liked having it in sight.

Hah! And they said she'd never walk again.

Through the hole cut in the thick plank flooring for the stairs, Elizabeth's music—real music, thank God—trickled, punctuated by the occasional thumping footfall. Light and lithe as a gymnast, yet the girl had a habit of walking on her heels. She made more noise coming and going than a troupe of clog dancers.

The noise, like the fortress of a house, was comforting. Elizabeth was safe. Anyone who wanted to harm her would have to cross half the continent, swim icy seas, scale cliffs, and pass through Heath's bedroom.

Lord knew, tonight, if they/he/it ran the gauntlet she wouldn't be asleep when they reached her room. Annoying, vaguely electrical twitches in her legs were driving her nuts. Horrid buggers felt nothing, were useless for anything but making laps for cats; still they leapt and kicked and jerked. Obviously they could move. They just wouldn't take orders. Most irritating.

Since sleep was off the menu, Heath sifted through the poisons someone was dripping into her daughter's world. After Tiffany Edleson fell through as the favored suspect, Heath, Anna, and Gwen had assumed the cyberstalker was one—or more—of Elizabeth's fellow students at Boulder High School.

Heath had spoken with E's high school principal and her English and geometry teachers. They'd been kind but useless. As it was when Heath was in high school, the phys ed teacher was the one to whom the kids opened up. Ms. Willis knew about the points game E had mentioned. The clique of boys who played the game boasted they wouldn't date any girl who couldn't be counted on for a friendly blow job.

"They're considered the cool boys, the BMOC, go figure," Heath told Gwen.

"They are nasty pieces of work," Gwen said succinctly. "Is oral sex de rigueur?"

They'd both looked at Elizabeth, who, by choice, was in on what they'd come to call the Cybercreep Councils. Heath and Gwen were reassured by the spontaneous "Gross, like way gross!

"The girls they get? You know, who hang with them and do the blow jobs and whatever? You'd think they'd be the school skanks, but they're not," Elizabeth told them. "They're real hotties. I think it's that Stockholm thing, where the hostages fall in love with the terrorists."

Heath hadn't thought of it that way, but she wouldn't be surprised if Elizabeth was on to something.

Gwen said, "The boys are the skanks, Elizabeth."

A sigh and an eye roll were her reward.

Could the jerk boys, the high school rotters who made a game of degrading girls have smelled Elizabeth's virgin soul, and set on the trail like hounds on the scent of a rabbit? Heath wondered as she listened to the tattoo of her daughter's feet on the planks overhead.

Bullies tended to pick on the strays, the oddballs. Though she'd never say so to Elizabeth, the child's peculiar upbringing didn't make it easy for her to blend in, be one of the crowd—an essential survival skill for a teenager.

From age four until she was nine E had lived in a polygamist compound that called itself Mormon, though the Mormon Church would have vehemently denied the relationship. Before kids in the cult reached puberty—the age when girl children were "married" off to the chosen elders, and boy children were run out of the community lest they become sexual rivals—they lived like the children of an enormous and amiable family circa 1898.

No Internet, no TV, no video games, newspapers, or magazines; they were seldom taken into the nearby town of Loveland. Their clothes were mostly homemade. All were homeschooled. They grew up knowing of the outside world only in a shadowy way. Though such an upbringing left them woefully unprepared for the challenges of the modern world, it did allow them an innocence denied children exposed from infancy to an overcommercialized, oversexualized, violent society careening into the future on laugh tracks and Big Macs.

Miraculously, Elizabeth still retained that aura of innocence. Once,

Heath had attributed it to her early cloistering. Now she believed Elizabeth would have been the same had she been raised in London during World War II, Berkeley in the sixties, or New York City in the new millennium. Nature winning over nurture.

Innocence was an almost irresistible target for kids who have lost theirs.

When Heath was in school, bullying had a bricks-and-mortar aspect: hallway taunts, locker vandalism, heads stuck in toilets. Bullies were a hands-on bunch; they liked to see the results of their work, enjoy the public humiliation, soak up the fear.

Since the Internet, things that used to be spray-painted under bridges were published for the world to see. Besides her personal electronic pages, a lot had been posted to a blog popular with Boulder kids, *whosewhoandwhocares.net*. The site was known for unflattering pictures with "funny" captions, outing romances, derogatory remarks about fashion, belittling football players who screwed up, and naming cheerleaders who—so said the blog—didn't wear panties.

Whoever was bullying Elizabeth was too cruel for a bulletin board invented for petty cruelty. The kids who ran the blog deleted the graphic attacks on Elizabeth the moment they saw them, then blocked the source. The bully got multiple URLs and reposted after every block.

Messages, fielded by the Boulder police while Elizabeth's phone was quarantined, leaned toward the threatening. Nothing overt; crawling, spiritual cockroaches afraid of the light. The wording got darker, the pictures more sadistic. Though sympathetic, the police considered cyber malice out of their jurisdiction.

Sam Edleson was in their jurisdiction, but without witnesses or evidence, there was little they could do. A couple of female cops went to the Edlesons' home and scared the stuffing out of Terry. Two of their male counterparts "had a talk" with Sam that left him the worse for wear. Or so said the kid who raked Heath's leaves.

The detective assigned to Elizabeth's case wasn't so user-friendly. He murmured about kids being kids, modern moms being oversensitive, letting 'em duke it out—a song that he should have known went out of fashion in the eighties.

Snug behind her castle walls on Boar Island, Heath pondered the metaphorical roaches. She was not being a hysterical overprotective mom. Heath had never been given to the vapors, not even during the dark days when she was newly disabled and Gwendolyn feared she'd off herself. Easier said than done when one can no longer access high places from which to leap.

At present Elizabeth was living on a rock made of nothing but high places and deadly falls. Heath thought of the messages urging her to kill herself. How many would it take to turn E's mind back to suicide? Ten? A hundred? After all that had happened, had the vicious words lost their ability to influence her? Heath hoped so. Hope and vigilance: Those were the only weapons she had.

Her thoughts left that miserable abyss and turned to the package of heroin and the anonymous tip, a tip given before the heroin had arrived. Obviously whoever tipped off the rangers sent the heroin. This attempt at a frame job was ludicrously amateurish. That fact would have been more reassuring had the excitement the district ranger evinced made her think he'd never smelled a three-day-old red herring before.

He'd scrutinized the contents of the box. It was filled with small rectangular packets wrapped in tinfoil. There had to be a hundred of the things. Heath had thought it was a box of toothpicks, two to a pack, the way they offer them in cheaper restaurants. With a look first at her, then at Anna, suggesting they might be in cahoots, Artie bundled the box into a paper bag, which he sealed and marked with a black Sharpie.

"Evidence," he said darkly.

Heath laughed remembering his barely concealed glee. The drug bust of the century, and he was on it! She doubted it would be as amusing if he got anyone else to take it seriously. In the justice system, things did go horribly awry now and again.

As soon as the rangers left, Heath jumped on the Internet. The tiny packages—if they even contained heroin and not baby powder or whatever—were probably one-twentieth of a gram and cost ten dollars on the street. Nicely set up for resale. An eight-ball was supposedly three grams. Eight-ball. Behind the eight ball? Was that the legal limit or something?

It was so absurd, so obviously part of the harassment of E, it had not crossed Heath's mind that the district ranger would consider her guilty. But he did. He might even have arrested her had Anna not laughed when he mentioned it. In the end he said, "Well, it shouldn't be hard to catch you."

Heath smiled to herself remembering Anna's muttered "That's what you think."

The package had no return address. The postmark was Walla Walla, Washington. A dead end, undoubtedly. Whoever was after E had spent God knew how much money to frame Heath for drug dealing. That was a lot of malice, a lot of planning—even if it was bad planning.

What they'd considered high school bullying was taking on a whole new level of threat.

Surely nothing would come of the drug charge. Surely Artie wasn't that stupid. Surely.

Idly, she wondered if jails were handicap accessible. In the movies they all had miles and miles of metal stairs.

Heath readjusted her pillow. Her shadow flashed on the tower's curving whitewashed walls. For a few minutes she amused herself making shadow puppets on the old plaster. A bunny, a duck, a wolf with its tongue lolling. At that, Wily groaned. Coincidence or not, Heath laughed. Taking that as an invitation, the dog jumped up onto the foot of her bed—not in one try, but he made it.

Doctor's orders were no lying down with dogs for Heath. Without sensation in her legs, the possibility of accidental damage was too great. Still, she didn't order Wily off. He'd worked too hard to get up, and she'd loved him too long to insist.

Scratching him between the ears, she felt the bed shake as he echoed the pleasure with a scratching hind leg. A year or more before, that leg had been broken, leaving Wily with a limp, but it still worked well enough. At least as well as Anna's left arm.

"If not Tiffany, then who?" Heath whispered the question to Wily. "Who would set me up—us, me and E—for a drug charge? Why? Ruin our reputations? Make us less believable to the powers that be? Make me look like an unfit mother?" That seemed most likely. If Heath was a drug dealer and her daughter a whore, then . . . Then what? No one would care when one or both of them disappeared? Or died?

A sudden and desperate need to see E flooded Heath. She sat up abruptly. Rather, her mind told her body to sit up abruptly. Not a great deal actually happened. She twitched like a landed fish, then pushed herself up on her elbows.

Having thrown off the covers, she shoved her legs over the edge of the bed, then laboriously worked her slippers onto her feet. Gone were the days when she could unthinkingly run around barefoot. How would she know if she injured herself? Caring for her legs often felt like caring for ungrateful children.

Wily whined from his place on the foot of the bed. "It's okay, pal. Nothing you've got to catch or kill," Heath reassured him. He thumped his tail on the coverlet.

Her electronic suit, with its gyroscope-that-wasn't-a-gyroscope thingy Leah was testing, was designed to be ultrastable. Even though there was a good sturdy handrail running up the curving wall, Heath had no desire to try the suit on the narrow stairway that corkscrewed up the tower.

The wheelchair, of course, was useless. There was no way she could climb the stairs in a dignified *Homo erectus* sort of way.

In the 1860s paraplegics were SOL.

Lowering herself to the cold stone floor, Heath scootched backward using her upper-body strength—a mode of travel at which she'd become quite proficient. If she could ever figure out how to do it without dragging her pants off, she would petition the Special Olympics to add the Backward Butt Traverse to their sports roster.

Wily was accustomed to Heath's unusual modes of locomotion. He eased off the bed, stretched, sketching a deep bow, and then padded over to collapse with a gusty sigh near the foot of the spiral stairway.

"Easy for you, my four-legged friend," Heath grunted.

At the bottom step she stopped, pulled up her pajama bottoms, positioned herself with her back to the step, legs out in front of her, and caught her breath. The Backward Butt Traverse might be the best way to move without mechanical aids, but it wasn't easy. Heartbeat returned to near normal, she began the long circuitous ascent. Elbows back, palms on the step behind her, push up, swing her fanny back, settle, palms on the step behind her: twenty-three steps, twenty-three ten-inch lifts.

I shall have the triceps of a god, she promised herself.

She could have simply hollered for Elizabeth to come down, or blown the whistle that E insisted she wear around her neck, but where was the challenge in that?

When she was about three-quarters of the way up—eighteen of the twenty-three steps, and sweating like a pig—the query "Mom?" came from above.

"Coming," Heath gasped back. The tower, with its coil of stairs, didn't allow for doors. As Heath looked up at the rectangle of golden light where the steps passed through the plank floor of Elizabeth's room, her daughter's face appeared, long, straight brown hair falling down around it like the tentacles of a particularly relaxed jellyfish. Whenever she caught a different angle of Elizabeth's face, Heath was struck all over again by the girl's beauty. Part of it, she suspected, was a lack of objectivity on her part. Regardless, Elizabeth was lovely, tall for her age, willowy, with flawless skin, eyes that seemed too big for her face and were the brown of expensive chocolate.

Pride in her child went cold with the realization that images of that sweet face were being defiled in the public forum. Facebook, MySpace, Google: Elizabeth's junior varsity girls soccer team made the state championships. Even though they didn't win, a team photo could have made its way into cyberspace. Elizabeth was in an online yearbook. Any pictures taken of her by her friends and posted on public media were out there. Every pervert in the world had access to her daughter's face.

"Privacy is dead," Heath said to the face floating above her.

"Yesterday's news. Can't a girl can go a whole evening without her mom bum-thumping up her stairs? Why didn't you call? I'd've come down."

The mixture of irritation and concern gave Heath the strength to make the last five steps, and even hide some of the strain as she did so.

"Did you have a reason for this, or is it just your version of jogging?" E asked as Heath levered herself onto Elizabeth's floor, her feet dangling over the dark stairs.

Heath hadn't much of a reason. *I had to see you with my own eyes, know you were real and alive* was too much emo to dump on one's child in the night. "I had a question," Heath said, hoping she'd think of one.

"Um . . . you lost one slipper and couldn't wait to ask me where it went?"

Heath looked down. During her ascent she'd lost a shoe. Damn. "I'm still better off than those with no slippers at all," she said unctuously, then admitted, "I just came up to see how you're doing."

"Okay, I guess." Elizabeth stared down between their dangling feet.

"You don't have to come up, Wily." Wily laid his chin on the bottom step and made a whuffing noise.

"Any more interesting slurs on your character?" Heath asked carefully.

"I asked Tiff to keep an eye out, and I've been to all the regular places. The porn gets cleared out by the websites after a while. The 'die bitch die' stuff isn't showing up too many places. I guess it's the personal touch. My phone only."

Heath was pleased E could still make jokes, and scared that she was using humor to cover uglier truths.

"Will you get arrested?" Elizabeth asked suddenly. "You know, as a drug dealer?"

"You'd think even a blind carpenter could see this was a frame job," Heath replied.

"Ha, ha," E said, then automatically corrected Heath. "Visually challenged."

Surprised, Heath asked, "Isn't 'blind' still okay?"

"I don't know what's okay anymore," Elizabeth said miserably. Heath knew she was talking about more than politically correct language.

"If I go to jail, would you bake me a cake with a file in it?" Heath asked to cheer her daughter up.

"So not funny."

"Anna doesn't think it will amount to anything," Heath said seriously. "We don't even know for sure if it is heroin until they test it. That ranger guy, Artie, and Peter Barnes were here when it came; they could see I wasn't expecting it. There was no return address. Juries like nice middle-aged ladies in wheelchairs. They'd never get a conviction. Besides, I don't even know where you could buy heroin."

"I do," Elizabeth said.

Heath cocked an eyebrow.

"I don't know it like been-there-done-that," her daughter amended, "but I've heard there used to be a place called the Silk Road on the Internet where you could get anything except hit men. There were codes and secret e-mails and special wallets—the whole bitcoin thing—all untraceable."

"I remember," Heath said. "Then they captured the Dread Pirate Roberts and it was shut down."

"Tiff says there's another Dread Pirate Roberts," Elizabeth said. "There's always another Dread Pirate Roberts."

The Princess Bride was one of Heath's favorite books. She'd read it to E when she was ten.

"Maybe there's another one up now where you could buy something and have it mailed to anybody you wanted," E said. "Maybe somebody did that with the package you got."

"What would be the point?"

"Maybe to get you out of the way. If you went to jail, who'd get me?" Elizabeth asked.

"Anna," Heath said. "That's what godmothers do."

"That's okay then," Elizabeth said.

Heath laughed. "Thanks a million."

"You know what I mean," E said. Heath did.

For a while they sat, each lost in her own thoughts. Then E asked, "Do you think the heroin sender guy was my stalker guy?"

Heath wanted to lie, say no, she didn't think it was in any way related, so she could save Elizabeth the angst of thinking herself a danger to her family. Parents lied to children all the time to calm their fears—or to increase them.

"You'll put your eye out with that."

"If you hold the knife that way, you'll cut your fingers off."

"If you make that face again it will stick forever."

"Girls who whistle come to some bad ends."

"Boys seldom make passes at girls who wear glasses."

Heath had been careful never to lie to Elizabeth. The girl had been brought up in a multilayered matrix of lies, half-truths, myths, and monsters. Their first two years together, Heath spent a lot of time sorting carefully through Elizabeth's tangled belief system trying to ascertain which lies the child needed to hang on to in order to feel secure, and which were increasingly damaging the longer they took root. Even the dangerous lies could not be snatched away. They had to be replaced by a truth that would fill the resulting hole, or heal the wound the old belief engendered.

Rescued children didn't come with baggage; they came with unexploded ordnance from former wars.

For a while neither of them spoke. Elizabeth, her long lovely legs hanging down the trap across from Heath's, was swinging her feet idly, a trick Heath would have given ten years of her life to be able to do again.

"I expect it's part of the same deal," Heath said finally. "Stalker/heroin guy is trying to make you feel responsible for the damage he's doing. It ties in with the kill yourself, kill yourself messages. He hurts me, you blame yourself, you get depressed, etcetera and so forth."

"In a way it is my fault," E said.

"If you go there, you're basically stalking yourself. We'll have to check with Anna on the legality of that," Heath said.

For a while Elizabeth said nothing. Heath couldn't tell if she was processing or sinking into the depression that had followed her around like a black dog waiting to be fed since the bullying began.

To Heath's immense relief, the girl screwed her face up, closed one eye, and looked at the ceiling with the other.

"Well, when you put it *that* way . . ." she said. Then they were both allowed to laugh. Laughter, even when forced, is a good thing.

"Aunt Gwen thinks this place might be haunted," Elizabeth said, clearly needing a change of subject. Heath wasn't sure ghosts were the best direction the conversation could take.

"She said it *ought* to be haunted," Heath corrected.

"It is," Elizabeth said sincerely. "I saw a light sort of flickering around in one of the dead wings."

E meant one of the two crumbling arms that swept back toward the northeastern crag.

"Are you making this up to scare me?" Heath asked.

"Nope."

"Broken glass, trick of the light, squatters, enterprising tourists, could be anything," Heath said.

"Or it could be a ghost," Elizabeth said.

"I think a few ghosts would be groovy," Heath said. "Maybe we could catch one."

E gave her an annoyed look. Elizabeth believed in ghosts. Sometimes Heath believed in ghosts. She'd read somewhere that forty-five percent of Americans believed in ghosts, spirits of the dead walking the earth. Ninety percent said they believed in God, which was more or less the same thing, but on an impersonal, galactic scale. Dead saints answering prayers, angels averting car accidents, the Virgin Mother healing a child: all were just ghosts costumed in robes and feathers. The cult E had been raised in was a bizarre mixture of rogue Mormonism, Christianity, spiritualism, and carnival act. The compound was funded by the myriad wives working what used to be called welfare scams: money for unwed mothers, orphans, food stamps, single-parent households; Medicaid, Medicare, any social service that could be conned, was.

The children were taught to hate the United States government, love their spiritual leader in the person of the prophet Father Dwayne Sheppard, and believe every single thing he told them. He told them if they left the compound, ghosts of late Latter-day Saints would get them. If they didn't say their prayers, Satan would reach right up through the floorboards and snatch them into a fiery pit. He told them God wanted them to serve Him by serving him—Dwayne Sheppard. He told them that the Mormon Church had the power to bring the dead into the Mormon faith, and that all their ancestors back to Adam and Eve stood by their beds at night watching them from the beyond.

Elizabeth had shaken a lot of that spiritual olio from her proverbial sandals, but, like most Americans, she'd never quite given up the feeling that Something Was Out There.

"Should we buy it some chains to clank, or have they evolved, like vampires, into cute boys with dietary issues?" Heath asked.

"Don't, Mom. Ghosts hate to be laughed at," Elizabeth said, superstitious fear lowering her voice so phantom ears wouldn't overhear.

At that, the lights went out.

No flickering, no browning down: a sudden plunge into darkness.

"Holy shit!" Heath squawked.

Elizabeth squeaked, then laughed nervously. Power on Boar Island was capricious.

"Gosh, I hate that!" Elizabeth whispered, as if an entity in the dark might be listening.

"It takes some getting used to," Heath admitted. Ghost stories around the campfire always put the fear of God into her. She could remember when she was a Girl Scout kneeling beside her sleeping bag in a tent praying as hard as she could to keep the guy with a hook for a hand, who escaped from the insane asylum, from getting her. Forcing herself to speak in a normal tone, she said, "Time for bed anyway."

"Right," E said. "You talk about ghosts, then, bang! The lights go out for no reason, in the middle of the night, in a haunted house, on a deserted island, and you think I'm going to go to my little bed? I at least get Wily."

"I get Wily," Heath insisted.

"You can't get downstairs without a light," Elizabeth retorted. "I won't help. Don't help her, Wily," she called down into the inky darkness.

Wily whined.

Down was harder than up. Moving up, Heath used her arms and

towed her legs along. Since she really couldn't push noodles, the only way to go down was on her belly like a reptile, the legs bumping along behind in more or less a controlled fall. In the dark it could be dangerous.

"Loan me a blanket and pillow," Heath said. "I'll bunk up here until the lights come back on."

"You can have my bed," Elizabeth said with a sigh. "I'll sleep on the cold hard floor with the rats."

Heath laughed. "Such a gracious invitation is hard to resist. I don't mind the floor. I'm used to hard beds. Better for my back."

A sniff in the darkness, then, "Yeah, right, and Aunt Gwen comes home from her big date and sees me all snuggled in a nice comfy bed and my poor old crippled mother in a heap of rags on the floor. Like I'd ever hear the end of that!"

Heath smiled as she listened to Elizabeth creep across the room toward her bed. Eyes recovered from the sudden onslaught of night, she could see stars through the two windows and yellow gleams from houses on shore. They had power. They always had power. Boar seemed to suffer from an intermittent short somewhere in the system between it and Mount Desert, the main island. A match was struck, the sharp smell of sulfur, then the steady warm glow of the kerosene lamp.

"I like the lamplight," Elizabeth said. Heath heard wistfulness in her daughter's voice. Had they had kerosene lamps at the compound where she'd spent her childhood? Did she ever feel homesick? Heath knew the compound had electricity. That Dwayne might have kept the electricity for the "elders" and the computer cons, and made the women and children use oil lamps, wasn't beyond the pale.

From downstairs came the sound of the door to the front room opening. Then a faint susurration, like the shush of waves against the cliffs, maybe footsteps. Elizabeth heard it as well. Before she could say anything, Heath put a finger to her lips. Boar was a private island. Still and all, Heath had been a fool not to check the doors. She didn't even know if they had locks on them.

"Blow out the lamp," she hissed.

Eyes, wide and frightened, shone above the glass chimney, and then Elizabeth and the world disappeared in a puff of breath.

Heath listened with all the intensity a dark house and surreptitious sounds can put into human ears. The lighthouse was thick-walled and nearly as solid as the granite upon which it was built. The windows, a modern addition, rattled gently in the onshore breeze. Through the open casement came the sound of the sea. Elizabeth's bare feet whispered over planks worn smooth by more than a century of use.

Kneeling beside Heath, she called down, "Aunt Gwen? Is that you?"

"The lift bell didn't ring," Heath breathed.

Nothing but darkness rose from the tower rooms below.

"Anybody there?" Heath called, since the sanctity of the silence had been broken.

A creak? A tiny scrape of leather on wood? The hushed thump of a door closing? Nothing?

"A trick of the wind," Heath said firmly. "Light the lamp before we scare ourselves silly."

Before Elizabeth could find the matches, the radio blared, lights snapped on, and both women screamed.

E had been right.

Ghosts didn't like being laughed at.

THIRTEEN

Statistically speaking, getting away with murder wasn't all that hard to do. The key was to murder someone who had no connection with your life. A stranger. The thing was, nobody but a psychopath would do that. Denise found it ironic that you could only kill with impunity people whom you had no reason to kill. Cops—even rangers—tended to be rational individuals. They liked there to be a reason for a crime. If they scented a reason, a motive, they sniffed and dug and pestered until they had enough for an arrest.

The drive-by shooters, freeway snipers, the people who put poison in Advil bottles at the drugstore—those with universal malice were almost impossible to catch. Even serial killers who kept on keeping on with their personal death marches were hard to get. Lots of evidence, lots of proof of crime, but no rhyme or reason behind it. At least not that a sane person could understand. When they did get caught it was because they wanted to. A younger, nicer, Denise had thought they wanted to get caught because they wanted to be stopped, felt a need to be punished. Now she guessed it was because they wanted credit for their work.

Because she was in law enforcement, and because America was a nation in love with serial killers, Denise had read interviews with those who had finally been captured and prosecuted. Never, not once, did one of them give a satisfactory answer to why they did what they did. Son of Sam's "The dog made me do it" was one of the clearer explanations.

That was why Patricia Highsmith's *Strangers on a Train* was such a brilliant concept. Had both men been true killers, they never would have gotten caught.

Was she a true killer? Denise had never thought about it. She'd thought about killing: thought about killing Peter, Lily, and for a brief— very brief—time, she'd even thought about killing Olivia, to hurt them as she had been hurt, to take from Peter what he had taken from her.

Thinking about killing was not the same as being a killer. Thinking was not doing. The Catholics were wrong; sinning in the heart didn't count.

As she sat in the hot airless dark of the nursery in the old shed, she went again through the plan she and her sister had come up with. Paulette would go to the old Acadian bar and stay there drinking from before Kurt's boat came in until after his body was discovered. Tuesday night was bowling night for him and his buddies, bowling and getting sloppy drunk on beer. Either Kurt would get a ride to the bowling alley with a guy named Lou, who lived a couple of houses away in the tiny town, or Kurt would pick Lou up. The pattern seldom varied.

That meant Kurt would come off the lobster boat about seven in the evening. He and his pals would hoist a few and eat burgers at a joint near the docks. Then home by nine thirty to shower, put on clean clothes, and be ready to fetch or be fetched by ten o'clock. Either way there was a half-hour window when he'd be home by himself.

Then the body would be discovered.

Lou would come to pick him up and find it, or Lou would come over to find out why Kurt hadn't picked him up and find it.

Paulette would stay in the Acadian, making sure the bartender noticed her, until eleven forty-five to be on the safe side. Then she'd come home and be surprised to find police cars all over the place. Not ranger cars— or maybe just a polite presence of green and gray in the background. The national park's law enforcement didn't have jurisdiction in Otter Creek. Who did have jurisdiction was complicated. On paper, the state of Maine and the national park (aka federal government) had concurrent jurisdiction. With Bar Harbor and other small-town police and fire departments figured in, it wasn't as straightforward as it might seem. That, too, would help. For a while state and local law enforcement might not be sure who had to do what.

It also helped that the chief ranger was out of the park. Artie was a joke. Gris was the real thing. Before he'd joined the Park Service he'd been a detective in D.C. Little Miss Bird Breath from out west would be gone in three weeks. She'd probably be only too happy to let the state do its job.

Nearly five hours in the bar at the Acadian for Paulette to establish an unbreakable alibi so she would be free and could inherit Kurt's property, thirty minutes for Denise to murder her brother-in-law.

Having greater expertise in the area of violent crime, Denise had worked out the details. After choosing the day and time, she and Paulette hadn't talked about it. Maybe identical twins didn't need to verbalize as much as other people. Certainly Denise's thoughts and her sister's seemed to run down identical channels. The killing was necessary, Denise assured herself for the umpteenth time. One, Kurt would eventually beat Paulette to death, and two, he would track her down if he wasn't dead, pursue them into their new lives for the sole purpose of ruining everything for his wife.

After the dust from the killing settled and Paulette inherited, she'd sell the property; then she and Denise would leave. Law enforcement rangers could retire after twenty years of service, just like real cops.

Denise could have retired six months ago. She only stayed on because she didn't want to move her hatred from Peter's field of vision. Being a thorn in his side, a shadow on his wall, a fly in his ointment, was better than having nothing. Hurting someone was something. You were there. Alive. Noticed. If she'd retired and quietly disappeared into the woodwork, what would have been left for her?

Now that was all changed. There was Paulette. There was Kurt's land to sell and, maybe, the "family legacy," if they were the twins referred to in the ads Paulette had saved. They would finish with the park. They would have the money from the land and Denise's pension.

Money was important. Denise had never been rich, but she had been dirt poor, and intended never to be that helpless and hopeless again. Besides, they would need new things; the family would need things. They would move somewhere nobody knew them and they would be able to be out in the open, two sisters, a family.

Unused to hope, Denise felt nervous entertaining the feathered thing. The picture was so pretty she wanted to stay in it, yet was afraid that would jinx it. The gods liked to snatch away hope. Accepting the risk, she allowed the movie to continue playing in her mind. They would both cut their hair short and style it the same way. Paulette could dye hers back to their natural brown—or Denise could go blond. Hard to picture that. Better brunette and short. Paulette's hair was in bad shape from all the bleach jobs. A cut would be good for it.

They wouldn't dress alike, not in public—too corny. In private they might. Denise would order her sister a pair of pajamas identical to the ones she always wore. No. She would order new pajamas for the both of them. A new start. Together. They'd settle in a small town, maybe in the hills of North Carolina or Georgia. Someplace warm; they had already suffered enough winters in their lives. Eighty-two years of winters between them; nearly a century of cold. A house in an old neighborhood full of mature trees; a neighborhood where no one would know who they had been. What they had done. A small house, maybe three bedrooms, one for each of them and one for . . .

Hoping.

Damn.

Denise knew better.

The dream winked out with the suddenness of a match dunked in water.

Pushing the tiny button on the side of her watch, she read the time by the faint green glow. Nine fifteen. Paulette would be nursing a beer at the Acadian by now. In half an hour she'd be sipping the next and Denise would be murdering Kurt.

Would she respect herself in the morning? Yes, Denise decided, she would. Being a victim shamed her. Taking charge, killing the man who beat her sister, so that she and Paulette might have a new life together almost made her proud. It did make her proud. It made her a hero.

She rose from the rocking chair, then crossed the hand-hooked throw rug to open the shed door. With ancient trees blocking a quarter moon and stars, the dark of the woods was as complete as the darkness inside the windowless room. In black jeans, black running shoes, and a black T-shirt, Denise scarcely disturbed the void. Wearing all black was kind of theatrical but practical, and these days everybody wore black a lot. If someone were to see her, it wouldn't be remarkable. Should Kurt see her, it wouldn't ring any alarm bells in her brother-in-law's booze-raddled head.

Stretching, readying herself to be quick and calm and deadly, she listened to the sounds of the island. Mosquitoes whined; car engines hummed faintly on the road; there was a distant whispering that sounded like the ocean but probably wasn't. A faint breeze in the treetops was more likely. With the quiet and the open door, she would be able to hear Kurt's car pull onto the gravel in front of the house. She and Paulette had tried it. It wasn't loud, but it was enough.

As soon as she heard the car on the gravel, she would walk softly toward the house, using Kurt's car and entry noises to cover what sounds she might make. The back porch light was already on. As long as she walked directly toward it there would be no obstacles. When she reached the back porch, she would stand with her back to the wall between the door into the kitchen and the window where the bathroom was. Though she would be in the light, the rear porch could not be seen by neighbors or from the road. After Kurt stepped into the shower, she would let herself in through the kitchen—the door was unlocked—slip through the bedroom, open the bathroom door, and shoot him. A shower scene, like in *Psycho*. Life mirrors art.

She would leave the same way she'd come, returning to the nursery. There she would collect the flashlight. Using it, she would walk cross-country the quarter mile to Otter Cove. Her blue runabout was moored in the reeds, invisible in the dark. In the runabout, she would row out about a hundred yards, start the engine, drop the pistol over the side, and be back at the dock in Somes Sound before eleven. No one would be there at that hour, and if they were, she was known for going out alone at night in her boat. They wouldn't give it a second thought.

From there she would drive home. For good measure she would burn her gloves and clothes in her tiny fireplace. No muss, no fuss, no motive, and the prime suspect in full view at the Acadian Lounge. A job well done, Denise would pour herself a double vodka, no ice, and order two pairs of pajamas from Victoria's Secret online. Not sleazy sexy ones; flannel would be better, cute and comfy.

An engine purred in the dark, got louder; tires crunched on the gravel.

Killing time, Denise thought.

FOURTEEN

Before she got under her own covers, Elizabeth helped Heath down the stairs to her bed. They had a system. Elizabeth sat with her back to Heath and one step below. She then folded Heath's legs—which weighed less than one would think—across her lap. This way they could descend step by step on a three count. "One, two, three, push up with the arms and the butts bump down."

Goofy as it was, Heath knew Elizabeth enjoyed working out new strange ways of locomotion with her. She would, of course, die of shame if anybody but Anna or Aunt Gwen saw them doing it. As long as there were no witnesses, E had fun. So did Heath. It was like being little kids, crawling around and wriggling. Better than being a kid, because what Elizabeth did really mattered; it mattered because compassion mattered. Compassion and courage.

As far as Heath was concerned, cowards were more dangerous than evil people. An evil person did an evil thing to get his evil way. It was focused, rational. If you didn't have what the bad guy wanted, you were safe.

Cowards were like broken safety rails or frayed climbing ropes. You counted on them, and one day, they gave way and down you went.

When she was a child of nine, Elizabeth had been slated to be married off to Father Dwayne Sheppard because E's mother was a coward. What happened to the biological father was a bit vague. Heath guessed the responsibility of a family scared him. He took off when E was an infant. At any rate, Elizabeth had no memory of him. Rather than to make it on her own, E's mom became Sheppard's fifth wife.

Though she'd been nine when she'd last seen her mother, E said she didn't remember her clearly. Heath did. Hard to forget a woman who had abandoned her child twice, once to Sheppard's demands and, finally, to Heath.

Even the all-powerful Prophet Sheppard had a yellow streak down his back. Why else work so hard to dominate weak people and children?

Cowards were dangerous.

Elizabeth was one of the bravest people Heath had ever known. Until this. This onslaught of threats and secrets and lies, and something E wasn't telling her or Gwen or Anna, was disabling her.

Heath knew herself to be a coward. Being disabled scared her. Being a mom terrified her. That she couldn't keep E safe made her blood run cold. As far as she was concerned her only saving grace was that she'd learned to hide what a big fat scaredy-cat she was. According to Aunt Gwen, that was courage, to be afraid and not let it stop you from doing what was right.

After what had happened to Elizabeth and the other girls when she was nine—what they had done, what had been done to them—it didn't surprise Heath that E's courage had holes in it. Being frightened was like getting a soft-tissue injury. Once, and you recovered. If injured again in the same place, it could cripple you. This web of mystery and unknown horrors was the third strike at the core of who Elizabeth was, how she fundamentally viewed herself.

The razor and the bath had been a call for help. It had also been an indicator of how deeply E had suffered—was suffering.

Elizabeth never spoke of the bad old days, not unless she talked about it with her therapist. As far as Heath knew, she'd never spoken to the other two victims about their experience, never contacted anyone from the old compound, never reached out to her mother, never even asked what became of them when the compound was shut down and the families scattered.

Once she'd admitted that sometimes she missed the compound. There were always lots of kids around. They played simple games like tag and Mother-may-I. All the girls played with dolls, handmade of rags and buttons. A lot of the dolls were pretty. The sister-wives took pride in their sewing. As an adult Heath understood that the simplicity and safety Father Sheppard promised were false, but to a little girl, they would have felt real.

For a little kid, it would all have been real: Sheppard's brand of religion, angels, plural wives, demons, pedophilia, ghosts.

For a long time after she'd moved in with Heath, E was afraid to sleep alone in her room at night for fear demons would get inside of her. Mormons—real Mormons—weren't big on ghosts or demons. Mormons were a practical people. Heath and Aunt Gwen explained over and over that Sheppard invented the evil spirits to use as another tool of control. Mostly she believed them.

Most wasn't all.

Then there were those damn ethereal footsteps. Given the situation, even Heath's skin had gone prickly and cold. Heath guessed that E, who still slept with every part of her under the covers because exposed bits were irresistible to monsters living beneath beds, had been more freaked out than she'd let on.

Elizabeth was hiding her emotions. Heath suspected it was a result of too much unconditional love. Gwen and Heath loved E way too much. Even Anna showed glimmers of it. None of them could hide the fact that they were bleeding to death behind their eyes, could diguise the great howling need to do something. If Elizabeth had said, "Hey, if you guys chop your hands off, I'll feel better," Heath would be rolling up her sleeves while Gwen ran for the surgical saw.

That kind of love had to be a burden. Like having a Dodge Ram parked on one's shoulders. Dealing with that, and the fact that she was being called a whore—with the pictures to prove it—to everybody she knew, and about a zillion people she didn't, that her social life was deader than roadkill, that there was no way she could go back to school in the fall without wearing a paper bag over her head so nobody would recognize her, and that some creep might actually be slithering out of his hole to lay his creepy hands on her to . . .

Take her, Heath thought suddenly. For a minute she thought she would vomit. Grabbing the bar over her bed, she dragged herself into a sitting position.

Take her.

The psycho who had taken her and the other little girls so long ago was dead, Heath reassured herself. Not imprisoned, not appealing his death sentence, not getting out for good behavior: dead. Good and dead.

Copycat.

She was definitely going to vomit.

Was E's stalker planning to re-create the Rocky Mountain horror?

Heath knew lightning did strike twice in the same place.

"Don't go there," Heath said out loud, but not so loudly E might hear and come down. "Not at night when there are ghosts whisking around." "There" was a place to be avoided. "There" was supposed to be where the bad things were. Tonight, "there" was here.

"Wily," she whispered. He was already awake and watching her, his eyebrows cocked. "Come up on the bed."

FIFTEEN

Using the noise of Kurt's tires crunching on gravel for cover, Denise moved through the dark as fast as she dared, heading toward the porch light. She cursed herself for not having gotten closer earlier. There were plenty of woods, plenty of darkness. It would have been safe enough to have halved the distance. More than that; she should have lain under the back porch or squatted behind the trash cans at the side of the house.

Paulette had timed the walk during the day, over country that was as familiar to her as the floor plan of her house. Denise should have timed it for herself, in the dark, with her lack of familiarity. There had been time to pace it off half a dozen times. Instead, she'd sat in the hot darkness of the nursery and toyed with the wicked imp called Hope.

The crunching stopped before she'd traveled thirty feet. Kurt's truck door screeched open, then slammed shut. One hand on a tree, a foot not yet fallen, Denise froze. The truck engine ticked as it cooled. A night bird called. She had no idea which one. She was law enforcement, not interpretation. An image of the Indians in old Westerns imitating birds to signal an attack struck her as horrifically funny. Hysterical. She held the laughter in with an effort, her chest twitching and her throat clenching.

No more sounds from the soon-to-be dead man. Was Kurt lighting a cigarette or checking his cell phone? Did he stand by the truck listening, sensing danger? Had Paulette accidentally tipped him off, and he was waiting for Denise with a knife or a pistol? Laughter dried up in her lungs, tickling like ashes when she breathed too deeply.

Denise really had to pee.

Crunch, crunch, crunch: gravel tread under heavy boots. He was coming for her. Fear paralyzed her mind, and Denise could not run. She could not even lower her raised foot, or draw in breath. Clomp, clomp, clomp: ascending the three wooden steps to the front door.

All was well.

Home, to the shower, to his death, just like it was supposed to be. As Kurt banged the screen and front doors, Denise sucked in a lungful of air, then ran lightly toward the lamp on the porch, her light in the darkness, her star of Bethlehem. The flame the moth incinerated itself in.

Panting as if she'd sprinted a hundred yards rather than crept thirty, she stopped short of the circle of light leaching into the dirt-bare yard.

Kurt was inside the house.

Maybe Kurt was inside. Denise had heard the front door slam. Was it possible he'd quietly opened it again, gone back to the truck for something? No, he wasn't the quiet type; she would have heard him. Maybe he'd only pretended to go inside. Maybe he'd heard her and slammed the doors to make her think he was inside when, all the while, he was sneaking around the side of the shack with an axe raised over his head.

Don't even think that, Denise commanded herself silently. They'd been careful. He suspected nothing.

He was in the house. That was the end of it.

The end of Kurt the baby killer.

Denise breathed in slowly to settle her nerves. Everything was as it was supposed to be. No muss, no fuss, like clockwork. That was the plan. So the trek from nursery to house had cost Denise a few minutes they hadn't counted on. There were plenty of minutes left to blow Kurt Duffy into the next world. Bullets were fast, just short of Superman-fast. Three seconds. Bang. Bang. Bang. Kurt is dead. Denise is headed for Otter Cove. Paulette is making eyes at the bartender miles away. Everyone lives happily ever after.

Stiffly, she started across the dusty yard. The scratch of her sneakered feet on the sand was as the grinding of boulders in the surf, an internal cacophony more sensation than sound. Step and step and step and no matter how many steps she took, the light didn't get any closer, the kitchen door looked tiny, wrong-end-of-a-telescope tiny, Alice in Wonderland tiny. Denise noticed her hands had balled into fists. Her vision was blurring, and sweat ran from her forehead in rivulets.

Suck it up, she ordered herself. It wasn't like Duffy didn't need killing. It wasn't like anybody would miss him. Killing him would be no worse than dropping a rock on a black widow or stomping a brown recluse. A spider, that's all Duffy was, spinning a web that caught her sister and held her paralyzed while it fed off her soul. It needed to be removed from the world. It needed to be crushed.

The porch, a couple of rickety steps up from the bare dirt of the backyard, cracked into her shins. Shocked, she blinked twice, confused by how she had closed the distance from not possible to bruising her legs. It was as if she'd gone to sleep for a while, her brain in Zombie Land while her body traversed the ground. How long had it taken her? How much racket had she made? Was Kurt in the shower yet? Paulette hadn't timed his showers. She'd just said he'd come home around nine, take a shower, and go out around ten.

Had he showered already and left to go bowling?

Denise dropped to her knees, hiding in the shadow of the raised porch. She rubbed her palms against the dirt, drying the sweat and working feeling back into her fingers. Forcing her lungs to obey, she began breathing slowly in and out through her nose. Sweat wiped from her brow with dirt-smeared hands, she put her brain back in its skull case and sat back on her heels. Nerve returned—or at least motivation. She pushed the tiny button on her watch.

Nine eleven. A good number for terrorists. A bad number for innocents. Was she both? Neither? It didn't matter. Nothing mattered but that she focused, stay on point. Back in the days when the government dared to let its officers shoot for scores, she'd been one of the best. Now there were no scores. Too many juries would want to know why an officer with a perfect score on the range didn't just shoot the gun out of the bad guy's hand since she was such an Annie Oakley.

With an act of will, Denise got to her feet. She unzipped the black nylon pack on her belt where she carried car keys and water when she went running. With two fingers she lifted out her .22 caliber Smith and Wesson revolver. The gun was untraceable. It had belonged to a foster mother's boyfriend. Denise had stolen it when she was thirteen. Ever since she'd had a nightstand that wouldn't be searched by some interfering do-gooder or rotten foster "family" member, she'd kept it in her bedside drawer.

As she eased the .22 from the rip-stop nylon, her wrist jerked as if hit by an electrical shock. Her fingers flew open, and the gun thudded into to the weeds beside the steps. For a moment she stared at the offending hand.

Nerves.

After she'd killed Kurt, when she and her sister were free of the spider, her nerves would heal. When they were free of the park and the state of Maine and settled in their cottage far away somewhere warm, the spastic nervous movements would stop.

She picked up the revolver, then checked the barrel to make sure it hadn't become jammed with detritus. Having squeegeed muddy sweat from her forehead with the side of her palm, she dried her hand on her jeans. Mentally she began singing "Itsy Bitsy Spider." On each syllable she took a small silent step. By the time the spider was up the waterspout, Denise was between the kitchen door and the bathroom window, her back pressed against the wood. Kurt was in the house, and was in the shower; she could see the water running through the clouded glass, and hear it through the thin walls of the shack.

Back on track. Back on point. Nerves back in alignment.

Once more she dried the palm of her gun hand on her trousers, then crept to the kitchen door and turned the knob. Bless Paulette! Not only was it unlocked, it was ajar. Not enough anyone could see, just enough the closing mechanism wouldn't catch. A gentle push and she was inside.

The kitchen was small, the linoleum old—real linoleum, not vinyl. Paulette had moved the scarred table—no bigger than most TV trays— and the two wooden ladder-backed chairs against the wall between stove and refrigerator.

Clearing the way for the exterminator coming to kill the spider.

Denise loved having a sister, a twin. Nobody, but nobody, had ever looked out for her the way Paulette did. Peter had pretended for a long time. Denise had been fooled for a long time. No more. Blood was the only thing you could count on. Family.

The door to the bedroom was open, the bedroom light off. Holding the gun at her side, Denise walked in. She didn't crouch, come in low or high, sweep the room, or step back against the wall. This wasn't like that. This was straightforward. A simple task: You walk in, you dispose of the spider, you walk out. She would touch nothing. When she'd been here before, she'd touched things. At the time she hadn't known finger-prints would matter.

Today Paulette had cleaned the house, scrubbed every surface, then touched them. No fingerprints was fishy. The wife's fingerprints were expected. Did twins have identical fingerprints? Denise would have to Google that.

The bathroom door stood half open. Light spilled onto the double bed, drawing up the one bit of color in the dim room, peach blossoms on a white background, branches cutting across in slashes of black. Denise moved to the foot of the bed, shoved the door to the bathroom open with the toe of her shoe, stepped over the sill, and, holding it with both hands, raised the .22.

The shower curtain wasn't the kind you could see through. Colorful fishes swam on a dark blue sea. The spider was big, though, and Denise could see his bulk where he elbowed and shouldered the curtain as he scrubbed himself.

Nerves were quiet. No ringing or crashing in her ears; she could hear the water striking the spider's skin. Her hands did not shake, and the sweat had dried on her face. Mind still and blank and clean, she aimed for center mass and squeezed off two neat rounds. The bullets cut so cleanly through the plastic they didn't even disturb the curtain.

The spider grunted.

Denise had expected a scream of pain, or death. She hadn't ever been shot. Probably what you'd feel first was the bullets punching you, like fists or a ball bat. It might be a while before the pain set in.

There was a loud wet thud. The spider falling down or back against the wall. The curtain pushed out as if he grasped at it for support. Denise pulled the trigger again. A hole appeared in the middle of a bright yellow fish.

Silence, roaring after the gunshots, filled the small space.

It was done. Denise lowered the gun.

The curtain exploded out. Kurt Duffy crashed into her with the force of a freight train. Air was knocked from her lungs. Plastic covered her face. Her spine cracked against the footboard of the bed. Kurt's weight threatened to snap her in two. Plastic, and a naked wet man, trapped her legs. Her arms were forced up over her head, her face smashed against his chest.

The only thought she could muster was that she should have brought the .357, something with stopping power. In the movies a .22 was the gun of choice for executions. The long bullets could spin, maximize brain damage. This was supposed to be an execution. She'd overlooked the fact that the man she was going to shoot wouldn't be on his knees with his back to her, the muzzle of her pistol pressed up against his skull.

Air rushed back into her lungs. The Smith and Wesson was still in her hand. She couldn't fire down at such a sharp angle without danger of losing the gun. She brought the grip down hard, not knowing what part of him she hit, only that the shock felt good up her arm.

He was grunting and pushing into her like a hog in rut. Disgust lent her strength. Bringing her right knee up into his groin with all the force she could muster, she simultaneously chopped down hard on his head with both elbows.

A beefy thigh took the brunt of the knee, but the pain of the elbows distracted him. Like a snake from under a boot, she coiled from beneath him, slid the rest of the way off the bed to land on hands and knees. Water and blood slicked the floor.

Blood was good. It had to be his. The more the merrier.

He should be dead. "You should be dead," she hissed.

Rearing up from the mess of the curtain, naked, hair on his chest and back and arms, streaming water, blood seeping from his shoulder, chest, and side, he growled.

Like a bear or a mad dog.

Like a monster in a horror movie.

Like a hog bent on eating long pig for lunch.

Like a bull ready to gore, his head swaying from side to side, he pushed himself up until he was kneeling. More hair blackened his groin and legs, his penis a pale worm in the matted nest. He was huge. On his knees he reached nearly to Denise's shoulder. His arms and legs were corded and muscled from a lifetime of working against the sea.

Three holes decorated his body: shoulder, left side of his belly, and, the last, nearly invisible in the hair on the right side of his chest. All were seeping blood. Seeping, for Christ's sake! They should be gushing. Great gouts of blood should be pouring out. Blood frothed on his lips. One had hit a lung. The big bastard could live to be ninety with those three bullets in him.

"Die, God damn you," Denise gasped. A paw the size of an oven mitt came up from the monster's side. "Die," she cried as she skittered sideways out of his reach. The corner of the bedpost banged her shoulder. The .22 flew from her hand and slid under the dressing table in front of which she and Paulette had so recently sat marveling at their twin features.

This was wrong; things weren't supposed to be this way. Spiders weren't supposed to be this hard to kill. "God damn it!" Denise threw herself flat and groped under the dresser after the pistol. Her fingers touched the barrel. A beefy paw curled around her ankle. A bellow of rage; spittle and blood spattered the floor. In the faint glow of the bathroom light the blood was startlingly beautiful, rubies cast upon the ground. Another bestial roar, and Denise was yanked backward like a rag doll in the hands of a psychotic toddler.

Hunching her shoulders and ducking her head, Denise rolled onto her side, stared into the bloodshot eyes of the spider, and kicked out with the force of thighs and butt. One foot connected with his hairy gut above the navel. She was rewarded with a woof! as the air was knocked out of him. Again she kicked, aiming higher, aiming for the bullet that had collapsed his right lung. Again she made a solid hit. He fell back on butt and heels, clutching at his chest as if he could force the lung to take in air. The next kick landed on the wound in his side. Screaming, he tried to sidle backward, escape her blows. The plastic shower curtain tangled between his feet and knees, and he fell back onto the plank flooring.

Quicker than she'd thought possible, Denise was on her feet. She caught up the bottom end of the plastic curtain and fell with it on top of the struggling man. He bucked, trying to throw her. Digging a thumb into the bullet hole in his shoulder, Denise rode him until pain and blood loss slowed his thrashing. Straddling him, knees on his upper arms, she shoved the plastic over his face, cramming what she could into his mouth as he screamed and fought for breath. Hands spread like starfish, pressing down on the plastic, Denise growled, "Die. Die, God damn you. Die. For God's sake, fucking die!"

Finally he grew still. Denise did not let up. Three minutes. She thought she remembered that from emergency medical training. Three minutes without air was enough. No. Couldn't be. She knew divers who could hold their breath three minutes.

Lights slashed across the room. Headlights from a car.

"Shit." Heart and lungs fought for ascendance, both in her throat.

A horn honked.

Denise rolled off Duffy, then stood, her legs shaking, knees wanting to fold. No time for feeling around. With one great heave she toppled the dressing table. Seven years of bad luck shattered around her feet. The Smith and Wesson was against the wall. She grabbed it up.

"Duff! Hey, Duff!" Pounding at the front door loud as a battering ram.

As the front door banged open, Denise was running through the kitchen.

She kept running into the black woods.

SIXTEEN

T his is Anna Pigeon, district ranger from Rocky. We go back a long time," Peter said, introducing Anna.

"Yes, I know. The acting chief." Denise's voice had the flat amiability of old enmity. Was it a not-so-subtle reminder that she and Peter shared old stories, old times, old friends? Anna wondered. Peter used to live with a woman named Denise. This had to be her.

"Denise Castle," the ranger introduced herself before Peter could.

Anna nodded. Gray-green circles, eerily matched to the Park Service uniform, puffed beneath Castle's eyes, and her skin had the desiccated look of someone who's just come off a three-day bender.

"There was a murder in Otter Creek last night," Peter went on. "The state has this one—not on federal land—but we should go to show the colors, see if we can lend a hand. Anna will go with you. Anna is an aficionado of bullet-riddled bodies."

Anna was not amused. The people she'd killed west of the Fox River had needed killing.

"Not exactly," she replied dryly. "Although they do seem rather fond of me."

"She's only acting chief," Denise said, ignoring the exchange. "I doubt she wants to look at a corpse."

"Beats paperwork," Anna said.

To Peter, Denise said, "I don't need help on this."

"Anna's your boss," Peter reminded her coolly. "Anna?"

Despite herself, Anna was interested. When someone else saw to the dirty work, a murder could be quite entertaining. Rather like turning over stones or poking around tide pools, digging around a murder turned up all sorts of interesting flora and fauna.

"Who knows," Anna said to Denise. "I've never been the chief ranger before. I might turn out to be helpful."

Denise's smile was on the watery side, as if she'd had to dredge it up from secret depths to meet the social norm. Then she said, "I'm retiring."

"Today?" Peter sounded confused.

The statement appeared to be as great a surprise to Denise as it was to Peter. She gasped a tiny gasp, then gusted it out on a laugh. "Soon," she said. The wavering smile firmed with what looked like smugness.

"Hop in," she said to Anna as she opened the door to her Crown Vic. "We might as well get this dog-and-pony show over with."

Anna slid into the passenger side of the patrol car, then buckled her seat belt. There was a reassuring sameness to Park Service vehicles, equipment, housing, even war stories. Six degrees of separation did not apply in the NPS. After a certain number of years, often there was scarcely one degree left. Everyone knew—or knew of—everyone, and had an opinion about them. Park people were like a hugely extended cantankerous family, complete with black sheep and heirs apparent. Some rangers felt claustrophobic in such an intrinsically small world. Anna felt at home.

Seldom did she get to ride shotgun. Rangers didn't work in pairs. She leaned back in the seat as Denise pulled out of the headquarters parking lot. It was a treat to relax and look at the scenery, enjoy the park tourist-style. A park existed for every mood, and Anna was a woman of many moods.

"What did Pete tell you about the murder?" Denise asked.

"Lobsterman shot sometime last night. Possibly a domestic. State and local police notified last night. The park, this morning. Concurrent jurisdiction. That's about it. No particulars."

"Ever heard of the lobster wars?" Denise asked.

"Sounds like a bad science fiction movie," Anna replied.

"It's serious business in these parts. Kind of like range wars in the Old West. Lobstermen are rough customers."

Anna had never known a lobsterman, but she'd worked with shrimpers out in the Dry Tortugas. Very rough customers.

"Do you think another lobsterman killed him? For lobster rustling?"

"Probably. Who cares? Otter Creek isn't on park land. The state guys, or the sheriff, whoever caught this one, probably cleared it last night. Duffy's—the lobsterman's name was Kurt Duffy—bowling pal found the body. May have been some bad blood there." Denise spoke in a bored monotone, her face a mask of indifference.

Anna watched her in the sideview mirror. Law enforcement rangers were never indifferent to murder. Parks were inconvenient places to deal drugs, host gang wars, or run prostitution rings. They were bucolic places filled with potato salad–eating people whose greatest crime was feeding the chipmunks. Most rangers never worked a single murder in an entire career. Wicked as it was—or sounded to outsiders—when a nice juicy murder did come along, the dilemma wasn't getting rangers to work the case but keeping them from trampling each other to get in on it.

"My guess is it's a lobster-war thing," Denise said as she conned the big Crown Vic along the narrow road. She was a skilled driver. She worked the mirrors with her eyes, and her hands loved the steering wheel. The only other person Anna had noticed driving with that kind of innate concentration was an ex-NASCAR racer who'd taught her defensive driving.

Really good drivers tended to drive fast. Yet Denise was poking along ten miles under the speed limit. Apparently she was not only bored by the prospect of a murder investigation but didn't want to reach the scene any time in the foreseeable future.

"We had a guy shot for robbing his neighbor's traps—Will Whitman," Denise went on with a bit more enthusiasm, warming to her subject. "Whitman's son was implicated along with his dad for poaching lobsters, but he's gone AWOL. It's probably what saved his life. These guys are the Hatfields and McCoys, Earps and Clantons—you name it, feuds go back four or five generations. There's a range war going on under the waters around here that makes Texas in the ranchers-and-farmers phase look tame."

"Did they catch the man who shot this Will Whitman?" Anna asked to be asking something.

"Sure. No problem. They threw him in jail, but he's out now. Shooting a man for robbing your traps in Maine is akin to the 'stand your ground' law in Florida."

"Whitman. Any relation to John Whitman?" John Whitman was the taxi man ferrying Heath and company around.

"John is—was—Will's father. When John retired, Will got his patch. Then there was the shooting. Since John's grandson ran off, the lobstermen have been haggling over who should get his territory."

"Any relation to Duffy?"

Denise started as if Anna had poked her with a pin, then settled. "Kurt Duffy? Probably. Everybody is somebody's cousin around here." On that she closed her mouth into a firm line that suggested the conversation was finished.

Anna let the subject drop. "Any news on the package sent to Heath Jarrod?" she asked.

"That's a strange story," Denise answered, seemingly more comfortable talking of drugs than of murder. "We field-tested a couple of the foil packs. Black tar from Mexico, the cheapest, nastiest sort. The rest we sent to the lab. If they all contain heroin there should be about three grams total. Dime bags, cut with something. I doubt the whole amount is worth more than a few hundred dollars."

Anna didn't know a lot about heroin. In the parks, other than visitors taking a tab of acid, munching a mushroom for the visuals, or smoking a little dope, drugs were urban problems. "Doesn't the stuff come in bulk?" she asked. "Then the dealer makes it up into packages?"

"I'd think so," Denise said. "I suppose there's people for that if you're willing to pay. Here we are."

As soon as they crested the gentle rise in the road, it became obvious where in Otter Creek the murder had taken place. Four cars—two police and one sheriff's and Artie's Crown Vic—were parked around a shiny blue pickup in front of a small cottage, little more than a square of weathered wood bisected by a door with a tiny pointed roof over the porch to keep the snow off the step. Two windows flanked the front door, both blinded by pull-down shades brown and curling with age. Yellow police tape crisscrossed the door. The front was not graveled, per se. It was simply stony soil that had suffered the sudden stops of too many tires.

It didn't strike Anna as the sort of home one would build on real estate that had to be worth more money than she'd ever see. Old, then, a homesteader from way back.

"Lobster fisherman and his wife," Denise said, as if reading Anna's mind. She parked the Crown Vic fifty yards from the house and made no move to get out. "Wouldn't you know it? Artie, on his day off. What a twerp."

Anna followed Denise's sour words to the district ranger, out of uniform but with a pistol in a holster at his belt.

"Not in the mood for a clusterfuck today," Denise said, switching off the ignition.

"Beats sitting in a hot car," Anna suggested.

"Not today it doesn't."

Anna didn't know what to say to that. Miss out on murder? Ridiculous. "Mind if I go?"

"Knock yourself out. Wait," Denise said suddenly. "I would like a look inside, at the murder scene."

That was more like the rangers Anna had known.

"Let's do it," Anna said.

A civilian around sixty, arms and hands scarred, face weather-beaten, sat smoking a cigarette on the downed tailgate of the pickup truck. A short distance away, not part of the group but near it, her back turned to the men, was a woman with too much bleached-blond hair. Oversized sunglasses hid her face. She was holding one elbow, her free hand keeping a long white cigarette close to her lips between drags.

Anna walked with Denise toward where the men were standing around the pickup's tailgate. Under concurrent, or shared, jurisdiction, if the incident was not actually on park land it was customary for the NPS to give way to the state. If it was on NPS soil, the state would usually take a secondary position. Since this wasn't exactly Acadia's jurisdiction—and Acadia wasn't even Anna's park—she didn't want to ruffle any feathers. "Just a tourist," she said as she glided up next to the district ranger.

"Anna Pigeon," Denise said.

"Right." Artie looked down at her from his considerable height. All Anna could see of his eyes was her own reflection in his mirrored sunglasses. The set of his mouth was not welcoming. Anna reminded herself to corner him about the heroin and Heath. Make sure he thought it stank to high heaven as he ought to.

"Hello, Ms. Pigeon," he said coolly. "This is Sheriff Cotter."

Anna gazed at Artie expectantly, a neutral smile on her lips, until he caved in and added, "Ranger Pigeon is acting chief while Gris is out west fighting fire."

Anna nodded to Sheriff Cotter, a red-faced man in a dun-colored uniform. His skin was the type that probably burned and peeled three months of the year. Blond stubble glittered on his jowls, and his eyebrows were nearly white.

"We got this one," he said.

"Peter told me," Anna replied. Cotter nodded. No territorial fights over this murder.

"And Deputy—"

"Dremmel, Jack Dremmel," the sheriff's exceedingly young companion answered, sticking out a bony hand for Anna to shake. Anna wondered if it was just her or if law enforcement personnel were getting younger. Jack appeared to be about fourteen. Acne still clustered on one side of his chin. She couldn't imagine him shaving.

"Bar Harbor police," Artie said.

Two middle-aged men in blue nodded at Anna. No names were exchanged. They were just being nosey.

"I'd like a look inside," Denise said. If the set of her jaw was any indication, the disinterest she'd shown in the car had transformed into a grim avidity.

"Crime techs are all done," Cotter said. "We're just waiting for the coroner to come claim the body. How about you?" he said to Anna. "You want to take a look around, too?"

"Might as well," Anna said.

Cotter removed the tape. He held the door open. Denise and Anna walked into one of the most depressing rooms she'd seen in a while, and it wasn't the one where the murder had taken place.

"The bedroom," the sheriff said, pointing to a door.

There was only one door off the cramped sitting room. The house was a shotgun: sitting room, then bedroom, then kitchen at the back, no halls. Anna crossed to the bedroom door but didn't go in. Denise pushed past her, eyes searching everything from walls to floors to under the bed and dresser.

"Guy was shot three times, then wound up in the shower curtain. Cause of death might be suffocation. The shower curtain was shoved halfway down his throat. The autopsy will let us know," Cotter told her.

"Find anything else?" Denise asked. "Murder weapon?"

"No such luck," Cotter said.

"Sounds like you got another victim in the wars," Denise said, then abruptly left the room. Anna heard the front door close seconds later.

She looked over the detritus of the bedroom: a dead man, naked, blood mixing with a thick pelt of hair on his chest, face in a rictus of death, overturned furniture, plastic curtain with bright fishes. Shards of mirror reflected shards of what had been, to all appearances, a miserable life ending in a miserable death.

Murder was so often pointless and pitiful. Anna lost her fascination with who murdered whom or why.

"I've seen enough," she said, and she had. All she wanted was to get back out into the sunlight with the living things of the park around her.

Cotter followed her out the front door. As he was replacing the crime scene tape, Artie asked, "Where did Denise go? She's the one on duty today."

Anna glanced around. Denise was already back in the Crown Vic, seated behind the wheel. Her enthusiasm had been short-lived. Obviously there were undercurrents Anna was not privy to: Peter, a surprise retirement, mood swings. She felt as if she'd walked in on the end of a family fight.

"In the car," Anna replied.

Artie's lips curled into a sneer, but he said nothing.

"I'm Lou," the guy on the tailgate volunteered. "I found the body. Me and Kurt were buddies."

Close up, Anna could tell she'd misguessed the man's age by at least fifteen years. Lou was closer to forty-five than sixty. His face reminded her of the men she'd met who worked shrimp boats all their lives, or rode with a motorcycle gang back before the gangs were comprised of lawyers and doctors on pastel Harleys. Hard lives made hard faces. Lou's was carved by exposure and, most likely, alcohol. Only his hair retained the softness of youth; brown and thick, it swept over his forehead, as jarring against his creased skin as the tresses of a bad wig.

Lou was obviously proud of having found the body. Lots of people were like that. Being part of a murder investigation was their fifteen minutes of fame. Though, given the speed the Internet churned out fame, the average dose was probably closer to sixty seconds.

Whether or not he was broken up over his pal's death, Anna couldn't tell. His face was not the kind to share warm fuzzy emotions with strangers.

"I'm sorry," Anna said. "That had to be a blow."

"Yeah," Lou said. He dropped his cigarette and shifted his butt closer to the edge of the tailgate so he could grind it out with the toe of his boot. The cigarette was only half smoked. Lou moved stiffly, his head ducked as if to hide his face. Manly grief?

"Sheriff here'll be looking for a big man, and strong," Lou said as he straightened up. "Kurt put up a hell of a fight. Tore the whole bedroom up. I'm surprised I didn't find two bodies. Kurt was tough, I'll say that for him. Tough as they come."

He lit another cigarette, sucked in a lungful of smoke, then spat between his knees, the smoke trickling out his nose. "Anyway," he said on the last wisps of smoke, "glad it was me as found him. Polly isn't much good at the hard stuff."

The woman with too much hair and the wraparound blue plastic sunglasses, standing with her back to the men, said over her shoulder,

"Paulette. My name is Paulette." Peeking from beneath the dark glasses was a patch of makeup, slightly off color and applied too thickly. Bruises were a bitch to cover.

Lou's lips pursed in annoyance. Paulette turned her head away quickly as if her boldness in correcting him frightened her.

"*Polly*," Lou said, hitting the word hard, "was Kurt's wife."

The spouse, always the number one suspect. A battered spouse, better yet.

"Hi, Paulette," Anna said, moseying over. "I'm Anna Pigeon." She smiled. Sensing the woman would be less forthcoming at a show of force, Anna downplayed her authority. "Don't be fooled by the uniform. I'm just passing through. The park brought me to cover for the chief ranger for a few weeks." She stuck out her hand. Shaking hands wasn't her favorite thing, and the modern penchant for hugging made her blood run cold, but it was a nonthreatening way to take somebody's temperature.

Paulette's hand was cold and clammy, limp as a three-day-old fish.

Before Anna loosed her grip, the fish came alive and jerked away.

"I haven't had much sleep," Paulette apologized. She took another drag on her cigarette. The hand holding the cigarette was shaking so badly she could hardly get the butt to her mouth. She didn't look Anna in the eye.

"I bet not," Anna said sympathetically.

"I was down at the Acadian Lodge from six until nearly midnight. I didn't know what had happened until I came home and the cops were here."

Getting her alibi out right up front; not a guilty reaction exactly. Battered spouse, she had to know the sheriff was thinking she was a suspect. Lou seemed fairly hostile toward his good buddy's wife. Regardless of his talk of searching for a big burly murderer, Anna wondered if he thought she'd killed Kurt.

The insistent *Polly* chimed in her head, and she doubted it. Lou would have more respect for a murderess.

Paulette dropped her cigarette on the dirt, then ground the filter into the gravel with the toe of her wedge sandal. Her legs were pretty. Shapely and slim. The mass of fried hair and bruised cheekbone had blinded Anna to the fact that Paulette was attractive and not much past forty. Fishing a pale blue crumpled pack of menthols from the pocket of her skirt, Paulette shook out another cigarette.

"Would you like one?" she asked politely.

"No thanks," Anna said. "I'm trying to cut down."

Paulette nodded, as if to say every smoker she knew was always trying to cut down.

"How are you holding up?" Anna asked. Just because her husband knocked her around—if it was the husband who blacked her eye—didn't mean the woman wouldn't be heartbroken at his demise. Women were funny like that.

Paulette Duffy shot her a sidelong glance from beneath the temple of the glasses. She seemed to think it was a trick question. Anna smiled back with bland concern.

"I'm okay," Paulette said. She lit the fresh cigarette and took in a deep lungful. "The house is going to be creepy for a while."

"Do you have anyone you can stay with? A brother? A sister?" Anna asked.

Paulette twitched as if Anna had poked her with a hot iron. The hand holding the cigarette flicked out. The newly lit cigarette went flying. Paulette dropped the lighter she held in her other hand. Moaning, she fell to her knees to gather her belongings up.

"I'm an only child," she said as she scrabbled in the dirt.

Anna hadn't meant to push any buttons. "I have a sister," she said as a peace offering.

"Would you mind asking Sheriff Cotter if I can have my house now?" Paulette begged without raising her eyes from the ground. Her fingers closed around the bright yellow Bic lighter, but she made no effort to rise.

With a creeping crunch, a white fender brushed Anna's thigh. Willing herself not to squeak and leap, she glanced back over the long gleaming hood. Denise. The car crept forward. If Denise hadn't braked when she did, Anna would have had to leap back to avoid being eviscerated by the sideview mirror.

The passenger-side window smoothed down with an electric hum. "Get in," Denise said shortly. "We're done here."

Paulette crawled—actually crawled on hands and knees, the tops of her canvas sandals and the front of her skirt gathering dirt as she went—several feet before rising. Without a backward look at Anna, she scurried toward the knot of men, brushing at her skirts as she walked. The lighter and the unsmoked cigarette were still on the ground.

Anna leaned down to retrieve the lighter and return it to her.

"Leave it," Denise snapped.

Straightening, Anna gave her a level stare. She considered reminding her who was the acting chief, and who was the badly behaved subordinate.

"Sorry," Denise said with a crooked smile. "Got a call. Gets my nerves crackling."

Anna decided to let whatever Denise was playing at play out. She climbed into the Crown Vic. "What's up?" she asked, and began buckling belt and harness.

"What do you mean?" Denise asked.

"The call," Anna said. "What is it?"

Denise laughed nervously. "If these guys don't need us anymore, maybe we could get a bite of lunch."

Anna gazed at her. Denise wasn't being a smartass. From what Anna could read on her face she had forgotten—more than forgotten—she'd said she had a call. Her eyes were a total blank, as if the moments before had been taken from her brain and destroyed.

Everyone reacted to violent death differently. Most people were inured to it by years of seeing it on television, on the news, in the movies. If it didn't happen to a personal friend, most people just clucked, "Oh my, how awful," and went about their business. Except in politics and football, people cared very little about anything that didn't apply to them directly.

But for the crime scene, Denise had evinced little interest in the incident. Anna realized she been braced for the usual discussion. How much blood? How many bullet holes? Denise didn't start the conversation.

Anna sighed. She had lost interest as well. The instinct for the hunt had vanished with the sight of the pathetic dead man in his pathetic bedroom. Maybe she was mellowing with age. Maybe she was just getting old.

"Lunch is good," she said.

SEVENTEEN

Heath wasn't sure whether she was making any headway or not. There was no end to sites, articles, and blogs about cyberstalking on the Internet. As often happened, there was not a lot of content in any of them. Most simply described the phenomenon: stalking via electronic media, the cell phone the most common method. As in the schoolyard, the incidents could be anything from a snide remark to a death threat. Sex and shame were favored tools, and, though she'd thought it unique to Elizabeth, children telling other children to kill themselves wasn't all that rare. School and government sites had tabs marked "Prevent Cyberbullying," but they were little more than advice columns on how to police your own children and teach them what to post and what not to.

Several sites were informative as to how to report the incidents and get them removed from personal media. She learned there were things called "bashboards," sites where visitors could vote on who was the fattest or ugliest or meanest kid in class. There was one for Elizabeth. Someone else had already reported it. It still existed, but Heath couldn't open it.

On the subject of how to track down a cyberbully—or stalker, as she thought of the individual tormenting E—was vague and spotty. There was no clear path through the ether if the sender was even halfway clever.

A scream snatched Heath out of cyberspace.

Shoving the laptop off her legs, she yelled, "Elizabeth, are you all right?" Then, "Aunt Gwen!" Moving as quickly as long practice allowed, she levered herself off her bed, where she'd been sitting working, and into Robo-butt parked next to it. "Gwen!" she yelled again as she rolled across the old painted concrete floor of the lighthouse and toward the archway leading to the newer part of the house.

In reality the archway was a tunnel cutting through walls thirteen feet thick. Ms. Zuckerberg had painted the sides and curved ceiling with Peach Dawn at floor level and Midnight Blue with stars overhead. Heath shot through it like a mechanized comet.

"Elizabeth!" she shouted.

Wily began barking frantically.

"I'm coming," she heard her aunt call from the top of the lighthouse.

A wide living room formed an arc around the base of the lighthouse. Curved windows gave views east and west. Large overstuffed chairs and sofas, backed by heavy dark wood tables, lent the peaceful air of an old library or a high-end lodge from the turn of the century.

Heath rolled through the charming room, seeing nothing except that her daughter was not in it.

The barking escalated.

Another scream cut across Wily's shrill cries.

"I'm coming!" Aunt Gwen again. Heath could hear her footsteps rattling down the circular stairs.

The nightmare sensation of moving in slow motion through an atmosphere as thick and unyielding as bread pudding caught Heath. She felt as if her hands could not spin the wheels of the chair, as if she couldn't see properly, her vision dusky at the edges. Had she not been able to hear rubber squeaking loudly on the tile floor as she took the corner from the living room into the kitchen, she would have thought herself trapped like a fly in invisible amber.

Ms. Zuckerberg's kitchen was spacious and modern, with antique touches tying it to the island's past. The floors were of wide planks, aged and scarred, either salvaged from old ships or made to look old by an artisan. A kitchen island stood in the middle of the space. The sides were of dull beaten tin, the top of dark marble. Beyond was the sink, and more counter space beneath cupboards built of dark wood with perforated tin where glass might have been in another home.

Elizabeth was on her hands and knees atop the utility island. Wily was on the floor, hind end up in the air, forelegs on the planks, barking like crazy at something Heath could not see between the island and the sink. Heath jerked her wheels to a stop, and her chair slid another couple of feet. The floor was covered in water.

"What in the hell is going on?" she roared, panic making her voice big and angry.

Elizabeth snatched her eyes from whatever Wily had cornered and, to Heath's relief and fury, began to laugh. She was laughing so hard she was holding her sides and gasping, feet dangling over the edge, rear end on the cutting board, when Gwen came running into the room. Before Heath could shout a warning, Gwen hit the water-slick and careened across the floor in a comic-book slide, arms windmilling, to fetch up against the island.

This sent E into another round of hysterical giggles.

"She could have fallen and broken a hip!" Heath shouted at her daughter. "We both could have been killed."

For reasons that Heath had no interest in, this struck not only E as funny, but Gwen as well.

"Damn it, Wily, shut up!" Heath roared. To her surprise he did. He grinned at her foolishly, then trotted over to her chair. Grabbing his collar, though he was the only one who appeared to be paying any attention to her, she waited with grim patience until Elizabeth and Gwen saw fit to stop snickering.

"Are you done?" she asked acidly when they'd quieted. Careful not to look at one another lest they burst out all over again, they both nodded.

"What the hell is going on?" Heath demanded.

"Elizabeth was playing with her food," Gwen said. That set them off again. Heath sat and fumed. She'd have lit a cigarette if she'd been anywhere but inside a house. There was nothing she could do when Gwen was encouraging E. Aunt Gwen was in her seventies, but when the two of them got going Heath could easily see what her aunt had been like when she was thirteen. Finally they wound down to intermittent giggles.

Wily whined.

A skritching of hard, sharp objects clawing at the floor emanated from behind the island, where now both E and her great-aunt sat swinging their legs, heels banging lightly against the tin sides. Gwen was in lime green capri pants and aqua tennis shoes, E in sweats, T-shirt, and purple flip-flops.

Brownish green and curved, a claw protruded from behind the island, then another, smaller, then the rest of the lobster.

"There are two," Gwen managed, fighting to keep her face straight. "John dropped them by for dinner tonight."

Gwen had come home at two in the morning. Heath had checked the time when the lift bell awakened her. Then she'd heard her aunt and John giggling in the kitchen. By the time Gwen had tiptoed through her bedroom and up to her tower room, Heath had been asleep. Now Gwen's paramour had come by to drop off gifts. Things were certainly moving along in that quarter, Heath thought sourly—the sourness of the proverbial grapes, she suspected.

"I took the lid off that bucket." E pointed to an overturned metal pail by the refrigerator. "And they just came out."

Again she and Gwen went into gales of giggles. Regardless of the shock of thinking her only child was being slaughtered by barbarian hordes, Heath could see the humor and allowed herself a smile.

Gwen hopped off the island. Expertly, she grabbed the first lobster behind its claws. After a lifetime of dealing with squirming children, lobsters evidently were no challenge. While E squealed, "Eeew!" Gwen dropped it in the bucket and then caught the second one.

"I've got to go down the lift and get a bucket of seawater. Our friends here will die if they stay out much longer."

"Aren't they supposed to die?" E asked. "They're food. Shouldn't they be in the refrigerator or somewhere? Not running around the kitchen frightening the children?"

"You cook them live," Gwen said.

Elizabeth's face went stiff with shock, her mouth open. "You do not!" she exclaimed.

"You do. It doesn't hurt them," Gwen said matter-of-factly. In her soggy sneakers, her pail of lobsters at her side, Gwen marched out of the kitchen toward the lift.

"It doesn't *hurt* them?" E asked incredulously. "How can being boiled alive not *hurt* them?"

Before Heath could think of an answer, Elizabeth had run out of the kitchen. Heath rolled to the doorway, but E was not standing at the lift waiting for her aunt to return. She was nowhere in sight,

Unexploded ordnance, Heath thought miserably. Gwen should have known. She didn't know who to pity most, Elizabeth for her memories, or Gwen when she realized what she had done.

EIGHTEEN

Elizabeth couldn't run far. There was no "far" on Boar. Besides, Maine wasn't flip-flop country; it was all rocky ups and downs. She wouldn't dare be gone for long. Because of her depression and suicidal impulse, she knew if she was out of Heath's sight for too long, Heath would call in the marines.

Worse. She'd call Anna.

Heath had tried to make E know she understood thinking one wanted to die, thinking what a relief it would be to let all the pain and ugly drain away while she went to sleep. She also tried to bring home to her daughter the fact that that sleep was forever. A permanent solution to a temporary problem. What life had taught Heath, and what she clung to, was that if you didn't die, things got better.

Then, of course, you did die, Heath thought as she tried to decide whether it would be better to shout for Elizabeth to come back or let her have a little time by herself. But that wasn't the point.

Heath wanted desperately to talk to E about the lobster thing, though she knew Elizabeth was drowning in talk, advice, reassurances, and platitudes. "Love claustrophobia," E had self-diagnosed, suffering from too much love in too small a space. Occasionally, Heath wondered if E couldn't take love at the level she and Gwen were dishing it out because she had gotten too little love as a child. At other times, she assumed she and Gwen were a tad overbearing, both having been childless until Elizabeth.

Parental EMO. Elizabeth insisted it was enough to shrivel a person into a Cheeto.

Heath smiled at that, then yelled, "Elizabeth! Come back! We need to talk!" despite her better judgment.

When E was nine, a psycho had captured her and two other girls. Jena, E's therapist, had helped her work through it. Fervently, Heath wished Jena were on Boar Island. Without giving advice or passing judgment, Jena had the gift of herding a patient's thoughts the way a dog would herd sheep until they were all going in the right direction, then keep the patient company until she reached the place she needed to be.

Heath knew she and Gwen committed the sin of listening too hard. They couldn't help themselves. Sometimes Heath listened so hard she could almost hear her eardrums cracking. Aunt Gwen's face looked like Wily's when somebody had a piece of cheese he really, really wanted but was too well behaved to beg for.

Because of conferences with Jena, Heath knew what the kidnapper had tried to do to Elizabeth and the other girls. Making them kill mice was only the half of it. What the kidnapper had tried to do—had done— was rob them of themselves, then implant a version of his horrific psycho self in their brains.

The cyberstalker was trying to do the same thing, Heath realized. Using filth and threats and shame to take away E's sense of who she was and replace it with horribleness. No wonder she wanted to kill herself.

"E! Come back! Let's talk!" Heath shouted.

Wily trotted across the natural stone patio in the direction of the landward wing of ruins behind the lighthouse.

"Thank God," Heath breathed. There was no hiding from the nose. Elizabeth would never jump off a cliff in front of Wily, and Wily wasn't fool enough to jump off a cliff just because the other kids did, Heath consoled herself.

Elizabeth might not want a fairy god-dog along. She might try to evade him. E thought she knew all Wily's tricks. She didn't. Nobody knew all Wily's tricks.

Heath rolled herself across the flat apron until she could see a sliver of what existed behind the imposing buttress of granite that backed the house. Huge blocks with deep fissured shelves tumbled down toward the ocean. Beyond was a light fog, breaking like liquid in pure white waves against the shore of Mount Desert Island, poking feathery fingers into low places and humping up over rocks.

The lift bell rang. Machinery clanked. Gwen returning with her freshly seawatered lobsters. The platform clanked into place, and silence fell.

"Elizabeth!" Heath cried again.

There was no sound but for the ocean murmuring its secrets to the rock.

Gwen, slopping water from the bucket, crossed to Heath. "Why are you shouting?" she demanded.

Heath told her.

"Maybe it won't be so bad." Gwen's optimism sounded strained. "Lobsters are just big brownish green spiders, after all."

"It was the alive part. Boiling them *alive*," Heath said dully. "I don't know if she still does, but back when she said her prayers aloud she prayed to mice—prayed to rodents—begging them to forgive her. I don't want to hear her praying to arachnids."

"And me fetching a bucket of saltwater, toting living sacrifices to toss in the pot like cannibals toss missionaries in old cartoons! How could I have been so stupid!" Gwen moaned.

On the tail of the moan rode silence, the kind that sets like concrete in the ear.

NINETEEN

Anna stood at the edge of Thunder Hole, a favorite tourist spot. A keyhole-shaped inlet in the granite cliffs forced waves into a narrow aperture, creating wondrous booming thunder and geysers of silver spray, some a hundred feet high. A walkway with metal handrails descended partway into the hole for those who wished to be misted—or drenched, as the sea saw fit.

Lunch with Denise—Subway sandwiches gobbled in the car—had been uphill work. Denise said little, showed no interest in talking of the park or the park personnel, yet the silences were not comfortable. Anna had the same feeling around Ranger Castle as she had around a kid with a balloon and a pin. Any minute there was liable to be a big bang that would scare her half to death.

As acting chief, there wasn't a whole lot to do in reality. An ambitious "acting" on a short-term assignment could louse up a lot of paperwork. Anna had stepped in for other district rangers often enough to know that unless something momentous occurred—and the state of Maine had snatched the only good murder on the books—general housekeeping was the rule.

With nothing important to do in the office, Anna opted for foot patrol, asking Denise to swing back around the Mount Desert Island loop to pick her up in a couple of hours.

Being free of the Crown Vic and Ranger Castle was more of a relief than it should have been. Castle put Anna on edge in some indefinable way. The woman wasn't right. She was out of sync. Anna was a great believer in vibes. The eye and the subconscious mind were often better at reading the small print, and making sense of it, than the conscious mind.

Leaves swirling on waters suggested deep and troubling currents. Denise had enough swirling leaves to make Anna's scalp prickle. It lent her a greater appreciation of having escaped to blue sea, golden sun, salt breezes, tourists to annoy, and cigarette butts to pick up.

She was happily ensconced with a trio of visitors, holding forth in excellent ranger style, adroitly avoiding admitting she knew zip about the flora and fauna on the coast of Maine, when her cell phone vibrated.

"Excuse me," she said as she took it from its wallet and glanced at the face. "It's a call I need to take," she apologized.

As she turned away, she heard the woman say, "Isn't that nice! She apologized!" The teenaged son said, "For what?"

"The stalker is here," Heath said without preamble.

Caller ID had done away with the need for most of the old rotary niceties, an advance Anna appreciated.

"In Maine. In the park. Or says he is," Heath said.

Phone to ear, Anna walked across the loop road and into the trees. Talking to a ranger in uniform was too great a temptation for visitors to resist, regardless of what the ranger was in the middle of. She switched the phone from her left to her right hand. Since she'd taken a bullet in her left bicep a year or so before, the arm had been opposed to remaining in static tension for any length of time. Unless she kept it moving, it stiffened and ached.

Oddly, that the stalker was in the park jolted Anna. With Heath sequestered on Boar, she'd fallen into the trap of feeling Elizabeth was safe, as if she were vacationing in a secure resort, and being stalked was no more real than a death at a Mystery Dinner.

Cybercreep was here.

"This is good news," she decided, settling cross-legged on the pine straw, careful not to lean against the tree. Sap was impossible to get out of polyester.

"You're kidding, right?" Heath asked.

"No. In cyberspace we had the chance of a snowball in hell of finding him. In a national park, it may be doable."

"Good point." Heath sounded relieved. "Except that he intends on doing more than slinging porn at E. He wants to meet with her."

Cybercreep had escalated. Anonymous bullies usually stayed anonymous. If this one was calling for a face-to-face, it was because he wanted to do something more than shame and frighten. He wanted a hands-on experience.

"Start at the beginning," Anna said.

"I got two texts—in reality, Elizabeth got the texts. Her phone buzzed. I grabbed it. I've saved them," Heath said unnecessarily. She, Anna, Gwen, and E had already had that talk. "The first says, 'I know where you are.' Not very original; we knew that from the heroin. The second says, 'Come to Cecelia's Coffee Shop today at six. Come by yourself if you want your real life back.' Cecelia's is in Bar Harbor on the town square. I Google-Mapped it."

"Better and better," Anna said. "A time and place." Silence followed that. Heath was no dummy. She would know the "better and better" could involve using E as bait at some point. Without knowing who the stalker was, or what he wanted—other than the obvious: rape, white slavery, psycho amusements of all sorts—there was danger in letting him within shooting distance of E. Then again, if they did use E as bait, at least they would be there when whatever trap he had planned began to unfold.

"This is not usual for a cyberbully, is it?" Heath asked. "More like a blackmailer, but so far nobody has asked us for anything."

"You're right," Anna said. "Poison pens and cyberstalkers thrive on being hidden, anonymous, watching the havoc they create from the safety of their webs—spider or otherwise. They wouldn't want to meet for coffee in public. Has E seen the texts?"

"Not yet. She and Wily are off somewhere licking their wounds."

"Wounds?"

"John gave Gwen two lobsters. She mentioned to E that they were boiled while alive."

"The mice," Anna said, remembering the little corpses nailed to the side of the outhouse at the cabin in Rocky. Nailed while they still lived. Not an image a young girl should have burned into her brain. Or a ranger of a certain age, for that matter.

"Get your real life back," she said, changing the subject. "What do you figure that means? If they're talking reputation, that ship has sailed."

Heath groaned. "God, don't say that."

"When I was in high school there was a girl all the boys called Rosie Rotten-crotch," Anna said, remembering. "Supposedly she was the school hump. At that age, I never thought to question it. Now I wonder if Rosie said yes, or maybe no, to the wrong boy. Or if a jealous girl started it. Rosie was an American Indian girl from the local Paiute tribe. Scapegoat. Nobody cared to dig any deeper." Anna felt a stab of guilt. She hadn't cared either. "Rosie was ruined. There's no way to rehabilitate this sort of reputation wreck."

"Yes there is," Heath insisted firmly.

Anna let that stand. If Heath said it, they'd figure out a way to make it true. Later. She glanced at her watch. "It's four thirty. Our stalker might know you're in Acadia, but I bet he doesn't know you're on Boar, or he'd have given E more lead time to make the meeting. I think I can make it."

"So can I," Heath said. "I'll call a water taxi and meet you in Bar Harbor."

"No," Anna said. "'Come alone if you want your life back.' Elizabeth was to come alone. We should assume this person knows something about you. We don't want to scare him off."

There was a long silence, then a gust of air that Anna suspected was tainted with tobacco smoke. "Right," Heath said finally. "A woman in a wheelchair is noticed. Then ignored."

"It's the first part that would wreck the surveillance."

TWENTY

Denise picked Anna up ten minutes after she called. Denise's unsettling aura, the one that made Anna's spine tingle, evaporated as Anna told her what she wanted. The abrupt loss of Denise's erratic hypervigilance made Anna wonder what she'd been expecting. What she'd been fearing. Given Ranger Castle's behavior, Anna didn't think "fear" was too strong a word. Maybe whatever had inspired her sudden retirement was still haunting her.

"So," Anna finished, "Elizabeth's stalker is here in Maine. Wants a meet-and-greet. E's off somewhere communing with the spirits, but we don't want to let the opportunity slip past."

Denise leaned forward until her chin was almost resting on the steering wheel. "Are all men such bastards?" she demanded. "Serial killing, child molesting, rape, bestiality—you name it, men do it."

"Women, too," Anna said because she was in the mood to poke a hornets' nest.

Denise sucked an audible breath through her nose, then puffed the air out of lips loose with scorn. "Sure. One, two maybe. Not enough for a decent statistic. Get real. Women do shitty things, no doubt about it, but the twisted male victimization of women is front page every day. Got a cult leader? What's the first thing he does? Makes all the women sleep with him. Got a God? First thing the guy says—and the gods are all guys nowadays—is 'Obey your husband. Put yourself in a black bag so nobody can see you.' Root of all evil, Eve and the goddamned apple my ass! More like Adam and his snake."

Anna laughed. "I like that. I have to remember to tell my husband. He's a priest."

Denise looked at her, her eyebrows in a shocked V. "Like defrocked?"

Anna laughed again. "Episcopal."

"Sorry I shot off my mouth," Denise said. She sounded more sulky than sorry. Rather like a child who got caught doing something she wasn't supposed to.

"Don't be," Anna said easily. "In this case, you're preaching to the choir. This victim is a particular friend of mine." She didn't mention that E was her goddaughter. Being married to a priest was condemnation enough to a cynical ear.

Having cleared the change in routine with Peter, Anna and Denise would swap out cars so they weren't in a marked NPS vehicle. Denise would accompany Anna to the coffee shop. It was unlikely, but whoever was behind the bullying might recognize Anna on sight. Denise had the advantage of being an unknown.

"Do you know anything about stalking via the Internet?" Anna asked as Denise pulled the patrol vehicle into the parking garage beneath her apartment building in Bar Harbor.

Denise's head jerked back as if Anna had flopped a nasty fish in her face.

"What are you implying?" she asked, an edge to her voice.

Maybe Denise had done a bit of cyberspying after the split with Peter. Before the Internet, dumped girlfriends had to drive by "his" house to see whose car was parked there. Now, armed with personal information, they could read credit reports, check Facebook. All manner of interesting new methods of self-torture were available.

"I'm pretty ignorant when it comes to this stuff," Anna replied mildly. "I hoped you might know more."

"Oh," Denise said. "No. I'm not into that. I don't even have a cell phone."

For a law enforcement officer not to have a cell phone was tantamount to dereliction of duty. More was the pity; a cell phone saw to it that no one was ever truly off duty, or home from work. Anna tossed this lack of modern technology onto the pile of Weird Denise Castle Things growing in the back of her mind.

With the nervous reluctance of a jeweler ushering in a cat burglar, Denise let Anna into her apartment. To Anna's eyes there was nothing to be ashamed of. The place was neat to a fault—no books, no magazines, no cats or dogs or dirty underpants on the floor. White walls were decorated with framed photographs in black and white of the park both above and below the surface of the Atlantic. The carpet was white, no off-color spots where beasties vomited or booted feet left dirt. The couch was white, black-and-white zebra-print pillows standing sentinel at either end. A glass coffee table and a flat-screen TV finished the decor.

With the air of a wary damsel inviting a vampire over the threshold, Denise said, "This way," and ushered Anna into the apartment's single bedroom. It was as monochromatic as the living room. Both rooms had the impersonal feel of having been "dressed" by a Realtor looking to sell.

"These should fit well enough," Denise said, pulling a pair of gray linen slacks and a white pleated-front blouse from the closet. A narrow black belt was hooked over the hanger by the buckle. The clothes in the closet were all arranged in outfits. She laid the clothes on the bed, then took a shoe box from a neat arrangement of shoe boxes on the closet floor. "Size seven and a half," she said.

"That will work," Anna replied.

Denise looked around the sparsely furnished room, then left reluctantly as if she thought Anna might pocket any valuables left lying around.

Having put on Denise's outfit, Anna studied herself in the mirror on the sliding closet door. In any mall in America she would have gone unremarked. Salespeople would trust her. PTAs would welcome her as a member. Anna felt deep, deep undercover. Still, it was good to be free of the Kevlar vest. Anna missed the days when they were an option, not a requirement, for law enforcement rangers.

In the mirror's reflection she noted the single personal item in this impersonal lair. A photograph stood on the black wooden nightstand. Drawn to it, Anna picked it up. A narrow rectangle, matted to fit the standard frame, showed a much younger Denise in her Park Service uniform. Three fingers wrapped around her right arm. It must have been taken when she was with Peter. He'd been cut out and the mat redone to cover the excision. Symbolic, this hiding of the past with a black mask. In the photo Denise was smiling, an expression Anna had seldom seen on her face. It had been taken before Denise had gotten her teeth capped. Her old incisors, the way they neatly overlapped, struck Anna as familiar.

"Are you done?" Denise demanded. She had entered without knocking and stood in the bedroom door radiating disapproval.

"Yes," Anna said. "Is this you?" she asked, holding up the photograph.

"It was," Denise said.

"You remind me of somebody," Anna said, turning the picture to study the image.

Denise laughed, a cartoon laugh, "Heh, heh, heh." In two steps, she'd crossed the small room and taken the picture from Anna's hands. "I have that kind of face. I always remind somebody of somebody else." Opening the drawer on the nightstand, she dropped it in facedown, then snapped the drawer closed again. "Let me get dressed."

Summarily dismissed, Anna slunk back into the living room. She'd thought the woman had been warming to her. Evidently that phase of their relationship was abruptly at an end. Why? Was Denise hiding something? Shame at having cut Peter from a picture? Embarrassment at having her crooked teeth on display? Her sudden iciness seemed overkill for such minor humiliations.

Unless Anna had stumbled on a sore spot, pushed an old button. Perhaps Denise had been teased about the teeth. One never knew which closets harbored a stranger's skeletons.

In moments Denise emerged from the bedroom in black slacks and a white sleeveless mock turtleneck. "Let's get on with it," she said as she walked to the door. Opening it, she held it, whisking Anna out with a sweep of her hand.

Door closed and locked, Denise relaxed marginally. By the time they'd traveled down the stairs to the garage, she seemed nearly her usual slightly weird self.

She opened the door of a forest green Mazda Miata. The top was down. "Cool," Anna said as she slid in.

"Not very practical," Denise said as if she quoted a stern and humorless mother.

Cecelia's Coffee Shop was on the town square in the heart of Bar Harbor's tourist district. Had the Miata not been so small, parking would have been a bitch; as it was, Denise slipped into a slot between two SUVs less than a block from the square.

She and Anna were intentionally early. They bought ice cream in small foam cups from a vendor in a pseudo-nineteenth-century cart complete with horse, then wandered to a bench in the square where they could watch the coffee shop.

"Your stalker can't have too sinister an intent on his mind," Denise said as she carved out a neat bite of ice cream with her tiny plastic spork.

"Not here," Anna agreed. This wasn't the haunted house at midnight.

There would be no kidnapping, raping, or pillaging. Café tables sat beneath a striped awning, mothers and students and tourists perching on the ironwork chairs. People in shorts and T-shirts carrying plastic bags emblazoned with the names of local shops entered. A few minutes later they exited, iced coffee or mochaccino in hand. Nothing fishy, nothing shady.

On such a sunny afternoon, in the middle of a town set above the glittering blue of the Atlantic, and Disneyesque in its adorability, kidnapping, raping, and pillaging seemed an alien concept. Surely a species that invented ice cream, kites, and flip-flops would be incapable of harming a hair on a puppy's head.

The mystery of humanity wasn't that people were starkly evil or magnificently good but that they were both all the time. Sanity and insanity dwelt side by side in the human brain. Only when one grew so big it overshadowed and starved the other was it noticed.

People tended to either keep their crazy to themselves or gather with others sharing the same delusion. Churches, synagogues, temples, covens, mosques: If enough people believed a thing, it was declared sane. One person speaking to invisible beings was a nutcase. A thousand was a cult. Ten thousand, a religion.

Fortunately, most human madness was harmless, creative even; it made life rich and memorable and annoyingly real.

"Any clue as to what we're looking for?" Denise asked, cutting into Anna's thoughts.

"Nope." Anna took a small bite of pistachio ice cream and let it melt on her tongue for a moment. "Early on I would have said teenage boys or girls, but they aren't the sort who track victims across land for a couple thousand miles. That takes money and autonomy."

"Any Dirty Uncle Ernies on the radar?" Denise asked.

"Not since she was nine."

"Goddamn sons of bitches," Denise said.

Two white high-school-aged girls and a woman who could have been their mother sat at one of the tables. Both girls were on iPhones. Mom, evidently old school, read a paperback novel. An older white male with a fat dachshund on a pink leash sat at another table and read a newspaper. Two boys came, opened their laptops on the third table, and ignored each other.

The older man finished his coffee. He and his hound ambled off. A barista cleared away his paper cup. Two middle-aged black women, both in capri pants and high-heeled sandals, took his place, sipping iced coffee. Obeying some psychic—or cyber—signal, the boys simultaneously folded up their laptops and left, still not speaking.

Time for the rendezvous came and went.

As afternoon on the square melted into evening on the square, Anna told Denise the details of the bullying. "At first we figured it must be a kid—or kids—in her school. As it turns out, if the victim doesn't know the bullies or the bullies don't ID themselves, or friends rat them out, there is virtually—and in this sense I mean virtually literally—no way to track them."

"There's got to be," Denise said, settling on a bench near an old cannon on a concrete slab. "They can hack into your computer and record every keystroke you make, redirect your browser to ad sites, turn on the volume when they want to sing you a slogan, pinpoint your position anywhere on the face of the earth, find out what color panties you're wearing, then try and sell you Viagra. How can they not track some pricks bullying a girl?"

"I guess we're talking different theys," Anna said as she spooned up a bit of the green dessert and laid it neatly on the end of her tongue, where it would melt over as many taste buds as possible on its journey to her esophagus.

"The capitalist theys are more motivated and tech-savvy than the don't-bully-children theys," Anna finished.

"And you can bet not one of them gives a flying fig about lost girls. Not one," Denise said as she savagely attacked the chocolate chunk with her spork. "What makes you think it isn't scumbag kids?" she asked around a mouthful of ice cream. "It stinks of scumbag kid fun to me."

"Asking for a face-to-face," Anna replied as she watched the people coming and going at the coffee shop. "To make a trip cross-country suggests an adult with the independence and money to travel."

"What does the girl . . . Elizabeth?"

Anna nodded.

"What does Elizabeth think of the new development?" Denise asked.

"She doesn't know yet. Her mother said she needed some time by herself. The combined concern of her mother, her great-aunt Gwen, and probably me can't be all that easy to deal with. Poor kid."

"Yeah, poor kid," Denise echoed dully.

Anna was thinking of her husband, Paul. Never had anyone loved her like he did. More than she deserved. More than she could accept sometimes. There were moments it was as if she dared not feel pain because he would feel it as well, when she could not choose to spend herself as she would like because of what it would cost him.

"Unconditional love, in large doses, can be a burden," she mused.

"I wouldn't know," Denise said.

Her tone snapped Anna out of her reverie. "There's an odd one," she said to deflect the feeling of guilt Denise's sudden exposure had awakened. Using her spork, she gestured toward a woman nearing the coffee shop. She was plump, tall in platform sandals. Screaming red hair was styled in a short curly cap and set off by oversized glasses framed in turquoise. An enormous straw bag flapped at her legs as she walked, gripped by a hand as round and dimpled as that of a child, though the woman was probably in her mid-to-late thirties.

"What's that in her bag?" Denise asked.

"Damn," Anna said, then laughed. "It looks like a welding glove."

"I think we've lost our window of opportunity," Denise said finally.

"Maybe a no-show," Anna said.

"Maybe," Denise replied.

"Got cold feet?" Anna wondered.

"Made us?" Denise suggested.

"More likely, we didn't make him." Two college boys online, one old guy with a dog, one fat guy with badly behaved offspring. Woman with a Bozo hairdo. Nothing screamed stalker.

"We're nowhere," Anna admitted. Her cell phone buzzed. "Excuse me," she said as she looked at the screen. "It's our victim's mother, probably wanting to know how we're doing." Anna poked the green phone icon and put the cell phone to her ear. "Heath," she said.

"Elizabeth has gone missing."

"You said she needed time alone," Anna said, surprised at the terror in Heath's voice.

"Hours ago, damn it! Hours ago. This island is the size of a postage stamp. She hasn't come back," Heath said.

Her fear awoke Anna's. This wasn't like E, to worry people she loved.

"Is Wily with her?" Anna demanded.

"I guess," Heath said distractedly.

Anna smothered the urge to say, "That's okay then." Absurd as it was, the fact that the old dog was with E reassured her. Anna and Wily had forged an odd connection in the North Woods of Minnesota. It wasn't something Anna chose to talk about. She doubted Wily did either.

"Anna, I'm pretty sure she's not on the island," Heath almost wailed. "I've looked everywhere I can, and called until I'm hoarse."

While Anna had been neatly occupied eating ice cream in Bar Harbor, E had disappeared. Were the two connected? Had Anna been made a patsy? "Is Gwen with you?"

"No, Gwen and John went to Bangor for the evening. Dinner and a visit with Chris Zuckerberg."

"I'm on my way. Give me half an hour," Anna said. It would take her that long to talk somebody out of a boat and get to the island. Elizabeth's body—Anna shuddered as she thought the word—would be found only by boat if she had fallen.

Or jumped.

TWENTY-ONE

Heath half crouched near the wall of boulders ringing the area that had been leveled to build the tower and house. She had on Dem Bones, her high-tech robotic walking suit, legs and belly strapped in, bright silver lozenge-shaped pieces of machinery on the outside of her thighs and calves, hinges at hip and knee. The arm-brace crutches lay fifteen feet away where she'd flung them in a rage when they got in the way of her attempts to get this so-called wonder of modern technology to complete the simple task of moving her bony ass up and over the chunks of stone calved off the granite wall.

"Goddamn useless piece of shit," she cried. Her hands clawed at the slick rock as the weight of her lower limbs, and the titanium skeleton, dragged her down. Using the motions available to her, she could only manage to kick uselessly at the rock with feet like senseless clubs, and knees not worth the effort it took technology to bend them.

As she slid back for the third time, leaving long white scratches on the glossy silver finish of the thigh and calf pieces, she screamed like a wounded panther.

Frustration consumed energy that, left alone, would turn to thoughts.

There was nothing Heath could think that wasn't insupportable, that wouldn't sear the marrow in her bones. Someone was stalking her daughter; now her daughter was missing. Heath had been a fool to think cyberfilth would be the sum total of it. She was a fool not to have taken E to London, put her into witness protection, hired bodyguards. Such was her arrogant stupidity, she had thought a cripple, an old dog, and a septuagenarian pediatrician could keep her child safe.

E hasn't been missing all that long, she told herself.

"Damned she hasn't," she said aloud. Only a few hours, but Boar Island wasn't a few hours' worth of adventure. Heath automatically reached down her right hand. No wheelchair, no saddlebags, no cigarettes. "Piece of shit," she muttered.

Never would E intentionally scare her or Gwen by staying away so long. Wily would have come back if he could have, if for no other reason than his dinner was served at five every day. If E was hurt, Wily would have howled when he heard Heath calling his name. There was no girl and no dog, and the only way that could happen was if they'd been taken.

Not jumped or fallen, Heath thought. E wouldn't take Wily with her into the grave, and Wily wasn't the type to leap off a fifty-foot cliff even if E did. Besides, Elizabeth was past suicide. She was.

The lift bell rang. Frankenstein-like, Heath turned, then lurched toward where the elevator would release its passenger. "It better be you, Anna," she shouted as she monstered across the level rock. Anna didn't deserve that. Scarcely thirty-five minutes had passed since Heath called. The superwoman suit didn't deserve to be called a piece of shit either, for that matter. Heath didn't care. Choices were limited: She could rage or she could fall apart.

The lift clattered into its dock with a groan that, no matter how often Heath heard it, seemed to presage immediate disaster. Anna stepped off. "It's me," she said unnecessarily. She was in her full ranger costume, gun and all. Heath was so glad to see her, she could have burst into tears.

"About time," she said.

Anna paid no attention to the snarling dog that had possessed Heath. Undoubtedly she'd seen that fear hound more times than she'd care to remember. Heath was grateful.

"Where have you looked?" Anna asked.

"Goddamn nowhere," Heath admitted. "I got back into the ruins a ways and called. There is so much crap on the ground and the floors are so rotten, I couldn't do much inside. The rest of this godforsaken rock might as well be Mars. I can't get out of this bear pit. I went up and down the lift a few times and saw what I could from the dock. I butted myself up the whole piece-of-shit tower, one hundred and seventy feet of metal stairs, and couldn't see a damn thing from the windows. Couldn't hold myself up to look over the sills for more than a second. That's it. That's it."

"How long has she been gone, and how did she go?" Anna asked.

Heath sputtered out the tale of the lobsters and Wily. "John picked Gwen up a few minutes later. It never occurred to us that E wouldn't be right back. I am an idiot," she finished.

Anna nodded as if Heath had given her a measured professional report of the search to date. She looked around the open space at the rocks and rubble, then up at the sky.

"Light's going," Anna said. "We'd better figure out where she headed and then get moving. You want to come?"

Heath wanted to. She wanted it so much she could feel her fingers curling around Anna's from where she stood.

"No," she said through stiff lips. "You'll move faster alone."

TWENTY-TWO

Denise sat behind the wheel of her car shaking. Not shaking. Twitching like a doll with its legs stuck in a garbage disposal. Tears—a luxury she seldom enjoyed—poured down her face. Before Paulette came and gave her permission to feel, one of the few times she'd cried was the day she heard Peter was engaged. Those tears had been turned to steam by white-hot anger before they'd reached the air. She'd almost missed the days when her tear ducts had been welded shut. Now great fat drops ran down the side of her nose to drip on the black linen of her trousers.

Ranger Pigeon was finally gone. She'd been in Denise's bedroom—again—changing out of Denise's clothes, then used Denise's bathroom, no doubt rummaging through the medicine cabinet, and the towel cupboard, and under the sink, looking for anything that would trigger the memory of who Denise's photo reminded her of. Her ferreting brain ticking like a bomb.

Denise had screwed up royally at the scene. She'd acted guilty as hell, searching the murder room for traces she might have left while the pigeon watched from the doorway, running back to the car and hiding, practically running the woman over to get her away from Paulette, going part postal over the old picture. Anna Pigeon was one of those people who saw, who looked and saw the person behind the eyes. Denise had run up about a dozen red flags.

"God damn me!" Denise cried and struck a fist against the steering wheel. "I didn't think. I didn't fucking think!" When she'd offered Anna a change of clothes, and the use of her car for the undercover stint, she hadn't thought of Paulette, of the plan. She had a family now. She had to think of them first, before the job, before cyberstalkers, before endangered citizens, before herself. Family came before everything. Family was everything.

"Don't screw this up," she muttered fiercely, then turned the key in the ignition, bringing the Miata to life. She had to see Paulette. They needed to talk this through. Denise was still in her civvies, still in the Miata, her radio on the passenger seat monitoring the traffic. It would be a risk, but the sense of urgency driving her made it imperative. She looked at her watch. Seven fifteen. Paulette was a nurse. Three days a week she worked the two-to-midnight shift in the infants ward at Mount Desert Hospital. This was one of her nights. Pulling out of the NPS headquarters' parking lot, Denise texted: *mt me H pking lot. 10 min.*

By the time she reached the hospital, the sun was going down. The long summer afternoons were golden, the light softening trees to a dark haze and turning the ocean to navy blue.

When she and her sister were ready, Denise decided, they would move somewhere there was no ocean, no winter, where the world wasn't made of rock and snow and ice water. Georgia maybe. Georgia in the pines, a little cabin. That would be perfect. Maybe a lake. Too dangerous, she decided as she parked the Miata in the darkest corner behind the building. Kids drowned in lakes all the time. In Georgia there might be alligators. Alligators liked children and little fluffy dogs. She'd read that somewhere.

Turning off the ignition, Denise lay back in her seat and waited. Paulette might not be able to get away instantly, but she'd come. Denise knew she would. They were twins. They had the exact same blood and bone and brain. They didn't have identical fingerprints. Had she ever Googled that in a hurry! What a drag it would have been if Paulette's fingerprints at the murder scene lit up Denise's own on IAFIS, the federal print identification base.

In everything that mattered, they were identical. Paulette would never let her down.

Ranger Pigeon and that damned picture. "Is this *you*? You remind me of *somebody*." The memory bit Denise in the butt again. In a fit of paranoia, she leapt from the car to put the top up. Nobody would be looking; still, it was best if she and Paulette were not seen together.

With the lowering of the sun, clouds came scudding from the southwest, and fog began to tease in from its hiding places out to sea. Good, Denise thought as she clipped the top securely down. Once she had hated the fog, hated the clammy dead touch of mist, and the confusion of veils across her eyes. Now it made her feel safer. To be hidden was calming, centering, like the world beneath the sea.

As she settled behind the wheel in the tiny car, a slash of light cut the deep shadow in the back of the building; the fire stairs, that was where the nurses left the building. There were no reserved spaces; their cars had to be parked in the back lot, the dark lot, the lot where bad things could happen.

"Screw men," Denise whispered. "Screw them all. Bastards."

She thought to flash the headlights to identify herself, but there was no need. Paulette would know where she was. She would feel her in the gray cloak of encroaching fog the way one hand felt the other in a game of cat's cradle. Such an old game. Denise couldn't remember anyone teaching it to her. No cheery childhood memories of doting grandmamas or loving aunts.

Poor little Anna Pigeon and her poor little Elizabeth suffering from a surfeit of love. "Such a burden!" Denise mocked, her voice pitched low. "God, how does one bear it!" She should have gouged Pigeon's eye out with a spork.

Nope, nobody had bothered teaching poor little Denise a nice game like cat's cradle.

Maybe it was a memory of Paulette's that had traveled into her head.

God damn Anna Pigeon. God damn Denise Castle for letting her into her apartment, leaving her alone in the bedroom, for not hiding the photograph.

Now she and Paulette were going to have to speed things up. The luxury of time was gone. It had drained away like water down a gopher hole during the time Anna Pigeon was with her. Beady eyes licking over everything, foxy ears perked, the pigeon watched and thought while Denise did everything but spray-paint GUILTY on the clean white walls of her apartment.

Paulette had to move faster on the land sale, and Denise on tracking down the legacy advertised in the papers. If there was a legacy. She also had to give the NPS notice and get her pension papers filed. Everything had to be in place so they could tie up the loose ends and be gone before anybody knew there was any reason to think there were two of them, that they had anything to do with Duffy's demise.

"I don't have long," Paulette said as she slid in the passenger door. "I said I was going out for a cigarette. The head nurse is cool with that. She smokes a pack and a half a day."

"We'll have to quit when the family is complete," Denise said, though she'd never smoked a cigarette in her life.

"Complete?" Paulette questioned.

That Paulette didn't inherently understand annoyed Denise. She pressed the sensation down hard. Paulette was her sister, her other self; she could never be annoyed with her. Not ever. "We're going be a family,"

Denise explained patiently. "Like we wanted. Like we are supposed to be. It's the last thing we have to do before we go. We got rid of Kurt. Now, as soon as we are complete, we can go. Have to go, and sooner rather than later."

Paulette looked confused. Or maybe Denise just felt her confusion. The little shards of streetlights and security lights refracting in the rear-view mirrors weren't sufficient to read a face.

"A family. More than just you and me?" Paulette asked.

Again the stab of irritation; again Denise shoved it down. "Families have children," Denise said too sharply.

"You said Peter had murdered your babies," Paulette said in a gentle voice. "Tell me how it was."

The irritation Denise was suffering wasn't for her sister, her twin. It was like the twitches, a case of nerves. She took hold of Paulette's hand and leaned back in the seat. The memory didn't come; it was always there, sharper and more detailed each time she revisited it.

"Four years ago I got pregnant," Denise said. "It was Peter's, of course. I loved my baby. I knew I wasn't getting any younger, and I loved my baby so much."

"Did Peter beat you?" Paulette asked. That was how her babies had been murdered.

"He said he didn't want our baby. He said he never wanted children. He said he couldn't face it. He made me get an abortion." He'd said he'd leave her if she didn't get an abortion, that's what he had said, but it was the same thing.

"Something went wrong," Denise said. "Something got ripped. I was told I couldn't have any more children. Then Peter left."

"And married Lily and had a baby," Paulette finished softly.

"My baby," Denise said.

Paulette squeezed her hand. "Is that why you came? To tell me about the baby?"

Denise opened her eyes, suddenly back from the ugly trip down Memory Lane. Peter had turned what should have been a sentimental journey into a nightmare on Elm Street. "No. I came to tell you we have to move faster. It's that ranger, Anna Pigeon. I caught her looking at a photo of us. Then she peers into me. Icepick eyes. I got that shivery feeling you get when something bad is about to happen."

"Who took the photo of us?" Alarmed, Paulette jerked her hand out of Denise's. Hot snaps of anger cracked up Denise's spine.

Not for Paulette. Nerves.

"It wasn't us exactly," Denise said. "It was me, before I got my teeth capped. My hair was blond then, and wild." For a moment she believed that, but it wasn't right. Her teeth hadn't been capped yet, true, but in the picture her hair wasn't like Paulette's. It was the same boring brown as it always was. For a moment, in her mind, she'd seen it blond and big like her sister's. Rubbing her face, she mumbled through her fingers, "Anna Pigeon knows. She stares at the picture, then gives me this smirky look and says, 'Is this *you*? You remind me of *somebody*.' She spent a lot of time with you at the house. She knows. Why would she say 'you remind me of somebody' unless she wanted me to know she knew I had a twin?"

There was a wrongness to her logic, Denise knew that; still and all, she felt it to be the truth. Knew it to be the truth. "Anna Pigeon will ruin everything."

Paulette sat quiet for a long time. Denise could feel twitches building in her hands, her feet. The sparks of anger flared in her esophagus until she thought she might breathe fire.

"Anna Pigeon, she's the ranger who came with you when the police were at my house?" Paulette asked, her words coming slowly, as if her mind were working hard between each utterance.

"That was her," Denise said. "Shit!" She slammed the heel of her hand against the steering wheel. "I never should have let the bitch out of the car. She's got a nose as long as a dachshund's, sticking it where it doesn't belong."

"I think maybe she knew I was me," Paulette admitted. "She looked at me like you said she looked at the picture, like she knew I was inside, there behind my eyes, and she was going to scrape me out like an oyster out of its shell."

Denise became still, no twitches, no angry motions. Staring at her sister, she let the awe that had been building since they'd found each other fill her whole being. Paulette knew everything that happened in Denise's head just as Denise knew everything that happened in Paulette's head. "Exactly like that. An oyster from its shell," Denise whispered.

"Oh God," Paulette moaned. "Maybe she looks at everybody like that. She's probably just the kind of person who really looks at things."

That wasn't it. Denise knew. Paulette knew, too; she just didn't want to admit it.

For a long time neither one of them spoke. Denise didn't feel alone in the silence. She felt *together* in the silence. Mostly.

"What do we do?" Paulette asked at last.

"I'll think of something. It's us against the world." Denise laughed because she knew it was true, the only truth.

TWENTY-THREE

The agony that stretched Heath's skin thin over the bones of her face fueled Anna's own fears. "Let's get started," she said, and turned away from her friend lest their terrors coalesce into panic. Eyes long since trained to look for spoor darted over the natural patio and the boulders surrounding it. A half-chewed bone—a project of Wily's, no doubt; flecks of brown tobacco, blowing in idle circles, eddying in the breeze where the walls formed a corner; faint tracks—the tread of Robo-butt's rubber wheels leaving bits of dried mud in the light burnishing of dust.

"It hasn't rained," Anna said.

"No. Why are we talking about the weather?" Heath was fighting tears. Anna could feel fear and shame and guilt boiling off of her like heat from pavement.

"Your wheelchair left tracks. See. Dry now, but you rolled through water. Why?" Anna asked. In the zone where spoor and prey are all that matters, Anna barely heard Heath's sputtered curses as she backtracked to where the wheels had found enough water to make mud.

"The lobsters," Heath cried suddenly. "They were in a bucket there. Gwen put them down, and we forgot all about them."

"No lobsters, no bucket," Anna said. "Do you think John Whitman took them? Maybe when he came for Gwen, he took them home to eat them himself?"

Heath thought for a moment, then said, "No. I watched Gwen and John go down the lift. Gwen had her little book-pack full of things for Ms. Zuckerberg, and her purse. John wasn't carrying anything. Both hands were empty. I'm sure of it."

"Somebody took lobsters and bucket. E? Returning to the scene of the crime to rescue the lobsters from the pot?" Anna suggested.

"Yes!" Heath almost shouted. "Yes! She would have come back and gotten them. She would want to set them free. Save their creepy crustacean lives out of the goodness of her heart. Yes. Oh, God. How long does it take to let a couple lobsters go? Ten minutes? We're in the middle of the goddamn ocean. Not even five. She's been gone three hours and twenty-three minutes," Heath wailed. She looked at her wristwatch. "Twenty-six minutes," she amended.

Anna didn't bother to ask Heath if she'd called 911, the Coast Guard, or the army. She knew the drill: Nobody looked for adults—and for this, E counted as an adult—until they'd been missing for forty-eight hours. Nobody looked for an emotional teenager out of sight for a few hours.

Heath's eyes filled with tears. Anna turned her back lest the contagion spread.

Elizabeth, worrying her mother into a state of frenzy, and risking Anna's wrath, by vanishing; that wasn't the child Anna had godparented. E cared what people thought of her, especially the people she loved. Often Anna had wondered if she cared too much, spent too much of her childhood being a parent to those around her, taking care of everybody at the expense of taking care of herself.

It would take a momentous event to lift that burden from E, to make her as thoughtless as the average person. Unless Barnum & Bailey had pitched a tent on Boar Island, or Brad Pitt made an unscheduled stop, Anna couldn't think what might distract E from her customary responsibilities.

If Brad, Barnum, and Bailey were out of the picture, the landscape became darker. Either E was not on the island or she was on the island but could not get back to the lighthouse. Anna tried to picture her curled up in the fetal position beneath the overhang of a boulder, Wily beside her. Asleep maybe.

Several hours was a long time to sleep on a rock.

A sixteen-year-old girl, possibly suicidal, definitely tormented, gone for hours on a rock not big enough to register on most charts.

That line of thought served no one.

"So, E came back and got the bucket with the lobsters," Anna said. "Describe it."

"It was a bucket. A regular bucket," Heath said. Then she threw her head back like a cat and yowled, "Elizabeth!"

Anna had seen Heath under pressure before. In life-and-death situations, physical stress and emotional pain, but she'd never seen her like this, losing control, becoming a victim herself.

"Think," she demanded. Then went on, "Bucket full of water and lobsters, the bucket would weigh close to thirty pounds. So E could lift it, but not carry it easily. Buckets are awkward. So she's got the lobsters, and she's planning on emancipating them. Elizabeth would know they'd die if she just turned them loose on a rock in the sun. Might as well go ahead and boil them, if she was going to do that. At least it would be faster." Anna followed a slopping trail where water had mixed with sand particles and dust, then been dragged through with a smooth shoe, probably Elizabeth's flip-flop. It led to the wall that protected the patio from the fifty-foot drop to the ocean. Anna leaned out and looked down the precipitous fall to the rocks below. "So she dragged the bucket to the cliff and looked over. That's a long way down. If she poured them over, the fall might kill them."

"The lift," Heath said.

"The bell ringing would bring you and Gwen running," Anna said.

"And she didn't want to see us. Didn't want to talk to us. Couldn't believe we would talk about boiling living things alive so we could watch them die." Heath's voice was climbing and diving as her mind drove it from self-hatred to despair.

"I need you to focus," Anna said. "Was the bucket metal or wood?"

"Metal," Heath managed, then pressed her lips together as if holding back a horde of wasps wanting to swarm out of her mouth.

"Five gallons or thereabout?" Anna asked. Five was a standard bucket size.

"About." Heath let the word out before resealing her lips.

"Full of lobsters and water," Anna said. "Heavy." She studied the granite above where the water had spilled, then dried. "There."

"I don't see anything," Heath said, coming so close she rolled one wheel half over Anna's toes.

Anna ignored the pain. Heath had enough on her mind. "There," she pointed. "See where the metal bucket scraped the rock. E hauled it up here. Dragging." Following the marks, Anna climbed the sloping face of the boulder on hands and feet. Her left arm ached. Since she'd been wounded it had never recovered its full strength. Physical therapy had only gotten it so far. After that, Anna treated it with denial.

Eyes to the ground, she climbed and boulder-hopped past the ruined wings of the old house and around the broken upthrust of granite.

The north side of the island, scarcely as big as two football fields, was formed of enormous chunks of granite that had cracked and worn over the eons until it created steep rounded steps descending in giant leaps to the sea. Sunlight caught shining facets, making them sparkle. Scrubby mosses and lichens grew between the rocks as if they'd been there forever. Anna smiled at the thought. Of course they'd been there forever. They were rocks.

Fissures wide enough to accommodate the passage of a slender girl and a skinny dog made a grid pattern. The lines were not straight or square enough to look man-made, but nearly so. Varying heights of rocks blocked any view of the island's shoreline.

As she stared into the distance over the swells, it struck Anna how much bigger the Atlantic seemed than the Pacific. The Atlantic and Pacific would be the only two oceans Elizabeth had ever seen. Before Heath found E, she knew nothing about the world. She was homeschooled. Her reading skills were strong, as were her math skills. She scored high on the IQ test the therapist Heath had hired gave her. Elizabeth could cook and sew better than most grown women. She knew the names of the major stars and constellations. But about the world's geography and sociology she'd been taught very little.

A lot of nine-year-olds at least knew there were seven seas. Elizabeth hadn't. She hadn't even known there were fifty states. Heath said she hadn't been aware there were people of different colors or who spoke different languages. She hadn't known people were gay or monogamous.

No television. No movies. No radio.

The world of the cult compound had little variety; everybody was considered a brother or sister or cousin whether they were blood relations or not. Polygamous, white, religious, and completely contained between the dusty gold walls of a canyon west of Loveland, Colorado, was the only life Elizabeth knew until Heath had adopted her. For the seven years since, she'd been in Boulder learning to be a twenty-first-century little girl. Then a high school girl.

Then a shamed and shunned pariah.

Now she was suddenly half a continent from Colorado, from her friends, marooned on an island. A lot for a person to deal with, Anna thought.

There was little in the way of earth or plants to mark the passage of girl and dog, but Elizabeth had not been trying to cover her tracks, so Anna followed the trail easily. The heavy bucket had slopped, leaving traces of disturbance in the fine dust. Where Elizabeth slid off of one boulder and onto to a lower one, the bucket left scrapes on the stone when she'd dragged it after her. Wily, probably not with the intention of helping Anna, but one never knew when it came to Wily, had lifted his leg several times, leaving a faint darker stain on the sparse dusty grasses that clung in the wisps of blown earth.

Following the trail, Anna wended her way downward in zigzags between boulders until she reached a point where she could finally see the edge of the little island. Twenty feet directly below where she'd stopped, water lapped the rugged shore. Anna stared at waves beating themselves to a froth on ragged rocks.

E wouldn't have dumped the lobsters here; there were too many rocks to ensure they'd have a safe landing.

As Anna picked her way through the maze of giant granite blocks tumbled together around the base of the island, she lost sight of both sea and mainland. In a slot between two great chunks of rock no more than six feet apart, the maze ended abruptly in a three-foot drop to dark water. The slot between the boulders continued several yards farther, creating a narrow inlet protected from the wind and much of the power of the sea.

Anna squatted, studying the lip of the stone above the water. The edge was sharp, squared off at a neat ninety degrees, the face making a straight line down toward the water. Getting to her hands and knees to take advantage of the low-angled afternoon light, Anna could see where Elizabeth had smudged the dust as she sat on the edge of the rock, her feet dangling over.

A wave rushed up the narrow channel and exploded against the island, coating Anna's skin with chilling spray. Beyond the mouth of the slot was a thin feathery line: fog cat-footing in.

The wave was sucked back into the gullet of the ocean, baring the boulders walling the slot. Along the stones at the waterline were scrapes of brown and a single sketch of blue. A small boat had docked here more than once.

Any legitimate visitor would bring his boat to the jetty, ring the bell, and walk in the front door.

As Anna leaned forward to study the marks, a wavering fishy silver flashed beneath the water. Fourteen inches beneath the water, on a ledge, lying on its side, was a bucket. The bucket.

This was the end of the trail. This was where E had loosed Gwen's dinner guests.

Anna lay down on her belly and reached into the water, icy even in the heat of summer, and managed to snag the handle of the bucket and haul it out of the water. Setting it carefully aside, where it wouldn't drip on anything vital, she made a minute inspection of the place from which E had vanished.

Tiny grasses were uprooted from a crack near where Elizabeth's left hand must have rested. Sand had been swept away on one side of the rocks bordering where the boat came into the island's embrace.

Elizabeth had not jumped or swum.

She'd been dragged off of Boar.

TWENTY-FOUR

Again Heath looked at her watch. Less than two minutes had passed since last time. Finally she held it up to her ear. Ticking. Time and its petty pace were making her crazy. At minute twenty-four, Anna slid back down the same rock she'd climbed out over.

"Bucket track," she said succinctly as she dropped the lobster pail to the ground. "I found where Elizabeth dumped the lobsters. There were skid marks in the loose gravel on the rock. A handful of plants were ripped from a crack as if she'd grabbed them to keep from being pulled into the water."

Heath felt her heart stop. When it started again each beat struck a blow to her rib cage from the inside. "Slipped and fell?" she croaked. "Drowned?" This had to be what dying felt like. Everything was going black but for Anna's face. Maybe Heath was falling. She couldn't tell.

"I don't think so," Anna said as she trotted toward the lift. "Wily is gone as well, and there were scrape marks on either side of the rock crack where she set the lobsters loose. A small boat is my guess."

"She took a boat?" Heath said stupidly. Her ears were hearing words.

She could see Anna's lips moving, but her brain was having a hard time making sense of things. "With Wily?"

"A boat took her, and I hope they took Wily and didn't just kill him and dump the body," Anna said as she opened the lift gate. "Coming?"

Leah said saltwater could damage Dem Bones's electronics. Leah said, "You break it, you buy it." She meant it. Leah was not a fanciful genius. To her a cliché was as good as a contract.

To hell with Leah. Heath couldn't take the time to get out of the thing and into Robo-butt.

"Of course I'm coming."

Anna turned and walked toward the lift.

Heath followed, the crutches giving her balance.

Anna was piloting the small NPS runabout, a single-engine boat with a canvas shelter over the steering wheel. Heath relinquished pride in favor of speed and let herself lean heavily on Anna's shoulder as the metal and electronics lifted her feet and legs from the dock and over the gunwale one at an excruciating time. With a push and a whirr, she was seated on the plastic bench that ran along the port side of the runabout. Anna held up an orange life jacket. Heath wanted to tell her to drop the thing, get a move on. Knowing it would take longer to argue, and she wouldn't win, she clenched her teeth and held her arms out so Anna could thread the PFD onto her shoulders.

"I'll get the straps," she insisted as Anna started to do up the front of the life preserver. Anna looked at her for a second.

"I will," Heath promised.

Evidently Anna believed her. She slipped into her own PFD, leapt out of the boat, untied the lines, leapt back in, and finally, finally, thankyou-babyjesus started the boat.

Breathe, Heath told herself. Breathe. Air came in through her nostrils. She seemed unable to force it down past the concrete closing off her throat.

"Where are we looking?" Heath asked. Her voice was nearly a whine. There was nowhere to look. Just ocean and drowned land.

"We'll start where the boat met up with Elizabeth and Wily. From there we will fan out in arcs. I will be looking for boats. You will be looking for anything, no matter how small, on the water. Every thirty seconds you will blow that whistle around your neck and shout Elizabeth's name and Wily's. When we lose the light, we assume they've made land somewhere—the boat was small, rowboat sized—and we stop. I call Peter, and the rangers start searching the park."

Heath nodded. Words were backed up behind her teeth, but not one of them meant a thing.

Evening, and the encroaching fog, rapidly cooled the air. As Anna pushed the throttle open, the rush of chill wind against Heath's overheated face felt like an acid wash until her skin became acclimated to the new element.

Darkness oozed in from all directions, the ocean, the edge of the sky, out from the islands, their skirts of rock turning black and ominous. Heath felt the world closing down, ending. "It's been hours, she's surely dead," she moaned. "I am such an idiot. I killed her."

Anna pulled the throttle to idle. Turning she stared down at Heath. "Do you want me to slap you?" she asked. "You know, the traditional cure for female hysterics?"

Heath blinked. Anna looked no softer than the granite, no warmer than the fog. Heath swallowed.

"Not necessary," she whispered.

"Good. Talk about something else. Tell me what Gwen's been up to. Anything. Watch and call and blow the whistle." Anna turned back to the control panel and pushed the throttle forward, not far enough to bring the boat up on plane, just above idle so voices could be heard over the engine noise and the wake wouldn't swamp anything that might be floating in the darkening waters.

Heath pulled the brass whistle Elizabeth had given her from under her shirt and life jacket. Sucking in as much air as her shriveled lungs would allow, she blew a long blast, then called weakly, "E! Elizabeth!"

"Good," Anna called over her shoulder. "Now talk to me for thirty seconds and do it again. Keep your eyes on the water."

Talk. About something else. Not the girl dying somewhere because Heath was a fool, a shit-for-brains fool. There was nothing else. Aunt Gwen, she thought, gone with John to Bangor. "Aunt Gwen delivered Ms. Zuckerberg's children." Heath said the words one by one like a not-so-bright schoolchild reciting a poem she didn't understand. When she'd done, she felt herself sinking, her eyes unfocused on the endless deadly expanse of water turning the color of ink. Under all that icy black was a child of light.

"And," Anna prodded. "Talk to me."

Slowly, Heath rose out of the depths and forced herself to think of anything else. "Ms. Zuckerberg isn't doing well. Heart weak. Transient ischemic attacks. She's lost the ability to talk, Gwen said."

"Good," Anna replied, as deaf to the words as Heath was. "Blow, call."

Heath blew the whistle and called Elizabeth's name. Her voice was stronger. The talking was keeping her mind off the horror that wanted to suffocate her as surely as the water had suffocated—

"Ms. Zuckerberg can't talk," Anna said sharply. "When she gets out of the hospital, is she going to her kids?"

"No," Heath said. She knew what Anna was doing. She knew she needed it, but, at the moment, she resented Anna for it. Despair pulled at her with an almost pleasurable force, the way a steep canyon would if she stood—rolled—too close to the edge. Part of her wanted to fall into the nothing that was offered. *Coward,* she cursed herself. Sucking in a lungful of breath, she forced herself to speak. "No. Her kids don't even—"

"Hush!" Anna said and cut the throttles to idle. "Listen."

Through the muffling of the coastal fog, now reaching halfway to

Boar, Heath heard what sounded like a dog's yip. Then nothing. She blew a blast on the whistle. "E!" she screamed. "Elizabeth! Answer me!"

A thin, reedy bark pierced the fog.

"There," Anna pointed to where the mother-of-pearl of the sea met the pearl of the mists. A dark shape, trapezoidal, about the size of an old shipping trunk, touched the water. Then an orange smudge showed above it. The smudge moved suddenly. As they heard the splash of a body hitting the water, a girl screamed.

Anna shoved full throttle.

TWENTY-FIVE

Denise sat at her small neat table in a space between the living room and kitchen called "the dining room" on the lease. In front of her, on the shining black wood, was a spiral notebook of college ruled paper. The cover was bright red.

She laughed. The sound startled her. Covering the notebook with her forearm, she glanced around as if the laughter had emanated from another source.

She was alone.

No. That was the old Denise Castle. *She* had been creakingly, hauntingly alone. An open wound walking through a world of salt and thorns, she'd not dared let anyone close.

Being alone was not being lonely.

People liked to say that. People were full of shit. Alone echoed down hallways of the mind, shrieking with the shrill voice of icy wind through winter-bare branches. Denise had thought that she would be alone forever, but that was just a lie the world told her. She wasn't even alone sitting by herself in her one-bedroom apartment in her single dining chair.

That was the first huge change. Massive. Making her not a ghost, but a guest, at the party. Better than a guest, family. For so many years she'd had to watch sisters and brothers, wives and husbands and children, being families while she was just herself, one hand clapping, a loose end, a fifth wheel. Families didn't even show her the courtesy of knowing they were the lucky ones. They fought and complained, disrespected each other, went years without speaking over a trifle, yelled at their children as if children were annoying pests they were forced to deal with.

Aborting babies.

Getting divorces.

Choosing not to be together on Christmas.

As if everybody had that choice, as if, for Denise, holidays hadn't been an inescapable nightmare, where, like a bird with no place to perch, she circled cold and alone high over lighted windows and laden tables, hoping that someone would invite her in, if even only for an evening. Then, if they did, it was worse because she knew she did not belong. They knew she did not belong. Once she was surrounded, all she wanted to do was get away, be by herself where the pain and shame wouldn't show.

Family cared enough to poke and nag, call too often and hug too tightly; they fell asleep with their head in another's lap, were carried to bed. They gossiped and worried and gave unwelcome advice. Family cared if you showed up for birthdays, chided if you forgot anniversaries, because your presence, mentally and physically, mattered. Family stimulated the psyche. Without it part of a person fell asleep, like a foot held in one position too long.

A part of Denise had gone to sleep like that. It was still alive, but didn't feel alive. It felt like concrete or asphalt. As time passed, the thought of trying to wake it, to suffer the miserable tingling of life returning, had become worse than knowing a portion of her being was as deadwood on a living tree.

Paulette had woken her without a twinge. Denise was fully alive for the first time in forever.

Then she'd killed a man.

Another huge new thing: life and death, both in her hands.

About life, she felt . . . That was it; that was the whole thing, she *felt*. Resentment, jealousy, spite: The stuff she'd been sustaining herself with for so long was not *feeling*. It was what replaced feeling, fake pain directed outward so the real pain would not eat the host alive. Becoming partially dead to keep the other parts from being flayed.

Life *felt* good. What did adults say when she was a kid? "You've got your whole life ahead of you." She'd thought they were idiots. Now she knew what it meant to have her whole life ahead of her.

About killing Kurt, she should feel something. Like sex, or reading *Siddhartha*, people were supposed to be changed by the experience, somehow different afterward. Killing another human being should be like that. One day she was Denise Castle who had never killed a person. The next she was Denise Castle who had taken a human life in sweat and blood and a plastic shower curtain with yellow fishes on it. Those two Denises should be different, but they weren't. Sex and *Siddhartha* had been like that for her as well. Not as big a deal as advertised.

For a moment she marveled at the things that had changed in the past week. Denise Castle: alive, feeling, killer, family woman.

Almost a family woman. That would come, she decided.

Alone and not alone, she returned to her notebook and her list, items that had to be checked off before the whole life she had ahead of her could officially commence.

> *Kill Kurt (Denise)*
> *Sell Land (Paulette)*
> *Quit NPS (retirement pension) (D)*
> *Find out about "Legacy" (if it exists) (P)*
> *Car, car seat, etc.*
> *Give landlord notice*

Arrange for family—Mt. Desert Hospital (D&P)
Leave MA for GA or SC or NC (D&P&O)
Rent (D&P&O)
Buy (D&P&O)

"Kill Kurt" was checked off.

"Sell Land" had a tentative pencil mark next to it. Kurt's house was worthless, but the land was not. The land was paid off; Kurt's parents were dead. He had no brothers and sisters, and no children. Paulette said it was to pass to her on his death. Ownership wasn't an issue. Denise figured Paulette could get around four or five hundred thousand for the place. They should take less if it would move the property more quickly. Timing was important.

They would skip the balancing act of selling and moving. There was no way to know if it would sell in a week or six months. Banks had gotten paranoid after the big savings-and-loan scandals, but given location, location, location, Denise guessed it would move fast. They'd have to find a way to do the paperwork from out of state. By the time it was all settled, they had to be long gone.

The land sale would mean a big infusion of cash, which was good. Denise had about a hundred thousand of her own in investments, and her pension should come to around forty thousand a year, less everything. Maybe a net of thirty. They had enough.

Again she bent over the list.

Between "Sell Land" and "Quit NPS" she penciled in in tiny letters "Remove Obstacle." Not that she'd forget to take care of that particular problem. Denise had an excellent memory—or had until her nerves started going bad. Still, the lists weren't a memory aid; she made lists so she could check things off, have the satisfaction of seeing in black and white what she had accomplished.

"Obstacle" was the second most complex item on the list.

Changing from a pencil to a pen, she underlined it in ink. Denise had hoped she could erase it as unnecessary. That hope was growing slim to nonexistent. There was no doubt in Denise's mind that Anna Pigeon would remember who the Denise in the photograph reminded her of. Those kinds of things tickled at the brain until they were solved. Anna would remember it was Paulette. Given what a nuisance the pigeon was, she would put two and two together and get Murder. If they could move the project along quickly, Anna would only have to be put off for a couple of days, three at most.

Denise overwrote the underlined word in ink. To the side, in parentheses, she wrote "triazolam." Google said triazolam was common enough. As a nurse, Paulette would be able to lay her hands on a few tabs at the hospital. Needed or not, it was important to have the drug option.

For a moment Denise stared at the wall, eyes unfocused.

"Family" was next on her list, the most difficult of all the tasks. She and her sister would be getting a family. Denise smiled. When she was a kid, people would say of a pregnant woman, "She's in a family way." There was something lovely about that. Denise and Paulette were going to be in a family way.

It was poetic justice that lovely fertile Lily was going to be their accomplice.

Lily took ergotamine for her migraines. Denise had Googled the side effects.

God, but Denise loved Google.

TWENTY-SIX

The surface of the sea had embraced the night. Foam and tendrils of mist sketched the waves with iridescence. There was no horizon; the line between water, earth, and air had been erased by the fog. As the boat leapt up onto plane, Heath, in her electronic bones, was thrown backward. Nothing looked real or solid, yet the hull of the boat slammed into the Atlantic as hard as if it traveled a surface of packed dirt. For a few heartbeats, half lying along the plastic bench, Heath thought she was falling, not just to onto the bench but out of the boat, into the sky or the sea.

Since fate or bad luck had decreed Heath had to have one part of her body that refused to work and play well with the others, she was glad it was her legs. Losing her wits—even for a few moments—scared her a whole hell of a lot more than not being able to run and jump.

Sudden silence snatched her mind back into the boat. Anna had shut the engine down. Sucking the quiet into her lungs and mind, Heath struggled to right herself, ears tuned to the sound of the yip, Wily's yip. The happiest sound in the world. Second happiest.

"Blow your whistle," Anna said. Her voice was steady, familiar; it poured into Heath's ears like a homing signal.

The whistle was clutched so tightly in Heath's hand it felt hot when she put it between her mist-chilled lips. She blew two short sharp blasts.

"Elizabeth!" Anna yelled. "E!"

A litany of prayers babbled through Heath's brain: Please God let me find her, please God, let her be okay, please God, please, please, please.

The only sound was the lapping of the waves against the hull like a beast lapping at the blood of its prey. Again Heath had the sensation of falling, but this time it had nothing to do with vertigo. The place she was tumbling into was where the mothers of dead children fell. It had no bottom and no way out.

"Wily!" Anna called. She turned on a spotlight mounted on the gunwale next to the steering wheel. The beacon lanced out, an impotent light-sword. In the fog and dusk it hid as much as it illuminated, the light catching particles of water and refracting back.

A tiny scrap of orange flared for an instant between the glazed obsidian of the water and the gray blanket of fog. "There!" Heath cried, pointing. "Move the light back. There!" A bit of orange flickered in, then out, of vision as the swells moved up and down. "Keep the light on it!" Heath shouted.

Anna didn't reply. Leaving the light where it was, she pushed the throttle gently forward and nosed the boat in the direction Heath was pointing, following the long bobbing finger from the floodlight.

The ocean heaved another great sigh, and the scrap came into sight fifty yards ahead and to the right. "One o'clock," Heath shouted.

"I see it," Anna replied.

Unfortunately, Heath did, too. Every cell in her body was straining toward that orange scrap. The apparition stayed in view a moment longer this time. Not a lovely child in a life jacket. A monster. Short truncated arms poked through holes too big for them. A misshapen skull was sunk into the body of the flotation device. It looked as if the thing were covered in rotting seaweed.

Heath opened her mouth to scream.

Anna beat her to it. "Wily!" she shouted again.

"Over here," came a faint reply.

"What the . . ." Heath's mind cleared. Wily, the dog, was in the life jacket. For an LSD moment, Heath thought Wily had called out, "Over here." Elizabeth! E was invisible in the dark water, but she must be swimming next to him. Alive.

"Coming! Hang on," Heath yelled as she pushed the button to lift herself into a standing position. At the faint whirr of the machinery Anna shot her such a repressive look she immediately whirred her butt back down onto the bench.

Anna had the spotlight on the dog in the life jacket. Heath could see the sleek head of Elizabeth beside Wily, her face a pale oval against the black water. At idle, Anna eased the boat toward them.

Heath's mental litany turned from "Please, please, please" to "Thank you, thank you, thank you," the two fundamental prayers of mankind.

As they neared, Anna ordered Heath to throw Elizabeth a life jacket. Heath pulled off her own and threw it hard in her daughter's direction. Her arms were stronger than they'd ever been, and, thanks to wheelchair basketball, her aim was good.

Elizabeth clung to the life jacket with one hand and to Wily's scruff with the other, her head barely above water. Anna picked Wily out of the water first and deposited him at Heath's feet with a slosh of cold seawater. Never had he looked so much like Wile E. Coyote as he did at that moment, water running from his ears and muzzle, orange vest hanging on his bony shoulders.

E was next, fished out and dumped on the deck with little more ceremony than Wily had received. The light was going fast, and Heath could not tell if Elizabeth or the dog was bloody or bruised.

"What happened? Are you hurt? We've been looking for hours." Questions and comments poured out of Heath so rapidly there was no time for answers. She knew it but could not help herself. Connection to her child demanded it of her, and, denied the luxury of grabbing the girl and holding her so tightly she could never escape again, words had to suffice. "Why is Wily wearing the life preserver!" she demanded as she ran out of breath.

Into the silence that followed, E said calmly, "He can't swim, Mom."

"He can swim," Anna stated flatly.

"Oh, yeah, right, *dog-paddle,*" E retorted.

Wily shook, spattering them with water and making the orange vest flap around his skinny form.

Elizabeth laughed.

How could she be so goddamned calm! Heath was shaking so badly she could hear her legs rattling in their shells. Her chest muscles contracted until drawing breath was nearly impossible, and she could feel her heart pounding so hard it shook her clothes.

"How did you get out here?" Anna demanded.

"A boat took me," E said.

Heath could almost hear the "Duh!" in her voice.

"Kidnapping is a federal offense," Anna said as she snatched the radio mike from its metal holder.

"No!" E cried. "Don't go all law enforcement on me. A friend took me on a boat ride. A nice person."

Anna stopped and stared hard at Elizabeth in the growing gloom. "And you forgot you weren't Jesus Christ and decided to walk home?" she asked.

"My friend wanted to take me back, but I insisted. When we heard you calling and I realized how long we'd been gone, I was afraid you'd arrest . . ."

Silence followed that.

"Why would I arrest a nice friend?" Anna asked.

A person. A friend. Heath could guess why this mysterious individual was genderless. The friend was a boy. Heath had been asking herself what would make a wonderful, considerate child like Elizabeth so forgetful that she would terrify her mother. A boy. A nice boy. A boy/friend. God was good. She was going to shackle E to the iron stair railing in the tower and feed her nothing but bread and water until she was forty years old.

For another moment, Anna just looked at E and said nothing. Elizabeth was hugging her arms, shivering. Anna opened the tiny door under the hull, pulled out a blanket that looked as if it was made of tinfoil, then tossed it to E. "We'll sort this out later. Wrap up. Both you and Wily." She shot Wily a hard look. "You should have known better," she said to the dog.

With that, Anna pushed the throttle to full and turned the boat back toward Boar Island.

Both Wily and E had bathed and toweled off. Anna built a small fire in the great hearth in the outer room skirting the tower. The evening was mild, but girl and dog had gotten thoroughly chilled. Anna also made tea. Elizabeth wrinkled her nose, then sighed. "Hot drinks, I know, the wilderness cure-all. Does Wily have to drink tea, too?"

Neither Heath nor Anna answered. Heath was seated in Robo-butt, her knees almost touching the overstuffed chair where her daughter was curled up. Elizabeth's feet peeked out from beneath a hand-knitted throw of purple and green. In T-shirt and sweatpants, her hair damp from the bath, and no makeup, she looked like a little girl. A delightful fact Heath knew better than to share aloud.

Sprawled in front of the hearth, Wily looked old and tired, his fur ragged and spiked with damp, his pointed ears at half-mast. Elizabeth might have deserved a ducking in icy water for being so thoughtless, but Wily didn't. The cold was hard on his old bones.

"Enough," she said to her daughter. "Tell us every single thing from the beginning of time."

"Billions and billions of years ago this was a vast inland sea," Elizabeth droned in a mockery of PBS specials.

"Don't," Heath warned. She wanted to be angry. It was spoiled by the fact that she had not heard such sauciness from Elizabeth since before the razor-in-the-tub incident. That, and the fact her daughter was alive and in one piece.

"Just tell it," Anna said quietly.

"Aunt Gwen was going to boil some lobsters alive," E said. Heath saw the wince in Anna's gaze at the same moment it clutched her own chest.

"I freaked," E apologized.

Heath had come to the conclusion it was she and Aunt Gwen who needed to apologize.

"I mean boiling alive, how rotten is that? So Wily and I took the lobsters in the bucket and went over to the far side of the island to turn them loose. We'd got ourselves down to the water and were dumping the lobsters into the ocean when, whoosh! This little rowboat rushes in between the rocks and almost smacks my feet." She laughed, and then shared the memory that brought the laughter. "I dumped the lobsters right in the boat and they started sliding all around."

She sobered. "It wasn't funny then, really, only now. What with the cyber stuff and everything, I got scared. Anyway. We became friends and I went for a boat ride, me and Wily."

"That's it?" Heath asked carefully. "You went for a ride with a friend?"

"I promised I wouldn't tell anybody," Elizabeth said.

Anna snorted.

Heath waited. E could occasionally keep secrets from her and Gwen, but never Anna.

"Wouldn't tell anybody what?" Anna asked innocently.

"You know, about him, and stuff." E had a pleading note in her voice. Anna ignored it.

"If there is something about him so dangerous that he made you promise not to divulge it to your mother, I think you'd better divulge it to your mother. And me," Anna said flatly.

"Not dangerous to me," E said. "Just him. He—oh God, I've told you he's a boy!" she almost wailed.

"Twice," Anna said. "Believe it or not, given we had a fifty-fifty chance of getting it right, we got that part right. We're betting a cute boy."

Elizabeth smiled and looked down.

"Now we know we got that part right," Anna said.

Heath said nothing. Anna was much better at this sort of thing than she was.

"So," Anna said. "You're on the back of Boar, down by the water, emancipating crustaceans, and a cute boy in a rowboat floods in. Merriment ensues, and you and Wily go for a ride."

"Yes," Elizabeth admitted.

"Being as he was adorable, and you're adorable, and everything is adorable, you become 'friends' and lose track of time," Anna said.

"I guess," E said.

"Then, when he realizes grown-ups are about to ruin this idyll, he chucks you and your poor old dog into the freezing ocean so he can save his sorry ass," Anna said.

"It wasn't like that," E protested. "I was the one who wanted to do it. To help."

"And he needed help because . . ." Anna said.

E's face took on a mulish cast. She studied her fingers. Wily licked his paw. Anna stared at E. Heath tried to fit the information E had shared into a coherent picture.

"I didn't hear a boat engine," Anna said. "And I didn't hear oars in oarlocks or paddles on the gunwale. So your new pal—who cannot be named—muffles his oars? Fishy."

Studying fingers, licking paws, staring into flames, thinking.

"You know I'll find out who fishy boy is," Anna threatened.

E said nothing.

Gradually it became clear that the boy's identity was one secret E was going to keep. At least for now. Heath quashed the urge to bargain or plead. E's new "friend" had not killed or molested her, and when she asked, he'd let her go free. That, and the fact that Elizabeth was happy, allowed Heath to keep her peace. In a bizarre way she was pleased that Elizabeth refused to divulge the boy's—and of course it had to be a boy—name. It showed backbone, honor, a sense of being in control of her own world that the Internet creep had stolen from her.

Quiet ticked by to the comforting sound of Wily working the salt from between the toes of his right paw with his tongue.

"Hey," Anna said finally. "On a lighter note, your stalker is here in Maine and wants to meet you."

Elizabeth toppled over on her side and pulled the afghan over her head.

TWENTY-SEVEN

Denise sat cross-legged on her bed. In front of her was a silver laptop. On the screen was a full-color fish-eye view of the nursery in Peter Barnes's home. Baby Olivia slept upstairs across the hall from Peter's room. Peter and *Lily's* room, she reminded herself. Where they slept on the bed that Denise had bought secondhand and refinished with such care.

Lit by the light of a Blue Fairy lamp, Olivia slept in a pink bundle. They'd let the room get too warm, Denise noticed with irritation. The baby was kicking her tiny feet, trying to get free of the rose-colored burrito *Lily* had thought suitable for swaddling. Why didn't the woman just stick Olivia in a papoose pack and lace it up tight?

It had been a week or more since Denise had allowed herself this particular torture. Paulette had taken her mind in other, more satisfactory directions. Directions that didn't all lead to a dead end. She'd missed watching Olivia. In a way, she was more a mother to the baby than Lily was. A couple of days after the baby was born, Lily had one of her migraines and checked herself back into the hospital. When she got out, though, of course Lily didn't have to work for a living; she went back to her "activities."

Not Denise. Denise had always been there.

The day Olivia was brought home, Denise stuck a Nice Lady No Bad Feelings face on the front of her skull and trotted right over to her old home, where Peter kept his family. In a beautifully wrapped box was an expensive fragile figurine of a guardian angel.

A smile pasted so tightly to her face that her lips stuck to her teeth, Denise told Lily it was to watch over the baby.

Nice, good, little Lily had put it on a table overlooking the baby's crib, right where the tiny camera hidden in the angel's armload of brightly painted flowers would capture the entire room.

Denise had invested in several snazzy little wireless cameras. This was the only one she'd planted in Peter's house, but it wasn't the limit of her knowledge of the Barnes family.

Before Paulette, when Denise had been scarcely more than a festering sore, barely able to keep her mind from pouring out through her eyes like molten lava, she'd kept herself alive by spying on the happy couple, then, when baby made three, the happy family.

She knew Lily's routine better than Peter did. Maybe better than Lily herself did. She knew when the baby napped and how often she was changed, when she was fed and what. She knew dear Lily was dry as an Arizona gully in August and never produced a drop of milk from her pert little tits to feed her child. Denise knew what kind of formula she used and where she kept it.

After he'd summarily thrown Denise out into the cold, thinking himself oh so clever, Peter had changed all the locks. He was too stupid to remember the dog door. Denise had been in that house dozens of times over the past three years. She knew Lily preferred Tampax tampons, the kind that looked like pink bullets; she knew when Lily's period was and how many days it lasted. She knew Lily suffered from migraines and what she took for them. She'd discovered Peter took Cialis. That had been a good day when she'd found those in his medicine cabinet. He also suffered from periodic constipation and kept *Playboy* magazines in the back of his closet.

During those awful times, all Denise thought about was revenge, years fantasizing about how she would get justice. As an employee of the American justice system, she'd thought justice was catching and punishing the bad guys. She had been wrong. What American law enforcement did was not justice, it was revenge, and revenge was for people who were helpless to obtain justice.

Paulette had taught her that.

Paulette coming into her life was the first justice Denise had ever experienced. Justice wasn't about the bad guy. It was about the victim. Justice made what was wrong right again. Justice made the victim whole. Justice put the jewelry back in the jewelry box, the car back in the rightful owner's garage. Justice was restoration. When Paulette came, Denise's lost soul was restored to her. That was justice.

Understanding this changed Denise's worldview. Revenge was not necessary—not even desirable—if justice could be had.

However, her years spying on Peter Barnes's family weren't wasted. It was serendipity—or fate, kismet—that she'd done this groundwork. At the time, she'd spied and pried because she couldn't help herself. Or so she'd thought. Some part of her brain must have realized that this information would become important to the planning of the whole life she had ahead of her now.

Not revenge; justice.

"Good night, baby girl," Denise said, and closed the laptop's cover.

She checked her watch. It was nearly three A.M. Time to leave to meet with her sister. Given how fast things were moving, and how small Acadia National Park was, meeting in the flesh, even in the dark of night in the woods, was risky, but after Denise had gotten off work she found a note Paulette had left in her mailbox; their cell phones neither texted nor took voice messages.

The note read *I have to see you. Please come tonight. We have to . . .* The last words were scribbled out.

Clutching the note, Denise feared she would have a heart attack in the foyer. Paulette had waltzed right up to the boxes in Denise's apartment building, in broad daylight, and popped a motherloving note, with her handwriting on it and, undoubtedly, slathered with fingerprints matching those at the crime scene, into Denise Castle, Law Enforcement Ranger and Identical Twin's mailbox.

Had Denise been a dog, she would have been mad enough to froth at the mouth. Thank God Paulette hadn't signed the thing. Might as well just add *P.S. We killed the prick. Love, the Bobbsey Twins.*

If anyone saw Paulette slip the note into her mailbox, Denise hoped they thought nothing of it. It had been with two bills and a flyer for used tires. Had Paulette come after the mailman, or had the mailman opened the box to put in the letters, seen the note, and read it?

"Doesn't matter," Denise said aloud. By the time the shit hit the fan, Paulette would be gone. One battered widow, no family, no friends, vanishes. A nonevent.

Denise changed out of her old pajamas. The new ones she'd ordered for her and her sister had arrived, but she didn't want to wear them until she and Paulette could wear them together.

Clad in dark clothes, she slipped quietly down the stairs and into her Miata. As on the night she'd disposed of Kurt, she would take the runabout to Otter Cove, then hike the short way overland. Covering the same ground more than once made her uneasy, but not as uneasy as taking the road. The inky shadow of the boathouse by the government dock on Somes was the only place she felt safe parking the Miata. Night diving was known to be her habit. If by chance the car was seen, no one would remark it there.

The NPS was understaffed and, at present, underfunded. Two weeks ago this would have pissed Denise off. Now park poverty was her friend. Acadia couldn't afford twenty-four-hour ranger coverage. On Friday and Saturday nights the last shift ended at midnight, on weeknights at ten P.M. Even Eager Artie would be abed by three A.M.

The Miata snugged into darkness by the boathouse, Denise rowed the runabout out a hundred yards. Probably an unnecessary precaution, but just because she was paranoid didn't mean somebody wasn't watching her. This was the downside of breaking the law—even when the law needed to be broken. Denise did not have a guilty conscience. In doing away with Duffy, she'd done the world a good turn, but it was like after she'd finished reading a mystery story. Once she knew exactly who, where, how, and when the crime was committed, it seemed it would be obvious to a two-year-old. To soothe her nerves she had to keep reminding herself that most people weren't all that bright. Better yet, most people didn't give a flying fuck unless it was a cop killed, or somebody they could use to make political hay.

Having shipped the oars, Denise fired up the engine and, at slightly better than idle, motored slowly down the sound. Air and water temperatures had reached sufficient equilibrium that the fog was shredding into thin feathers along the coast, eerie fingers given life by the light of a waning moon.

Boat firm beneath her, cool, fresh sea air in her lungs, Denise felt the iron band that Paulette's hand-delivered note had locked around her lungs loosen sufficiently to let her breathe deeply.

Please come tonight. We have to . . . Then the tangle of ink lines crossing out whatever it was Paulette decided they had to do. What could she have thought of that Denise hadn't? A few days before, Denise would have answered, "Nothing." The note and a few other things Paulette had done lately led her to believe identical twins weren't identical, as in *exactly* the same.

Denise shoved that thought aside. She and her twin were two sides of the same coin, peas in a pod, identical DNA. In everything that mattered there wasn't a particle of difference between them. She patted the front pocket of her black jeans where she had the list she'd made. Tonight they should be able to check off the meds and maybe the house. Paulette had had time to contact a Realtor, as well as two entire shifts to pinch the drugs.

Calmed by the eternal strength of the Atlantic surrounding her, Denise decided she wouldn't say anything about the hand-delivered note. Too many years in law enforcement had made her hypervigilant. That was all. Paulette, an infant-care nurse, couldn't be expected to see threats lurking behind every set of eyes. Denise loved that about her sister. Or she would, once there weren't threats lurking behind every set of eyes.

Denise expertly docked the runabout out of sight between two rocks, then followed the narrow beam of her tiny flashlight over the familiar ground between Otter and the old shed that Paulette had made into a nursery and was now their sanctuary from the world.

No light showed under the door. Clicking off her flashlight, Denise stepped beneath the roof overhang and put her ear against the wood of the door. Not a sound. Tapping softly, she whispered, "Paulette?" No answer.

Turning, Denise stared toward dead Kurt's shack. The back porch light was a blazing beacon through the trees. Paulette got off work at three A.M. She should have beat Denise to the nursery. Why was she in that rotting tomb of a house instead of in their secret place?

Paulette had been arrested for stealing drugs.

She'd collapsed of a heart attack.

Been run down by an SUV full of drunken tourists.

Panic drowning caution, Denise sprinted to where the porch hung precariously on the rear of the house. She leapt up the two steps, then stopped. The police might be inside, rangers, the sheriff, anybody. Denise stepped softly to the door. The knob turned easily. With three fingers, she pushed the door open a crack so she could see inside.

Paulette was sitting in a straight-backed chair at the small, beat-up kitchen table. Overprocessed blond hair was caught back in a purple scrunchie. She'd chewed off all of her lipstick. In pink scrubs, figured with Pooh-bears and daisies, she looked very young and helpless. A cup of coffee was between her hands. She was gazing into it as if the dregs would foretell her future.

"Hey," Denise said.

With a shriek, Paulette jumped to her feet. The mug toppled. Coffee poured over the edge of the table, dripping onto the dirty linoleum floor.

"God, but you scared me half to death," Paulette said with a shaky laugh. Before Denise had time to do more than blink, her sister had thrown herself into her arms and was hugging her with such force Denise could hardly move.

A rush of sensation overwhelmed her. Since Peter, three and more years ago, no one had touched her except strangers shaking her hand, or drunks bumping into her on their way to the men's room at the Acadian.

Babies needed to be touched. She'd read that. If they weren't touched they could fail to thrive, outright die.

Maybe adults were no different. Touch was life.

"Sorry I scared you," Denise apologized, all thought of the ill-considered note gone from her mind.

Paulette stepped away to grab a roll of paper towels off the counter. Ripping off half a dozen, she let them flutter to the floor, then used her foot to push them around, sopping up the coffee. The towels didn't get it all. What was left mingled with the yuck on the floor.

Perhaps not all the squalor had been Kurt's doing, Denise thought uneasily.

Didn't matter. They weren't going to be here much longer.

"Why didn't you wait in the nursery?" Denise asked as Paulette dropped the towels on top of a bunch of other trash in an open-topped can near the refrigerator.

"Oh, I don't know," Paulette said vaguely. "I wanted a cup of coffee. I thought this would be more comfortable."

The sordid kitchen in the murder house more comfortable? More comfortable than the nursery, with its art and painted furniture and promise of things to come?

Denise let it go, just like she'd let the leaving of the note in her box go. "Why did you need to see me?" she asked.

Paulette pinched up a packet of Nescafé, shook it, ripped off the top, and dumped the contents into a plastic mug. Taking the kettle from the stove, she offered, "Coffee?"

Instant.

"I'm good," Denise said, and waited. Her nerves weren't in shape for waiting, not in the wee hours of the morning in a trailer-trash kitchen. Her knee began bouncing, her heel never quite hitting the floor.

Paulette sat down across from her and repeated her gazing-into-the-cup routine. The spill on the scarred vinyl tabletop wasn't quite dry. Denise watched a tiny finger of it being absorbed into the cuff of the pink long-sleeved T-shirt Paulette wore under her scrubs.

"Did you have trouble getting the triazolam?" Denise asked, forcing an end to what was becoming an awkward silence.

Paulette hung her head. "I didn't get it," she murmured.

"Why the hell not?" Denise demanded, shocking herself with the outburst.

Paulette reached into the pocket of her scrubs and pulled out a handful of hypodermics with capped needles, each in its sanitary packet. "I got the needles," she offered pitifully.

Afraid to speak lest she batter her twin with abuse a second time, Denise stared at the empty hypodermic needles and nodded slowly.

When she felt she could speak normally, she asked, more gently, "Did you put the house on the market?"

Paulette shook her head.

Gentleness vaporized.

Paulette hadn't done anything. Nothing. Anger geysered up Denise's throat, hot and sulfurous as the fumes of hell. Given that Denise had shot Paulette's husband up close and personal three times, pilfering a few pills didn't seem like a big deal. Denise tried to force the bile down, calm herself. Pilfering a few pills, no big deal; Paulette would see it that way after Denise explained it.

The problem was Denise shouldn't have to explain it.

How could Paulette be sitting like a lump of raw dough in this filthy kitchen and not see how important this stuff was? Crucial.

Paulette, Denise reminded herself, was the gentle aspect of them. Of course she wasn't as capable of stealing or killing as Denise was. But not to put the property on the market? How much nerve did it take to call a Realtor?

Probably Paulette was afraid it wouldn't sell, afraid of being disappointed. Denise understood that. Better to pretend you don't hope than be made to look a fool when you don't get.

Denise decided that was all there was to it. She knew Paulette's lack of faith in their *themness* would have annoyed her, had it been possible for her to be annoyed with Paulette, genuinely annoyed, not just bitchy because her nerves were bad.

"I started on our legacy thing," Paulette said with a brightness Denise knew was false, and a smile that had been perfected to ward off the blows of her ham-handed hubby. Almost as if Paulette were afraid of Denise's displeasure.

Would that be bad? Denise wondered. Or good? Good, Denise decided. It showed Paulette cared, loved her.

"I used those old newspaper ads and sent postcards to the two PO boxes, the one listed in the original ad and the one listed four years later in that ad I showed you. Of course, even that was nearly a year old, but it could be something. It could be our mother," Paulette said, looking hopeful.

"Whoever put the ads in asking for twin girls separated at birth might have died or moved on," Denise said repressively. "More likely, good old Mom has decided nothing has changed, and she doesn't want us any more now than when she decided to chuck us out like so much garbage." Denise didn't think of the person who'd given them birth as "their" mother, just "the" mother.

Paulette twitched as if Denise had struck her. Unaccountably it made Denise angry. Guilt should have been what she felt, but she didn't. The cringing made her mad. "Please don't tell me you put this house as your return address," she growled.

"I put General Delivery like you told me," Paulette said softly, not looking up from her coffee. "Tomorrow I'll check. We could have got replies by then."

It was possible, Denise thought. Not probable, but possible. The legacy thing was just gravy, at any rate. They had enough. Counting on anybody or anything one couldn't control oneself was never a wise thing. Denise sighed, reined in her fraying nerves. Folding hands sticky with cold coffee from the tabletop one inside the other on her lap where they wouldn't betray her emotional turmoil, she said, "That's good. That's real good, Paulette. I'm sorry I got . . . Things are hard right now. Why did you drop the note by my apartment? What did you need to see me about?"

For a long moment Paulette said nothing. Denise could hear the wind soughing through the pines and imagined she could hear the surf breaking. Peaceful sounds, sounds she'd gone to sleep to for many years. This night they rasped over her eardrums like sandpaper over a sunburn.

"We have to stop," Paulette finally said, in such a tiny voice Denise had to lean halfway across the table to hear it, then couldn't believe it. A total non sequitur. Nausea washed through her. The overhead light, in its inverted bowl of dead flies, dimmed, then grew bright again.

Too weird.

Not a sudden onset of the flu or a brownout. Nerves. Putting both palms on the table to steady herself, Denise managed to say, "Stop what?"

"Oh, honey, everything. Everything!" Tears welled up in Paulette's eyes and spilled over her lids, rolling fat and oily down her cheeks. In their wake were gray trails of mascara.

Desperately, Denise reached across the little table and took both her sister's hands. "No!" she cried, not knowing what she was saying no to precisely, but aware that she needed to stop whatever tide was washing her sister away from her. Though the tide was not of water, not of physical stuff, she held just as tightly as if Paulette were caught in an undertow. Almost, Denise could see her growing smaller and smaller as the distance swallowed her. "No!" Denise gasped.

"I love working with the babies. I can't do anything else," Paulette sobbed, her tears so copious they dripped from her jaw, plopping onto Denise's forearms. "If anybody at the hospital thought I was even thinking about stealing drugs I would lose my job."

"What difference does that make?" Denise nearly shouted. The room was spinning around them. She had to hold tight lest she and her sister be flung away from the table by the centrifugal force. "We're leaving. We're going to get another house in another town and you can get another job. We've been over it and over it, Paulette. We're going to have a life, be a family."

"If we leave Acadia—you quit your job and I quit mine—and we sell and we move, they will know!" Paulette said brokenly. "That woman, that ranger lady—I was out shopping this morning and I came home and she was here! Right here at this house. She was coming out from the back where the nursery is. First she sees that picture where you look like me, then she comes here and sees the nursery and God knows what else. Why would she be snooping around here unless she thinks I killed Kurt or she thinks we are related? This isn't even her job. She's a park ranger. She knows we are doing things. We have to stop, just stop everything, don't do anything, just be quiet and normal and do our work and not be noticed. Maybe later . . ."

"Maybe the pigeon knows something, but that doesn't mean we stop. We stop her. That's all. I have a plan. We just distract her for a couple of days. No big deal. We just give her something else to think about, then we get our ducks in a row quick as anything, and we're done. No muss, no fuss," Denise pleaded.

Denise wanted to shake Paulette until her teeth rattled. How could she not realize there wouldn't be a later? They couldn't afford a maybe. This was their one shot; this was the brass ring, the lottery, the planets in alignment. It was a once-in-a-lifetime thing. And it had to be accomplished before Anna Pigeon could put two and two together and get twins.

How could Paulette be so stupid that she didn't get that?

All at once Denise understood why Kurt Duffy slapped his wife around.

TWENTY-EIGHT

Anna sat with Wily, Gwen, and Heath on the stone apron overlooking the sea. The sky was scattered with a herd of ephemeral sheep, as small and puffy and regular as if a child had drawn them. The sea was impossibly blue, navy in the shallow troughs and teal where the water thinned at the crests of the waves. This far north, the afternoons slipped into evening with exquisite slowness, the sunlight, rich as wild honey, striking diamonds from both the ocean and the granite.

Anna found it hard to believe that people bothered to torment and injure one another when there were so many better ways of spending one's time. Given the choice of a moment such as this or trolling the Internet, or shooting a hairy naked man, why would anyone choose the troll or the hairy man?

"Have you recovered from E's going AWOL?" Anna asked.

Heath sipped her bourbon. "Like it never happened," she said.

"She's lying," Gwen said mildly. Gwen was fortified with a glass of white wine, her feet resting on the rounded footrest of a classic Adirondack deck chair. "After much consultation, she has decided to pretend it is okay. I have not. In my day—and I very much think today is still my day, thank you very much—boys come to the door and meet the family."

"The boy remains a state secret?" Anna asked. "Do we even know for sure it is a boy?"

"Of course it's a boy," Gwen said. "Don't be ridiculous."

Anna smiled. Of course it was a boy.

"I wanted to forbid E ever to see the little bastard again," Heath said. "But I actually think she would have disobeyed. Yesterday E asked to 'go out' for a while. Like there was a mall nearby. Jesus. I managed to say yes without spitting."

"You get points for that," Anna said.

"Fortunately I was gone," Gwen said. "I think I should have spit."

"You were in Bangor with the owner of the island?" Anna asked to be polite.

"Yes. Christine has had several heart attacks. This last was accompanied by another stroke. She can't speak, and her left side is completely paralyzed. It's hard to see her so agitated. She fell trying to get out of bed. Dez said she had scribbled something about wanting to see her children."

"Elizabeth came back from her second 'date,'" Gwen said. "You were probably right to let her go."

"Right. Because she came back when she said she would, I should get Mother of the Year," Heath said. "If she hadn't . . ."

Heath didn't finish that thought. She didn't need to.

Maternal fear, so palpable Anna could almost see it, curled like fog around the wheels of Heath's wheelchair. "E didn't let any interesting information slip?" Anna asked, hoping to distract her friend from the nightmare possibilities.

"Nope. If she wasn't happier than I've seen her for a long time, I might consider thumbscrews," Heath said. "E is sticking with the basic 'nice friend' description of Boat Boy."

Anna would have liked to see Boat Boy behind bars, if for no other reason than that he took her goddaughter out in a boat that had but a single personal flotation device, muffled his oars, and refused to meet the parents for fear of being arrested.

"If I was trawling for a sixteen-year-old girl, a cute boy would be my bait of choice," Anna said.

"Don't think I haven't obsessed on that. And mentioned it to E about six hundred times. She insists that's not it. The child smirks and hums to herself," Heath said sourly. "If he's a pervert I will skin him with a dull Boy Scout knife, one square inch at a time, drench him with gasoline, and set him on fire." Abruptly Heath went silent.

"You two are scaring me," Gwen said mildly. "Talk about something joyful."

"Murder, then. Murder is always entertaining," Anna suggested.

"The murdered lobsterman—the second lobsterman killed recently, right? The first was shot with a rifle for stealing . . . poaching?" Heath asked.

"There's nothing to indicate the two killings are related—" Anna began.

"Smells fishy to me," Heath said.

"John says the two incidents have nothing to do with each other," Gwen said. Both Heath and Anna looked at her.

"And John knows this why?" Anna asked.

"It turns out—and this just breaks my heart—that the first lobsterman, the one shot because he and his son were suspected of robbing traps, was Will Whitman, John's son," Gwen said.

"God," Heath groaned. Her compassion ground deep. Anna knew she was thinking of losing Elizabeth. Anna could imagine, if only intellectually, what it must be like to lose a child, like losing a particularly magical cat or a dog one had bonded with. Maybe worse.

"John says his son is innocent, for what it's worth," Gwen added. "His grandson is still missing, trying to clear his father's name and keep himself out of the line of fire, I guess."

"John is probably right about Will Whitman's and Kurt Duffy's deaths being unrelated. Whoever killed this guy Duffy appeared to be a little more personally involved than a man gunning down a poacher. Duffy was shot three times—twice through the shower curtain—"

"And, one assumes, other parts of his anatomy," Gwen said.

"With a small-caliber weapon," Anna finished. "Then apparently smothered with the shower curtain. Since us 'acting' chiefs haven't much to keep us occupied, I cruised by the widow's house. It's not exactly park jurisdiction, but I thought I'd interview her just for the hell of it. Nobody answered the door. I walked around to see if Ms. Duffy was hanging out clothes or sunbathing.

"Talk about depressing. The yard is packed dirt with a broken swing set. The chain on one of the swings was banging against the metal pole in the wind. It was like a scene from Edgar Allan Poe, if Poe had been born in a trailer park in 1967."

"For whom the bell tolls," Heath said amiably. "Isn't the spouse the first suspect? An abused spouse in this case, wasn't she?"

"When all else fails, it's the wife," Anna said. "But I doubt that was the case this time. From the state the bedroom and the deceased were in, there was an all-out battle. Ms. Duffy doesn't seem to be the kind who could fight a sick puppy and win. What possesses a woman to marry a Kurt Duffy?" she wondered aloud. "Move into his hovel, cook his dinners, launder his sweaty fish-smelling undershorts?"

"As my father used to say, 'Perhaps Mr. Duffy has talents we are not privy to,'" Aunt Gwen said.

Anna grunted.

Heath struck a match to light her cigarette.

Elizabeth emerged from the house, "He's back," she announced.

From the sound of her voice, Anna knew it wasn't the boy with the boat.

"Read it out loud," Heath said to her daughter.

Elizabeth held the phone in front of her at eye level. " 'You didn't show up you lousy pig-faced C asterisk asterisk T,' " she articulated carefully.

"You're kidding!" Heath exclaimed. "A filthy cyberstalker who balks at the C-word?"

"He also misspelled 'lousy.' L-O-W-Z-Y. Loh-zeee," she said in the tones of a demented Hollywood Chinaman. "Sheesh! Even in text-speak we have our pride."

Then she laughed.

Anna sighed. No matter how old a woman grew, there wasn't much a cute boy couldn't cure.

At least for a while.

Anna hoped Boat Boy wouldn't break E's heart. At sixteen heartbreak was a miserable thing. Age did nothing but make it worse. Hearts that didn't grow harder as the years passed acquired an ability to love that young people could only imagine.

The text didn't prove the boy with the muffled oars, and the fear of law enforcement, wasn't a monster. It did suggest that he was not the cybercreep. Unfortunately there was more than one kind of monster in the world.

Heath lit the cigarette before the match burned her fingers, breathed in a lungful of smoke, blew it out. "Our Fox River thug ruined the F-word forever. Now this toad is going to ruin all the other bad words."

"Pig-faced asterisk asterisk is my favorite so far," Elizabeth said.

Heath shot her a sideways look, squinting through the smoke from her cigarette. "I think you're beginning to enjoy this," she said.

Anna heard the joy beneath the pretense. No one could miss how much happier Elizabeth was since her ersatz abduction, and E's happiness was Heath's happiness. "Anything else in the text?" Anna asked.

E's eyes tracked back to the cell phone. "'Same place, same time, day after tomorrow or else.' 'Or else' is in all caps."

"Are you being stalked by a ten-year-old?" Heath growled. "What does 'else' mean?"

"I don't think I want to find out," Elizabeth said, her good humor gone, anxiety dragging down her cheeks.

Anna thought for a moment, her fingers absently ruffling the feathers of Wily's tail; he'd flopped down between Robo-butt and Anna's chair. Threats were tricky things. Most went unfulfilled. Most. However, if the stalker wanted to meet with E, it was not to do her a kindness. "Or else" could be nothing. It could also be an ugly bit of business.

It was tempting to think the stalker would be mollified by contacting his victim in the flesh. He would say what he needed to say, be heard if he needed to be heard. Anna suspected that more than one person who climbed into a clock tower with a repeating rifle did so because they felt they could not be seen, could not be heard, could not break through the indifference of the world—or the bureaucracy—any other way.

One might be tempted to believe that a meeting would cancel out the "or else." Not Anna. To stalk and bully with the intensity this creep had shown was to prove oneself beyond the pale of society. Now that he was demanding to move from the ether into the corporeal world, he went from a psychological threat to a physical threat.

Resources were limited. Jurisdictions, considering the crime was instigated in Colorado and conducted from the cloud, were a mess. Stalking was illegal, but cyberstalking? That had yet to be dealt with in any definitive way.

Information was limited. None of them had a clue as to who this was. It could be someone connected to E's past in the compound, someone connected with the kidnapper who had taken her and the other girls, an enemy of Heath's—or even Anna's—or a random psychopath. He might recognize them or not. They might recognize him or not.

"We need to set a trap," Anna said.

"Anything to end the suspense," Heath said.

"What can I do?" E asked.

"Nothing," Anna told her. "You're the bait."

TWENTY-NINE

Until Peter, the parks had been Denise's salvation. At thirteen she'd gotten drawn out of the bleak misery that was her life to become a junior ranger and never gone back. During college she worked as a summer seasonal. After graduation she got her permanent status as a GS-3 taking fees at the entrance booth. From there she'd moved on and up. Until Peter Barnes had stopped time.

Ranger Castle, that's who she'd been, who she'd respected, who she showed the world. Ranger Castle was the only persona available to her that she'd ever been able to stomach. Now she was Denise Castle, civilian: no green and gray, no flat-brimmed hat, no badge, no cordovan-colored leather belt or boots.

Denise had quit the NPS, stepped out of her life, away from the things that had once defined her, and it had been easy. So very, very, insultingly easy. It pissed Denise off just remembering it. During the drive to headquarters to start the paperwork for her retirement, she'd wasted brain energy trying to think of plausible answers to the inevitable "Why so sudden? Why now? We'll need at least two months' notice. Who can take your place? We'll need time to hire a replacement. We have to plan a retirement party! You'll need to stay to train your replacement. If you stay another three years you'll get blah, blah, blah."

Nope.

Basically it was "Don't let the screen door slap your ass on the way out."

Her whole life, and no gold watch, nothing but a bunch of forms to sign, a couple of brochures, and a teensy wad of cash every month. She'd cleaned out her office in a matter of minutes. The only thing she'd left behind was an oversized model of an outrigger canoe Peter had bought her on a trip to Hawaii. She hated the thing. She'd only taken it because he wanted it. Well, he could have it.

Shitheads. Let them rot. The NPS, potlucks on the lawn, campfire talks, scraping tourists' automobiles off rocks was not her whole life anymore. Her whole life was ahead of her. Her real life.

Bastards. Pricks. The lot of them.

At least the fact that the NPS was no longer her good buddy lessened the guilt she felt at raiding the evidence room for a couple of rufies—Rohypnol, the date rape drug. They had been taken off, of all people, a gynecologist—Denise would have thought he'd have had his fill of women's parts—up from Boston, who'd gotten himself arrested in the park a few years back. It had yet to go to trial. Probably never would. The guy was a rich doctor.

Rohypnol, added to a dash of Valium she'd had in the bottom of her medicine cabinet, should work as well as or better than the triazolam. Paulette hadn't been able to lay her hands on any at Mount Desert Hospital. At least she said she hadn't. Denise suspected her sister lacked the gumption to steal it.

Or maybe the motivation.

No, Paulette wanted this new life as much as Denise. Maybe she didn't know it quite yet, but she would. Until then, Denise could do the heavy lifting. She was used to that. Once they had a home, were a family, Paulette would come into her own. Denise was sure of it.

For the second time in as many days, Denise crept up to the shed-become-nursery behind her sister's house. Her brain fizzed with the plan she'd come up with, loose ends popping like bubbles in a Scotch and soda. Rushing these things was never good. That was when mistakes were made.

No choice, she told herself.

Denise had insisted they meet in the nursery this time. Tapping on the door, she called Paulette's name softly.

"Come in," Paulette answered. Denise slipped through the door. Paulette had a single kerosene lamp lit. She was sitting in the low rocking chair. Her clothes were all in dark colors, and she wore lace-up sneakers. Good. Denise had been afraid she'd get here and Paulette would have disobeyed her. Paulette had asked why Denise wanted her to dress all in black, and Denise hadn't answered. Her plan wasn't something to be dealt with over the phone.

Denise dumped the heavy sack she was carrying as she folded down onto the hand-hooked rug at her sister's feet.

The sense that time was running out for them was driving Denise too hard for her to put off what she had to say. "I have been thinking about what you said, Paulette, about Ranger Pigeon being on to the fact we're twins, and then you finding her snooping around the nursery," she said without preamble.

"Not exactly around the nursery," Paulette said. "Just behind the house, really."

"Oyster out of a shell, that's how she looked at you. That's what you said."

"I guess," Paulette admitted.

Denise stared at her.

"Yes," Paulette said in a firmer voice. "I think she's been around the nursery. I felt it."

"Right," Denise approved. "You can see how that makes the death of good old Kurt not as simple as we thought. What had been a perfect murder now has a big fat hairy flaw in the ointment."

"Fly," Paulette said.

"Whatever. Anna Pigeon is that fly, that big hairy flaw. She's an obstacle," Denise insisted. "A serious stumbling block on the road to our new life."

"Oh." Paulette looked away. She stood, crossed to the crib, and picked up the little bear, her back to Denise. "If she's been back here, I haven't seen her. She hasn't tried to talk to me or anything. Maybe she was just, you know, poking around like rangers like to do." She set the bear down carefully in precisely the same place it had been before.

Why was Paulette being obstinate? "She might not have come back; more likely she did and you didn't see. The pigeon has all the pieces to you and me and Kurt dead and you at the Acadian. She's not stupid. She's an obstacle, and the obstacle has to be removed," Denise insisted.

Paulette spun around, her hands to her cheeks like a cartoon of "noooooo." "Do you mean kill her?" Paulette exclaimed. "Miss Pigeon is a ranger, law enforcement, like you. I've seen it in every movie. If a cop is killed—probably even a tree cop—the CIA and FBI and everybody start a huge manhunt!"

Denise stifled a sigh. "It's not like that. I know you're scared. I'd be, too. But we're not going to do anything drastic," she said, forcing a smile and a soothing timbre to her voice. "What I've got planned is more like a prank. It'll be seen like a prank. Ha ha, no big deal. You'll see. Rangers play pranks on each other all the time. Nobody gets their panties in a wad. We'll snatch the pigeon—like frat boys snatch each other for a joke. We'll keep her in here for a couple of days, then, when we've finished, we'll call somebody to let her out. Nobody gets hurt. We get what we deserve."

"You're sure?" Paulette asked. Denise's twin appeared to be growing younger and younger as Denise watched. Years dropping from her voice and face. Denise was growing older. At present she felt they weren't identical twins at all, that she was the much older sister and had to take care of Paulette.

"I'm sure," she said warmly. "We need more time, just a few days more to get everything we need. If we can . . . pull our prank on Anna Pigeon, it will buy us that time. We'll finish everything on our list, then we'll buy a nice big car and we'll go south until it's spring all year around, and we'll buy a nice house."

Paulette smiled wistfully. "It would be wonderful to have a nice new house," she said. "One that was clean and pretty, where nothing was broken or patched."

"That's what we're going to have," Denise promised. "Tonight we'll remove the obstacle. Over the next few days we'll tidy up, then off we'll go. An adventure."

Paulette's smile firmed up, her age steadied at about fourteen, or so it seemed to Denise. Fourteen would have to do.

"I got water for her," Denise said, pulling three liter bottles from her canvas sack. Without a word, Paulette gathered them up and carried them to a shelf next to the crib, where she arranged them in a neat row. "I brought these." Denise dug in her bag. "MREs from the fire cache. The park will never miss them. And these." She pulled two pairs of handcuffs from her belt. "Anna Pigeon will be fine. Just for a couple of days. I hoped you had an old bucket around somewhere."

"A bucket? What for?" Paulette asked as she piled the MREs in a tidy stack beside the water bottles.

"No bathroom," Denise explained.

"Yuck!" Paulette made a face. "Wait." Dropping to her hands and knees, she felt around under the crib. "If it's only for a couple days . . ." She dragged out a pink potty-training toilet. "It's nicer than a bucket." For a moment she studied it, then turned to Denise. "It's awfully small."

Paulette was so naïve, so sweet, like a little kid untouched by the whole real, nasty, shitty world. At times Denise thought maybe Paulette wasn't all there, wasn't quite right in the head. That would mean Denise wasn't right in the head either. They were identical twins. Being crazy wasn't a new thought. Things had gotten blurry and odd in the last while, maybe a year, maybe more.

Nerves.

"Anna Pigeon has a skinny butt," Denise said. "The potty is perfect. We do it tonight."

"I didn't get the triazolam," Paulette confessed. "I can look again tomorrow. We could do it tomorrow, couldn't we?"

Denise knew Paulette wouldn't have gotten the drug. Of course she knew. There wasn't anything she didn't know about her identical twin. To Paulette this was just talk, just a game. Paulette didn't think this was going to happen; she didn't think they deserved a life together. Kurt had beat that out of her.

Denise knew better. This had to happen.

"Not a problem," Denise assured her. "I got it all worked out. You don't have to worry about a thing."

"I did get this," Paulette said, brightening. "It's about the legacy. It came to General Delivery this morning." She held an envelope out to Denise. It had been opened. That irked Denise. The legacy was something they shared—or should share. Paulette should have waited until they could open it together.

Having unfolded the single slip of paper from the envelope, Denise turned it to the lamp so she could read the letters. *The woman who put the ad in the paper regarding the twins is very ill at present. I would not want to see her hurt or disappointed. To that end, I would like to meet with you before I share your card with her. There is a legacy, two to be accurate. We can talk about that when we meet.* The number of a cell phone followed.

"Sounds like a con," Denise said. "People run all kinds of con games.

This sounds like one of them. Did you call her?" she demanded. Her tone was too rough. Paulette aged a little more, and her mouth turned harder. Ugly, Denise thought.

"I didn't," Paulette said. "But I want to. I think it's real."

Paulette wanted to get back with their biological mommy, Denise thought bitterly. No matter that Mommy was obviously a heartless tramp. Paulette would probably want to hang around and nurse Mommy back to health, and to hell with her sister, her identical twin sister.

Denise rode a wave of anger until it subsided, leaving her tired and determined. "We'll do whatever you want," she said. "First let's get tonight out of the way, okay? Please?"

"Tonight?"

Denise said nothing, just kept a half smile pasted on her face. Paulette looked at her for long enough that Denise thought she was going to come up with another argument, distraction, or reason to postpone what they had to do.

"Just for a couple days, then we let her go," Paulette said.

Denise felt a rush of relief as great as the anger had been. "I love having a sister," she said.

"Me, too," Paulette said.

THIRTY

Paulette was in the boat; she had the needle with the mixture. Denise had explained what needed to be done, and Paulette had understood and seemed confident she could do her part. The sea was flat, and there was a gentle onshore breeze. Everything was as it should be, Denise told herself for the hundredth time. Once, like the whine of a mosquito near her ear, the thought surfaced that this part of the plan, disabling Anna Pigeon, wasn't crucial. A flash of the pigeon's eyes over the picture frame, or the tilt of her head as she'd interrogated Paulette, pulled the thought back into the depths. This was not a time to take even the slightest risk. If they failed, there would be no time to recover.

Since Kurt had died and Ranger Pigeon started poking her nose in, Denise had had that awful feeling she got as a child when she tried to balance a broom on her nose. Never could she run fast enough to keep it from falling down.

This was the second-to-last major step; then they were home free, free to have a home. She concentrated on that to keep the noise of the boat engine from bouncing off her sensitized eardrums with the force of a cataclysm.

Denise had coddled and pampered the little runabout's motor until it was as quiet as a fifteen-horsepower Evinrude could get. Unfortunately, on a still night, its high-pitched growl carried across the water like the wailing of an infant.

Before she could clearly see Schoodic's rocky point in the ambient light of a moonless sea, Denise cut the engine. For a minute she breathed, letting the magnificent silence erase their trespass.

The water was flat—or as flat as the restless Atlantic ever was. This was good. High seas would have postponed this adventure. Time had become a creature of three dimensions, slippery and short and sliding fast through Denise's fingers.

Having pried off the lens covers, she lifted the binoculars to her eyes.

Schoodic Point, as advertised, was pointed. It was a peninsula on the end of a peninsula that ended in a spade-shaped stone skirt digging into the ocean at the mainland's southernmost shore. Schoodic was a bleak beauty of rock, stone, sea, and sky. Fashion shoots favored it for high-end clothes, the emaciated models teetering over the round rocks in high heels, believing that people were staring because they were pretty and not because they looked like idiots. Weddings were often booked at Schoodic Point.

A hard, uncompromising beginning to married life, Denise thought as she swept the shore with the binoculars. An ugly parking lot scraped a flat place above the beach and nearly ruined the aesthetics. This night Denise forgave its existence because it had the decency to be empty. It was after three in the morning, and RVs weren't allowed to park overnight, but they often tried to get away with it.

No RVs. No sedans with thrashing bodies in the backseat.

"We're clear," she whispered to Paulette. "We paddle from here."

Frizzled blond hair tucked under a black watch cap, small body hidden under a black long-sleeved T-shirt, black sweatpants, and black running shoes, Paulette was merely a shadow in the bow. Denise thought of herself as a strong, strapping woman. She saw Paulette as fine-boned and delicate. Odd that she and her sister were the same height and weight, same shoe, glove, and bra size. Paulette's shoulders were hunched, and her chin was down, as if she tried to disappear into her own skeleton. Black ops were not her forte. Well, Denise thought, they weren't hers either. She just did what she had to do. Paulette would see that. After the fact, when done was done, she would understand.

Both women had blackened their faces with makeup. Denise didn't know what the Delta Force guys or the Navy SEALs used, or what football players put under their eyes, but she and her sister had made do with a mix of Paulette's black, gray, and dark blue eye shadows. The effect was all she could have wished for. But for her hands, Paulette looked to be little more than a texture on the night seascape.

As did Denise. Invisible twins. Could invisible people still be identical? Sort of the visual equivalent of the tree falling in the forest: Could one no-thing be exactly the same as another no-thing? Denise wondered as she watched Paulette's white hands float up like the ghosts of long-dead starfish and close around the handle of a paddle.

In an inexpert attempt to get the paddle in position she struck the blade against the gunwale. The clunk was loud enough to wake sleepers in Nova Scotia.

Maybe Denise suffered from nervous twitches, but she was beginning to think her sister was just clumsy. She swallowed an oath.

"I'll paddle," she whispered, making her voice extra kind to stifle the traitorous thoughts about her twin.

The runabout was a bitch to paddle. Denise had done it enough that she could make it work. Work was the key word. Outboards weren't meant to run on manpower. Or, in her case, womanpower. By the time she managed to catch the crest of a good wave, and ride the surf into the rocky beach on the point below the parking lot, sweat was pouring down from her temples and between her breasts.

As the swell that beached them retreated, it dragged small stones along with it, clattering back toward the ocean floor. If she timed it right, the racket of the stony surf would cover the racket of beaching the boat.

Denise was over the side in a second. Even in midsummer the water off the coast of Maine was cold. She was used to wearing a wet suit complete with booties. Cold feet were the least of the dangers, she reminded herself as she shoved hard on the stern to move the boat out of the reach of the surf before the Atlantic could turn it into flotsam. Paulette sat like a statue in the bow, making the going that much tougher. Again Denise felt irritation rise up her spine to scratch like a metal rasp on the back of her brain.

Lot of stress, she reminded herself. Lot on our plates. "Us against the world" was not as romantic as fiction writers would have it. "Us" could get real bitchy. Things would be better—like they used to be those first few times they were together—once they got straightened away, got the legacy, the pension, the money from the sale of the house . . .

Denise slammed her mind shut against the list. It grew longer every minute she dwelt on it, longer and heavier, each chore another lead weight on her metaphorical dive belt threatening to drag her down, drown her.

Paulette jumped from the boat, grabbed the bow with both hands, and began to help drag it up on shore.

See, Denise told herself. Not irritating. Good and right.

The previous day Denise had driven to the peninsula on reconnaissance to find a secluded spot to cache the boat. It didn't need to be totally hidden, just out of casual sight should a ranger be on patrol—not likely; there weren't enough green-and-gray bodies for round-the-clock coverage on Schoodic either. More likely would be a nosy insomniac out for a ride.

She'd found a shallow dry creek to the side of the point not too long a walk from the employee housing area and the old US Navy base—now a rotting hulk of dorm rooms and hallways—but far enough so that the sounds of their arrival wouldn't wake any of the summer seasonals, or the sculptors on Schoodic for an artists' retreat.

Psychically speaking, killing Kurt had been no big deal. He was a lout and a bastard, and even his best friend was over it in a beer or two. Even without killing, this would be different. Paulette was right. There would be cops all over a federal law enforcement officer going missing. Since Pigeon was "acting" chief, Denise hoped there'd be a time lag before the NPS declared her disappearance officially suspicious. Then Denise wasn't sure who-all would descend, but she was sure it was going to be a big deal. Hence: black clothes, black face, surgical gloves for the event, and a getaway boat hidden in the scrub.

Leave No Trace.

That was a Park Service motto. Good old NPS, Denise thought with a smile. Good old Superintendent Peter, moldy green and moth-eaten gray down to his grubby little soul. This was going to look bad on Happy Daddy's résumé. A perk she'd not considered before.

Paulette was making a lot of racket puffing and grunting as they dragged the boat into the wash. After they'd settled the runabout, Denise could still hear her breathing. Paulette hadn't kept herself in shape. Denise stared over the dark shape of the hull between them. Despite the black makeup and the brim of the ball cap, she could see that Paulette's face was crumpled like a little kid's before it starts to shriek.

"Are you okay?" she asked softly.

"I have to pee," Paulette said. A nervous titter escaped her lips.

"Because you're scared?" Denise asked.

"I guess." To Denise's surprise, tears started cutting white stripes through the powder on Paulette's face. All her irritation was blown away on a gust of pity. Paulette was the softer Denise, the gentle Denise she could have been if not for the foster homes and other bullshit. Tonight was going to be hard on Paulette because of her tender heart. As soon as she could afford the luxury, Denise decided, she would have the compassion

Paulette had. For now, she was grateful that her heart was hard as flint, that it had been pounded and tormented until it barely beat. Right now, tonight, that hardening was going to pay off. Paulette would understand how it had to be, if not right away, then when they were in their new house and their new lives.

Sitting on the keel of the boat, Denise patted the wet fiberglass beside her. Obediently, Paulette came around the stern to sit next to her. Denise took her sister's hand between both of her own.

"This isn't like it was with Kurt," Paulette snuffled. "It's hard to take someone when you don't want to hurt them, when they're not bad, just too smart and in the way."

"It is," Denise admitted. "I can do it without you if you like," she offered, though, in truth, she didn't think she could. "We're not doing alibis or anything."

"No alibis because we both live alone, it's the middle of the night, and no one will suspect us anyway," Paulette said, repeating exactly the words and intonations Denise had used when they discussed the venture in the boat. Denise looked at her hard, trying to figure out if she was being mocked.

No, of course she wasn't. Paulette would never do that. Twin souls would sound the same, would speak as one. Of course. Same DNA.

"Can't we just not do it? Turn around and go home?" Paulette pleaded, glancing up at Denise from under the ball cap.

Denise felt as if she towered over her sister, like a Goliath, a monster. This was as much for Paulette as it was for her. More. Compassion burned out on sudden unexpected anger. Jolted by the intensity of the fury, Denise's tongue clove to the roof of her mouth.

They had been through this. "It's just for a couple of days." Denise forced herself to go through it again. "She'll sleep through most of it. Then we tell somebody where to find her. No harm, no foul."

"Sorry, sorry," Paulette said before Denise could say any wrong words and ruin everything forever. "Of course we can't just not do it. Let's do it. Let's go. Right now."

"Don't have to pee anymore?" Denise asked as Paulette rose.

"I couldn't if I wanted to. All my sphincters are slammed shut," Paulette said, and produced a wan smile.

Denise smiled back. Paulette was trying. Paulette was a trouper.

"We'll be fine," Denise promised. "Do you have the stuff?"

Paulette unzipped her waist pack and checked the contents as Denise had seen her do half a dozen times since the boat left Somes Sound.

Paulette lifted out a syringe with a plastic safety cap over the needle. Holding it near her ear, she shook it. Paulette had crushed the rufies to powder using the bowl of a teaspoon to mash the tablets against the bowl of a soup spoon. Denise had thrown in a Valium for good measure. When the powder was as fine as they could make it, they mixed it with tap water and drew the resulting liquid into a syringe.

Denise remembered how Paulette's hands shook, setting up a tiny tempest in the spoon, how her own had shaken so much they lost some of the precious stuff.

Two street-made rufies, 1.0 mg of Valium. There wasn't anything on the Internet about the mix, but enough Rohypnol could cause unconsciousness and even coma. Coma would be good, Denise thought, startling herself. She didn't want to kill the pigeon any more than Paulette did. Still, a coma would be a whole lot easier for everybody concerned.

"Two rufies and a Valium is a lot," Paulette said. "Maybe too much."

"You should know. You're the RN," Denise said. She'd meant to sound complimentary. It came out waspish.

"LPN," Paulette said in a barely audible voice.

For a moment the letters made no sense to Denise. Paulette was a nurse. Nurses were RNs, registered nurses. Then she remembered. LPN meant licensed practical nurse. No better than an EMT.

"A Candy Striper?" Denise demanded, aghast.

"It takes a year to get accredited. RNs take four or five years." Paulette hung her head so low her forehead nearly touched her knees. "Some of us do injections, but there's always a doctor's okay, or an RN to help. I don't know whether injecting Rohypnol instead of swallowing it will make a difference. What if she ODs?"

"Shit." Denise forced herself not to roll her eyes. What if she did OD? Would it be worse than if she didn't? Worse, of course, in the sense of murder, but worse all around? For her and Paulette?

"It can't kill her," Denise said firmly. "I Googled it."

THIRTY-ONE

Anna's sleeping mind conjured up a wasp. The insect was stinging her bicep. Instantly she was awake, but, for a moment, she
couldn't remember where she was. Not Rocky. Acadia. No Paul,
no roommates, yet a shadow, as wide as it was tall, clotted the vague light
between her eyes and the ceiling.

"Hey!" Anna barked. Squeaking like a colony of bats, the shadow
changed shape and squeezed toward the door. Not a shadow—this in-
vader was corporeal in nature. Shadows were the stuff of silence. This
apparition was making a hell of a racket.

"Who are you?" Anna yelled as she threw off her covers. There was a
brief scuffle as the night creature tried to shove itself through an opening half its size.

Leaping free of the bedclothes, Anna yelled: "Stop!"

The black shape wrestled with itself for a moment, then popped
through the bedroom door into the living room. Anna scrambled for the
light switch. In the unfamiliar room, she was slow. By the time she'd flicked
the light on, she could hear the sound of feet pounding down wooden
stairs. More than one person, two, maybe three. A wave of dizziness

overtook her; sound was behaving oddly; the light seemed to shimmer. She brushed her wrist over her eyes.

Hers was one of four apartments in the building used for employee housing on Schoodic Peninsula. The structure was divided in half, two floors on each side, an apartment on each floor, the two halves connected by an open-air breezeway and stairs. Though it often happened in cookie-cutter dwellings, these weren't drunken neighbors wandering in the wrong door. Drunken neighbors wouldn't run; besides, at present, Anna's was the only apartment occupied.

It could be park visitors. As far as vacationers were concerned, rangers were always on duty, always there to stanch the bleeding or lend a cup of sugar. Since Anna—like a lot of the old guard—still refused to lock her doors, a couple might have wandered in and been scared into running when she awakened.

"Hey!" she shouted again. "Hold up."

In three strides she'd crossed the small living room. As she reached the head of the stairs, two humanoid shapes careened through the downstairs breezeway, running out into the parking lot with more speed than grace.

Not tourists with bad manners. Sinister miscreants. "Damn!" Anna muttered. She staggered, caught herself on the railing, then turned and ran back into her apartment. For an instant, she stood beside her bed, trying to remember why she'd come back. "Intruders," she said, and she pulled on her cordovan boots, grabbed her SIG Sauer from the drawer in the nightstand, and, stark naked but for boots and gun, hurtled out of the apartment, down the stairs, and into the night.

In the middle of the employee-housing parking lot, she stopped, eyes wide, ears open. Without warning a blackness as heavy and dark as igneous rock rolled over her brain, crushed her vision, and clogged her ears. Anna's joints turned to water. She fell hard on her knees.

Pain cleared her mind. She could hear sneakered feet scratching on pavement; the intruders were headed across the access road toward the renovated Rockefeller building used as the Schoodic Education and Research Center. Beyond the Rockefeller building were the crumbling ruins of an old navy base's housing wings.

Currently the research center was home to granite sculptors doing a summer workshop. Possibly her wee-hours visitation was from feral artists, but Anna was more worried about the artists as victims or hostages than as perpetrators. Though one or two of the huge, labor-intensive granite monoliths did look like the work of troubled minds.

As her vision cleared, she saw the two figures running hard toward the plaza where the sculptures were being carved. She heaved herself to her feet and, boots ringing on the asphalt, sprinted after them.

"Stop or I'll shoot!" she yelled. She wouldn't shoot. Rangers didn't shoot fleeing suspects even if they had slithered up to one's bedside in the dead of night.

The dreamlike sensation of running ever slower through air viscous as mud dragged at her legs. Distance—or her perception of it—underwent a sea change. The ruined barracks wavered, retreating in an undulating wreck of roof lines. The Rockefeller building, no more than two hundred yards from her apartment, refused to move closer as she ran; then, suddenly, the immense granite sculptures were looming over her.

Anna didn't so much stop with intent as simply cease to move because her body chose stagnation regardless of what her mind ordered it to do. The retreating human-shaped fragments of darkness had run past the sculptures. Immobile, she watched as they reached the barracks where the wings of the ruined building came together. Her eyes told her they vanished like smoke; her mind suggested they'd probably run down one of the stairwells that let into the basement level.

Even if her legs had not ceased to function properly, and the night had not broken all the laws of physics to become a nauseating, undulating mess, Anna would not have given chase. Nothing short of a shrieking child or a mewling kitten could induce her to pursue bad guys into that haunted hulk in the dark.

The abandoned barracks was two stories of smashed desks, shattered walls, mirror shards, falling staircases, and other sharp-edged detritus. In that place, if fleeing felons didn't kill you, tumbling down stairs or broken glass would.

Broken glass would what?

With sudden alarm, Anna wondered why she was naked, why she was standing in the shadow of lowering chunks of granite with her gun in her hand. She had no recollection of kneeling, yet she was on her knees on the stone.

Stinging in her upper arm claimed her attention.

Clumsily, she brushed at it. Something clinked to the paving stones of the sculpture yard. Stupidly, Anna stared down at it, eyes and mind disconnected. Part of her brain knew she should recognize the shape. Most of her brain was atomized, loose dust blowing in a windy night.

A syringe. The item that fell from her arm was a syringe. There was quarter of an inch of liquid in it.

Evidence of something.

She picked it up, holding it like a dagger. Forget evidence. Two weapons were better than one. Weapons against what?

People were hiding in the old barracks; she'd been chasing them. They had stuck the needle in her arm while she was sleeping.

Light. She needed light if she was going to go into the garbage- and rat-infested derelict building. Light and backup; she had to get a flashlight and a radio and a pair of underpants.

First she had to get up off of her knees. At one time she knew how human legs bent and flexed to execute this intricate maneuver. No more. She wasn't even sure where her feet were. She could neither see nor feel them.

A clunk startled her in a vague way. Rolling her head carefully to the side, she looked down. Somebody had dropped a gun—a SIG Sauer—beside her right knee. Careless bastard. What kind of idiot dropped a gun?

Me, she thought. My gun. Bending at the waist to pick it up, she fell face-first onto the granite paving. A cracking jarred the interior of her skull. Nothing hurt. Her skull felt as if it had been hurled against a wall, but nothing hurt. Or if it did, she couldn't feel it.

Straightening her arms, she forced her head and shoulders up from the ground. Sculpted works in progress, high as houses and cut into fantastic shapes, moved slowly around her, waving and leaning like grasses in a breeze. The brick and stone facade of the beautiful old building beyond rose as high as Half Dome, its many windows blank and lifeless.

"Help," she creaked. The noise she made was so thin and tiny she thought of the Woozy in *The Patchwork Girl of Oz*, the creature whose roar was supposed to bring down mountains but in reality was a teeny squeak. It didn't matter. Sculptors were artists. Artists didn't go around rescuing people. When the shit hit the proverbial, nobody ever yelled, "Is there an artist in the house!"

Anna pulled her knees under her to sit on her heels. In an attempt to scrape off the toxic fog devouring her brain, she scrubbed at her face. Pain that should have come when she fell blindsided her. She cried out feebly. One hand came away black and wet. Blood was pouring down over her left eye, blinding her.

Paul will still love me, even if the corner of my head is smashed, she thought. The image of her husband, Paul, in all his strength and calm, centered her. She was able to find her feet and push to a standing position. Her pistol was still on the ground, an infinite distance from her eyes. Teetering sickeningly back and forth in her boots, she tried to decide if it would be worse to leave her gun and go find a radio or stay with her gun and . . . what?

Just stay with her gun.

Besides, she was naked. She'd been reminded of that when she looked way, way down at the gun. No clothes. Naked outside in the weird with no clothes. This had to be a dream. That was a relief. Peculiar dreams were not strangers to Anna. There was a foolproof test to see whether one was dreaming or not. It wasn't pinching. That was silly. It was flying. If she could fly, that was proof positive she was dreaming.

Anna tried to lift her arms. They did not reach Superman-in-flight position, only zombie-seeking-edible-brain position.

No flying.

Not a dream.

Again she looked toward the ruins. The stairwell was disgorging its recent meal, bipedal shapes bulging forth to be delineated by the faint light of the stars. The creatures who'd put a wasp in her dream, a drug in her veins.

Anna raised her gun hand. "No further," she said. "Move and I soowt." She'd meant to say "shoot." The bonk on the head, or the chemical they'd injected, turned her lips to rubber. The figures halted, murmured, then came toward her.

Anna pulled the trigger. Nothing. Her hand was empty, the gun ever so far away on the ground by her foot.

The figures separated, moving slowly in her direction. Ninjas, black clothes and hoods and faces, with four white hands, fake as plastic mannequins' hands, floating along beside them. They were wearing surgical gloves.

Coming to butcher the kill, Anna thought as she tipped into nothingness.

THIRTY-TWO

Denise couldn't take her eyes off the fallen woman. In the starlight, Anna Pigeon was faintly luminescent, as if she'd been swimming in phosphorescent plankton. The boots, incongruously dark, made it appear as if her legs had been lopped off just below the knee, leaving white stumps. Anna's hair, always in a single fat braid, was spread out around her in a dark fan shot with silver, a protective cape that reached to her waist.

Denise didn't know what she had expected to happen when they'd set out on this venture, but this wasn't it. Despite the fact that three of her bullets were in him, Kurt Duffy had roared and fought. That made it self-defense in a way. Killing should be a positive or negative choice, not made in hot blood, necessarily—cold blood was fine—but with a real sense of commitment. One *committed* murder; murder didn't just happen. The gun didn't just go off; the victim didn't just run into the knife seven times.

Since she wasn't murdering Anna Pigeon, just removing an obstacle for a while, she'd pictured it happening in a prosaic, workaday kind of way. Or peacefully, like taking out the garbage on a Sunday afternoon. The unconscious body would lie in its own snug little bed, drifting quietly into deeper and deeper sleep. Then Denise and Paulette would wrap her tidily in one of her blankets and haul her to the runabout.

Not this blood-and-snot-filled gun-toting drama.

Also, in her mental picture, Anna Pigeon would wear a pair of pajamas, for Christ's sake, or a T-shirt and panties. What kind of lunatic leaps up and gives chase wearing nothing but a pair of cordovan NPS boots, even if she is drugged?

Naked was bad in an unsettling way. Naked was vulnerable and very female. Naked gave a body a gender and an age. "She should wear fucking pajamas," Denise hissed. "Rangers get called out at night."

Paulette said nothing.

The shushing sibilance of the sea washed between Denise and her sister. Usually the sounds of the ocean soothed Denise. These rasped. The clacking of rocks as they were rolled by the receding waves clattered like a plague of demented cicadas.

Anna Pigeon's hand twitched. Passed out on major drugs, the woman seemed to still be reaching for her gun.

"Oh God," Paulette whispered. "What do we do now?"

Trained to the call of "Gun!" Denise ran forward quickly and kicked the SIG out of the reach of the weak and groping hand. At a safe distance from the moribund ranger, she retrieved the weapon and shoved it into the waistband of her pants at the small of her back. Unlike Paulette, Denise had opted for black Levi's instead of sweatpants. The denim waistband held the gun firmly.

"We get her to the boat," Denise said.

"Shouldn't we get her some clothes first?" Paulette asked plaintively.

The toe of Denise's sneaker twitched out and struck the downed woman in the shoulder.

"Don't kick her!" Paulette exclaimed.

Like that was worse than drugging and snatching her.

Denise made no reply. She hadn't meant to kick her. Her foot had jerked out of its own accord. Nerves.

"We can lend her some of our clothes," Denise said. "She won't need much. She won't be there for long. Help me pick her up."

Paulette didn't move. She was looking past the naked ranger toward the housing area. "Maybe we should go back to her room. She's going to need some things. Maybe she takes medication . . . and toothpaste . . . that kind of thing," Paulette said.

Denise thought about that for an instant—not the meds or the toiletries, a blanket to cover her up. Anna had made it fifty or sixty yards from her apartment. There was nothing but open road and parking lot between where she lay and her bed. A sculptor up late smoking dope, or doing whatever sculptors did in the dead of night, might see them. "Too risky," she decided. "I'll take her arms, you take her legs. Put a hand under each knee; it'll be easier that way."

Paulette tiptoed gingerly around the crumpled form on the paving stones. Leaning down, she lifted one of the booted feet and pulled the leg. With the leverage, the senseless woman rolled to lie upon her back, hair veiling her breasts. Half of her face was covered in a black mask. Denise stared until she realized that it was not a mask; it was blood.

"She's bleeding!" Paulette exclaimed. "Why is she bleeding?"

To Denise, it sounded as if her sister blamed her, suggested she'd kicked Anna Pigeon in the face. Her toe had only just tapped the woman's shoulder. "She must have cut her head when she fell," Denise said curtly. "Get her legs." Moving briskly to give herself more courage and authority than she felt, Denise grabbed a limp wrist in each hand and lifted the upper body.

The used syringe fell from Anna's lax fingers. Denise dropped the hands. Flesh thudded against the ground.

"Careful," Paulette whispered. "We don't want to hurt her."

Denise grunted. Stepping on the needle, she pried the plastic up until the needle snapped off. She put the syringe in the front pocket of her jacket. Both she and Paulette had worn surgical gloves when they filled it; still, forensics would be able to tell what drugs were used, maybe match them to the rufies missing from the park's evidence locker. If anybody even thought to check there. The syringe itself might be a special kind Mount Desert used exclusively. One never knew what mattered and what didn't until it was too late.

The bit of evidence secured, Denise grabbed Anna's wrists again and whispered, "Grab her legs."

Paulette grabbed the top of the boots and pulled Anna's naked legs up and apart. A whimper escaped her as she slowly lowered them again, boot heels carefully together. "I can't!" she wailed softly. "It's like rape. Please, let's get her some clothes. Or put her back in her bed and leave. She won't remember us. You said she won't remember anything."

Denise wanted to lash out at Paulette, but a part of her felt as her sister did. Not about putting Ranger Pigeon back and pretending it never happened, but about one woman prying apart another woman's legs and stepping between them when that woman was naked. It was icky. The worst kind of icky, the kind that stuck to the inside of your skull for years.

"Right," she said to herself; then, to her sister, "But we can't go back. We're way beyond that. We can't leave her. Let's do this. Come take an arm. We'll drag her so her feet stay together and we're not . . . you know, looking at her that way. We don't have to drag her far. Jumping out of bed and chasing us, she did half our work for us. Another couple hundred yards and we're good to go. All the hard part over."

Paulette came up beside Denise but made no move to help. Denise shoved one of Pigeon's arms into her hands.

"Ranger Pigeon was nice to me the morning Kurt was found," Paulette said, looking into the bloody mask of a face.

Denise heard faint accusation in her sister's tone and bit back a harsh response. Paulette was her gentler self; she had to respect the Paulette half of her personality even when it was a huge pain in the butt. "Everything is going to be fine," she said calmly. "We've come so far. We do this and we're almost free. Think of our house in the pines somewhere warm. Think of being a family and never being cold or alone again."

Paulette took in a deep breath. "Okay," she said. "You're right."

Denise exhaled in relief. "Here we go," she whispered.

Both of them pulling moved the body at a snail's pace. Anna Pigeon couldn't have weighed more than a hundred and ten pounds, a hundred and fifteen at most, yet she apparently had made a deal with gravity; the earth seemed to hold her fast. Agonizing minutes passed as they dragged her from the granite apron in front of the Education Center onto the road to Schoodic Point, where the boat was stashed.

"Shit," Denise muttered as one of Anna's boots came off. Half a yard more and her heel was red with blood. Or, in the moonlight, black with blood. Denise was imagining the red color.

"We have to stop," Paulette said. "We're scratching her bottom and her legs all up."

"We're making a ton of noise," Denise said. Dumb and Dumber move a body, she thought. Murder wasn't glamorous; she knew that from killing Kurt. Neither was kidnapping, but it shouldn't be stupid. This was stupid, like a bad movie.

For an awful moment, Denise flew free of her body. From twenty feet up in the air she looked down at herself and her sister dragging the drugged ranger. They were ludicrous, absurd. Minuscule black ants, intent on abduction, hauling along a naked human. Insane. The picture whirled, and Denise crashed back into her own skull.

Not absurd, necessary.

Okay, absurd, but necessary, Denise admitted to herself. They had to do this to get what was owed them. She was sorry about Anna Pigeon, but Anna would have sided with the Peter Barneses and the Kurt Duffys and stripped Denise and her twin of everything. Again. Thrown them out to rot with the garbage. Again.

On second thought, she wasn't that sorry about Anna Pigeon. She should have kept her nosy little pigeon beak out of things that were none of her business, kept her beady little birdy eyes off of other people's things.

"Let's get her up," Denise said as she dragged the ranger's limp arm around her neck, hoisting her half of the inert form. "Like this, like we're walking a drunk. Then we won't be scratching her. It'll be okay. Put her arm around your neck." After more fumbling clown antics, they had the unconscious woman between them and were moving forward. Denise cursed herself. Anybody with half a brain would have worked all this bullshit out before doing the deed. The pigeon was to blame. If she hadn't nosed around they wouldn't be in such a rush, moving too fast to think things through properly.

With Anna draped around their necks, they traveled at a fairly good pace. Pigeon's toes dragged, but there was nothing Denise could do about that.

Within minutes they had trundled their catch over the rough cobble-sized stones of the point to the wash where they'd hidden the runabout. Unseen. Unheard. Like they'd never been to Schoodic. Like none of it had ever happened.

"We're good, we're good," Denise gasped, breathing in gusts as much from fear as exercise. Together they lowered the body, laying it out on the stones. "Catch your breath," Denise told her sister. "Almost done." Leaving Paulette standing over their captive, Denise went to turn the runabout right side up. The boat and outboard motor were heavy, but, unlike handling dead humans, Denise was accustomed to handling the runabout. She pried it up onto her knees, then flipped it easily over onto its keel.

Looking back over the gunwales, she expected to see Paulette getting the pigeon ready to drag over the side and into the boat. Instead, Paulette was sitting on the ground, in the rocks, her palms held to her cheeks and her feet in front of her like a little kid.

"We can't do it," Paulette said, eyes fixed on the prone naked ranger. "The shed won't be a good prison. She'll get out. Everybody will be swarming the island looking for her. Kidnapping is a serious crime. We could get the death sentence."

Like murder wasn't a serious crime—but then, Paulette hadn't murdered anybody. Denise had.

"How can we can we keep her quiet, even for a day or two?" Paulette wailed, her voice rising too high, too loud. "Hikers and tourists go in the woods, they could hear. Handcuffed, how can she get to the toilet? Feed herself? If we do it, she'll see us. Or hear us. We should have thought this through. Keeping her drugged all that time could hurt her. She could OD or dehydrate or something. I won't."

Paulette sounded mulish. More than that. She sounded firm.

What a miserable time for my sister to develop a spine, Denise thought. What a miserable time to get a conscience. Rage of the kind she thought she only held for Peter and his ilk rose up in her gorge hot as lava.

Paulette was staring up at her beseechingly, the ruined blond hair wisping out from beneath the black ball cap. Though they had been born only minutes, maybe seconds, apart, Denise realized Paulette was much younger than she was. Denise had to take care of her. You didn't rage at a child. Especially not if that child was you when you were little, back before they ruined you. Besides, Paulette was right. A nutcase who would run after you naked with a gun wasn't a person who would be easy to keep as a pet for an hour, let alone a couple of days.

Swallowing the molten anger, Denise walked around to where her sister sat beside Anna Pigeon. Crouching, she lifted one of Pigeon's arms, then laid two fingers over the pulse point at her wrist. For thirty seconds she concentrated. Having laid the hand back on the stones, she shifted, put her first and second finger on the ranger's trachea, and let them slide down into the hollow where the jugular vein was closest to the skin. Again she concentrated on feeling for a pulse.

It was there, thready and faint.

Making an executive decision, Denise removed her hand.

"Too late, Paulette," she said. "She's dead. You killed her."

"Oh God," Paulette murmured, and began to rock back and forth.

Denise sat next to her and put her arms around her. "Shh, shh," she whispered. "It's all good. This is how it was meant to be. I killed Kurt; you injected the pigeon and it killed her. That's how it had to be. We did nothing that wasn't supposed to happen. Things are just happening to help us now instead of hurt us. I'm going to take care of everything. No need to worry. Shh." She laid her cheek against her sister's. Paulette was calming at her touch. Denise savored the sensation of being of use, of value, to another human being.

"Are we done?" Paulette sniffed.

"Almost," Denise said. "I just need to find a garbage bag."

THIRTY-THREE

There was sensation of a sort. Anna didn't know if it was life, death, dreams, or something altogether different. As in a dream, occurrences that would have been staggeringly bizarre to the waking mind, felt ordinary.

Zen.

That thought wafted through the utter darkness inside Anna's skull. In dreams one was truly in the moment: no worries for the future, no regrets from the past, no expectations, therefore no surprises. The entire universe created in the mind, and the mind created in that universe.

A sliding sensation followed by a hard whack to the small of her back startled Anna free of philosophy. Pain was real and actual. Pain made a person care, and damn quick, what was going to happen next, and what had happened a second ago. Pain meant she wasn't dead and she wasn't dreaming. Life was happening.

Further than that, she couldn't fathom. "Breathe," she told herself.

ABCs: airway, blood, circulation. Breathing was first. Of course she was breathing. Alive, one did that sort of thing. But it wasn't easy. Almost, she had to tell her diaphragm to drop, her lungs to expand. Not an out-of-body experience; more a trapped-in-a-worthless-body experience.

As consciousness and breath fluttered in and out, pictures came back fleetingly: the jab, the wasp, the chase. Like old Polaroids, colors were muted and images fading like ghosts at sunrise.

Shadows had come to her room and pricked her arm. She had chased the shadows. Now she was blind and couldn't move. By the slick fabric clinging to her face, and the faint rubbery smell, she guessed she was in a big plastic sack. So, perhaps not blind, merely temporarily unable to see.

Drugged. Paralyzed. In a sack.

But not scared or unhappy. To the contrary, Anna felt fairly chipper. The drug, though powerful and paralyzing, had potential as a recreational drug. Nice of her kidnappers to think of her feelings. For a moment, Anna felt warm and fuzzy toward her shadows.

Then one of them stomped on her ankle. Roaring filled her ears. The two happenings were unrelated. The roar was an engine. Her sack and she were in a boat, or had been dumped in the backseat of a car. Boat. No car had that high whiny sound. A go-cart maybe.

Who kidnapped anybody with a go-cart?

For a while Anna faded. She knew she existed, she knew she was cold, but she had little opinion regarding these things. On some level she knew she was in deep trouble. People were not drugged and bagged and carted out to sea in a go-cart unless they were going to be disposed of.

Oddly, she didn't care overmuch.

Then the whining growl of the engine was gone. Anna's mind rose from the depths as if the harsh noise had been holding it under. Silence was a balm. Opening her mouth, she tried to breathe it in. Plastic stuck to her lips and tongue. Hands grabbed at her, latex screeching on plastic as fingers plucked and slipped on her shroud, then pinched and clutched, trying for better purchase. Heavy breathing and grunts filtered through the bag, but no voices. Not that it mattered. There would be no harm in her identifying the voices. The dead tell no tales and all that.

Dead. That sounded so melodramatic.

Anna would have liked to fight, just to say she had, that she'd gone down swinging and taken a few of the bastards with her, but she was unable to lift a hand or make her lips form a word.

As she was manhandled up to where her belly pressed hard against the gunwale, the boat rocked dangerously. Just as she was thinking how grand it would be if it capsized, and her shadows had to escort her to Davy Jones's locker, her head plunged into the cold. Plastic form-fitted itself around her mouth and nose, and she couldn't breathe.

Another heave and the rest of her followed out of the boat. Every inch of Anna was pressed with cold plastic. The ocean was too cold. Anna didn't want to die in the cold. Maybe she'd suffocate or die of hypothermia before she drowned.

"It's not sinking," came a shrill voice.

Well, that was good news.

In the fetal position inside the garbage bag, Anna felt the sea roll her onto her back; then she spun weightless into the sucking cold.

"There she goes," a calmer voice said.

Not much of an epitaph, Anna thought.

THIRTY-FOUR

They motored back to Somes Sound, Paulette as uncommunicative and dark as a lump of coal in the bow of the boat, Denise's mind fixated on Ranger Pigeon's demise. Not her drowning or suffocating or ODing or whatever finally took her out, but how weighty deadweight was. Manhandling the body was much harder than she would have believed. In the gym, Denise could bench press her own weight, one hundred twenty-five pounds—or could when she was in her early thirties. Yet moving a soon-to-be-dead body that weighed a bit less than that had been backbreaking, even though there were two of them doing the manhandling. Dead—or deadish—people were denser than living people, physically speaking, and just as uncooperative.

Denise was glad that the killing portion of her new life was at an end—maybe at an end. One thing did tend to lead to another. Obstacles would always pop up when one least expected it. Kurt had been a given, but the Pigeon thing, that was extemporaneous. Either way, Denise had reached the conclusion that killing people was more work than it was worth in a lot of ways. Hitler probably would have won World War II if he hadn't wasted so much time and energy killing people who didn't need killing.

Kurt had needed it. That hadn't made it any easier. Anna Pigeon hadn't needed it; things just got away from them, choices lopped off, until killing her was the only good one left. That didn't make it any easier.

Paulette, too, wasn't making things any easier. Denise watched her sitting in a heap as the boat cut neatly through the gentle swells. Paulette was more delicate than Denise had thought anyone who shared her DNA could be. It must be that nature made them both the same, but nurture had toughened Denise up. Nurture for Denise had been a brutal series of beatings and betrayals. Of course Paulette had been abused by her husband. Probably she was too old by then for the abuse to have any effect other than beating her down, Denise thought, whereas she—what? Had been beaten up?

However it worked, it was obvious that the removal of Anna Pigeon, though it had given them more time—a day, maybe a day and a half— had been harder on Paulette than it had been on her. Maybe it had broken some bit of her sister that could compromise the plan. Denise sensed that waiting while feds, rangers, and whoever else swarmed around looking for the missing Pigeon would be a bad idea. Paulette would fold under the pressure. Denise didn't like to think it, but she herself might have issues. Her nerves, once as strong as steel cables, had begun to fray. Age might account for it. Or Peter Barnes. Everything. Not that she'd fold under pressure, but she might explode. Either would mean disaster.

Time, in this case, would not heal all. It was a bomb. Denise could feel it ticking. Paulette or Fate or dumb luck was going to trigger the explosion soon. That this was so was felt in her viscera, as palpable as an electric current. Even with Pigeon out of the picture, things would have to be moved up. Way up. The sale of the Duffy shack, the so-called legacy, and family.

Tomorrow night they would tick "family" off the list, then get the hell out of Dodge. Do the rest long distance. Denise had no doubt that once they were out of sight, they'd be out of mind. A has-been ranger retires and moves. A bleached-blond housewife, with an iron-clad alibi for her husband's murder, sells the house where he was killed and leaves town. Nobody would connect those nonevents to a missing acting chief ranger from Rocky Mountain National Park. No connection between Denise and Anna, Anna and Paulette, Denise and Kurt, or Paulette and Denise.

All that could screw the pooch now was Paulette babbling or Denise going postal. So: tick, tick, tick.

For Denise that meant the night, though nearly spent, was not yet over.

By the time she got the runabout moored, and Paulette headed for her bed in the shack, only fifty-six minutes remained before dawn. Sunrise would be at 5:03 A.M. At five Peter would get out of bed and go to the bathroom to pee. At 5:04 he would be pulling on his running clothes; 5:10 and he'd be out the front door swinging his hands side to side and jogging in place. He would run 4.5 miles. Depending on how he was feeling, he would be gone thirty to thirty-six minutes, getting back to the house around quarter to six.

Rather than sleeping in like a sane woman, little Lily flower got her lovely little ass out of bed at 5:15 every morning, checked on the baby— didn't pee, she did that between midnight and three—and went down to make her darling hubby coffee.

Like Peter couldn't poke the button on the coffee machine before he left.

She'd poke the button, then, while she waited for it to brew, prepare Olivia's first bottle of the day, setting it in a pan of water to heat. Microwaving wasn't good enough for Lily's baby. No nuked fake milk for Olivia.

After the burner was on low, Lily would go upstairs and brush her teeth and comb her hair so she'd be all nice and minty fresh for that big sweaty kiss Peter would plant on her when he came huffing back for his coffee.

That gave Denise a four-minute window when nobody would be in the kitchen.

Years of covert surveillance were paying off big-time, Denise thought with satisfaction. Those long nights with binoculars, the skulking in the woods, following in rental cars, hadn't been insanity, it had been foresight. A lot of what she'd seen as problems were turning out to be plusses.

She'd been going to tell Paulette about this step in the plan. Then she learned her twin wasn't a real nurse, just a nursemaid. If she'd been a real RN it would have been good because Denise would have been more confident about the dosage. Since she wasn't, Denise hadn't said anything out of spite. Now she was glad. Given how shaken the Pigeon thing had left Paulette, the less she knew of the sordid details, the better.

Originally, Denise had planned to do this when she could take her time and make sure she got everything just right, not have to rush things to get it all done in a four-minute time slot. Most days, at two fifteen, Lily put the baby's food on to warm, then went upstairs to make the bed. Picturing it, Denise shook her head in the dark as she climbed into her Miata. What kind of a nitwit makes the bed at two in the afternoon?

Still, that left a seven-minute window. Tons of time. Denise should wait until two fifteen, but she wouldn't. Couldn't.

Tick, tick, tick.

Four minutes would have to do.

Five A.M. sharp, Denise pulled the Miata into its customary space, the place she parked for her breaking-and-entering activities. A dirt road, a quarter of a mile down from Peter and Lily's house, led to a construction boneyard no more than a hundred yards behind their property. One day a home would be built there. For the past several years it had been from whence Denise's forays into the Barnes family homestead had been staged. Car tracks could link her to the place if anybody got that far into the investigation, but she wasn't too worried. Big machinery was in and out during working hours: trucks, bulldozers, front-loaders. By noon the tracks of the Miata would be well and thoroughly squashed.

She popped the trunk, walked around to the back of the car, and unerringly laid her hands on the crumpled McDonald's bag half wedged beneath the first aid kit. Inside, wadded in a used napkin, were three white pills, crushed to a powder. Having retrieved one of the unused Mount Desert syringes, Denise filled it half full from her water bottle, poured the powder in, shook it a few times for good measure, then stowed it carefully in her jacket pocket.

"What the hell," she whispered, and threw the bag onto the ground. Maybe she'd get lucky and the litter would blow into Peter's backyard.

THIRTY-FIVE

eath's eyes opened to unremitting black. Where in hell was she? Clearly not in her bed in Boulder. Momentary panic from watching *Premature Burial* too many times as a kid engulfed her. The adrenaline rush brought her to full alert.

This wasn't the first time she'd woken up and not known where she was. After the accident, when she was on medications and changed hospital rooms or therapy venues, it often happened. The amnesia seldom lasted more than a second or two. A calming thought.

Ah, lucidity!

She lay in her little bed on Boar Island, and the black was not unremitting. At ground level, the tower had little in the way of natural light, but halfway up the winding stairs was a bar of living dark, dark like the midnight sky or the surface of a lake on a moonless night. There was a difference between living dark and the dark, she presumed, of a coffin six feet under.

What had wakened her?

In a second, it came to her. The lift bell had rung. Or a bell on a buoy in the ocean. Heath had seen those but never knew what they were for.

To let fish know the wind was blowing? As far as she knew, both Elizabeth and Gwen were asleep in the rooms above. It was possible they could have descended the iron stairs and slipped through her room undetected. Possible but unlikely; the old stairs complained bitterly when they were used.

Heath switched on the bedside lamp, found her phone, and pinched it on. Dawn had not yet creaked. Surely John Whitman had more sense than to come calling on his lady love at this hour. She smiled, imagining the crusty old seaman serenading Gwen as she leaned over the rail around the top of the lighthouse.

Wily opened his eyes from his chosen spot at the foot of the stairs, where his charges would trip over him should they try to elude his vigilance.

"I've got ringing in my ears," Heath said to the dog.

Wily thumped his tail.

The ring must have been from a buoy, or a ship's bell. Ships did have bells, Heath remembered from old books. They told time by them. Probably they now set all the sailors' cell phones to ring at the appropriate hours. Heath turned off the light and settled down to go back to sleep.

Again the bell rang.

Definitely the lift bell.

The lift bell rang when it was called down to the jetty, and it rang when it was sent—or called—to the top of the cliff. When they'd retired for the night, it had been at the top of the cliff. Two bells; somebody had called the lift down, gotten on, then sent it up. That somebody was now on the island.

In the wee hours.

"Damn," Heath muttered. Wake E? Call Gwen? Flash an SOS to the mainland? "Why aren't you barking?" she suddenly demanded of Wily. He swept his tail over the wide boards of the floor.

Since Wily wasn't alarmed, Heath felt safe enough to see what was happening before she roused the house. The last thing she wanted was to make this ivory tower—such as it was—feel unsafe when Elizabeth was experiencing just how unsafe most of the world was.

A metal bar on legs, like a spare clothing rack, but narrower and much stronger, stood over the head of the bed. One of Leah's designs, it was lightweight, stable, and easily broken down into a civilized-sized carrying package. It was a great help when Heath overnighted away from home.

Using the bar, she hoisted herself upright, then pushed her legs free of the covers and the mattress. From there it was a fairly easy swing into Robo-butt, parked next to the bed. In one of Robo-butt's saddlebags, among other things, was a small Maglight. Heath took it out, clicked the switch a couple of times. Satisfied the batteries hadn't gone dead, she dropped it into her lap.

Rolling toward the long tunnel through the tower wall of the lighthouse, she asked, "Coming, Wily?"

The steady pad-pad of his paws on the flooring behind her was reassuring.

Though there was no moon, the arc-shaped main room of the tower, with its floor-to-ceiling windows, was surprisingly light. The sea seemed to maximize ambient light, catching the stars on the whitecaps. The granite Maine was built on had that same reflective quality, thousands of tiny facets polished by the centuries until they shone like mirrors.

Heath twisted the dead bolt, then shoved open the door with the foot of her wheelchair. Still showing no signs of alarm, Wily trotted out in front of her onto the apron of granite. Warily, she rolled after him. Halfway across the natural patio the lift platform came into view. A pile of pale stuff lay on it.

Wily trotted toward it.

"Wait," Heath called, afraid whatever had been sent up at this ungodly hour was dangerous, poisonous, or vile in some other way.

Wily ignored her, stepped delicately from the landing onto the platform, sniffed the pile, and whined. Heath clicked on the tiny flashlight, shoved the butt end into her mouth, and rolled slowly toward the dog and his catch.

It looked like a mess of fish caught in a net. Another gift from the sea provided by Gwen's beau? Wouldn't fish be nasty after even a few hours lying about? Heath rolled nearer. Saliva drooled down her chin. Since she needed both hands to roll in a straight line, she ignored it. Wily wouldn't mind. He'd been known to drool a time or two in his life.

The dog turned in a tight circle, sat down, threw his head back, and howled.

It wasn't a net of dead fish. It was a dead woman. She lay on one shoulder. Both arms were stretched above her head, the wrists tied to one of the rings used to secure cargo to the lift floor. She was naked but for one boot and the wild netting of red and silver hair.

Anna.

For a heartbeat, Heath denied it was she. Anna didn't lose, didn't die, didn't quit. Anna wasn't beaten and trussed and delivered like the morning paper. If Anna wasn't invincible, what chance did ordinary people have?

Reality snapped back.

"Gwen! Elizabeth!" Heath shouted, the Maglight falling from her jaws to her lap. She jerked the brass whistle free of the neck of her pajama top, put it to her lips, and blew for all she was worth, three piercing blasts.

"Oh my God, Anna!" She rolled until one of Robo-butt's wheels was on the lift. Having put the brakes on, she levered herself out and slid down next to the body of her friend. The Maglight rolled onto the lift platform to lodge against Anna's naked breast, the light shining ghoulishly up beneath her chin.

Heath laid a hand on Anna's bare shoulder. The skin was ice cold and felt firmer than it should. "No, no, no," Heath was whispering. "Gwen!" she shouted again. Gwen was a doctor. Gwen would make it okay.

"Anna," Heath said. "Can you hear me? You're going to be just fine. Fine and dandy, damn you." As Heath murmured in a kind, reassuring voice, a voice designed to bring kittens out from under houses and rangers back from the dead, she lifted the hair from Anna's face and neck. A mass of it was pasted to her back with blood. Blood showed dark on her butt and the heel of her left foot.

"What have you been up to?" Heath asked as she felt for the carotid pulse. "You're alive," she said, more for Anna than because she was positive the weak flutter against the pads of her index and middle fingers was blood being pumped through veins.

"What is it?"

Heath turned to see Gwen, tying a robe around her, trotting toward where she sat with Anna. E, in tank top and pajama bottoms, followed close behind, her small narrow feet silent against the rock.

"Move aside," Gwen said the moment she identified the incident as medical. "Elizabeth, run for blankets."

As Gwen fell to her knees beside Anna, Heath wormed herself into a position where she could attend to the binding around Anna's wrists. The ties were cut lengths of yellow line, the kind used in boats. They weren't tied tightly. Circulation wasn't compromised, and had Anna been conscious, she could easily have escaped the bonds. Balancing as best she could on her hind end, Heath untied Anna's wrists and began massaging her cold limp hands.

"She has a pulse," Gwen said, "but it is weak and too slow." Heath said nothing. Elizabeth was sprinting from the house with an armload of blankets. Gwen was running her hands over Anna's body, palpating for injuries, breaks, and bruises.

Elizabeth dumped three down comforters onto the ground. Heath pulled one over and began covering Anna.

Gwen sat back on her knees. "Nothing I can find. Hypothermic probably. Contusions on back, buttocks, and right heel. One lump above her left temple. That might account for the unconsciousness, but it could be any number of things. We have to get her inside and get her warmed up, then get her to a hospital as soon as possible."

"She's awake," Elizabeth whispered.

Heath leaned down so she could see Anna's eyes. They were half open.

"Hi," Anna said in a voice as creaky as a rusted gate hinge.

The eyes drifted closed again.

"That was informative," Heath growled. Seeing Anna helpless frightened her. Heath had always been a person who turned fear into anger. At the moment, she was furious and terrified. Laserlike heat burned inside her skull. Heath half believed that if she ever saw whoever did this to Anna, she could flay him using just her eyes.

For a quarter of an hour there was no talking. A comforter was ruined as the three of them dragged Anna in from the lift. Gently, they hoisted her up onto the couch, then packed down quilts around her naked body. Without being told to, Elizabeth found heating pads in one of the closets.

With a last look at Anna, she slipped into the kitchen, to microwave the pads and boil water for hot drinks, Heath assumed. While Gwen was Velcroing a blood pressure cuff around Anna's upper arm, Heath was searching the contacts list on her phone for Peter Barnes's home number.

The silence was broken by Anna.

"Stop," she croaked.

"Hey!" Heath said with relief as she put the phone to her ear.

"No calls. Not yet," Anna managed, and, "Help me up."

Sitting up was perhaps not the best of ideas, but both Gwen and Heath had known Anna too long to think telling her to stay still would be efficacious. Gwen left the pump bulb on the cuff dangling to put an arm around Anna's shoulders, helping her into a semisitting position against the pillows piled on the arm of the sofa.

"You need to go to the hospital," Gwen said as Heath was asking, "What happened?"

Anna clutched the sides of her head as if the two soft voices were a cacophony. "What happened," she echoed. "Before you . . . Tell me what happened. I'm so cold."

With use, her voice was normalizing, but the words were slightly blurred—not the slur of a drunk so much as the drawl of a person from a very, very deep South.

"A man said he thought I was a lobster," Anna mumbled, shaking her head. "No. That can't be right. Yes. He thought I was a lobster. Said he thought I was . . . And now I'm here." She dropped her hands to her lap and looked hard first at Gwen, then at Heath.

"What are you guys doing here?" she asked with a certain petulance.

"We heard the lift bell," Heath told her. "Wily and I found you on the platform."

Heath watched, letting the information sink in through whatever was clouding Anna's perception. Anna's eyes roved the room as if to see where she'd washed up. "Boar," she said finally. Heath, Gwen, and Elizabeth, drawn in from the kitchen by Anna's voice, nodded like bobblehead dolls. Gwen took two heating pads from E. Having peeled back the blankets, she began arranging them along Anna's ribs.

Anna watched her for a long moment. "I'm naked," she observed.

"That's how we found you. Wearing only one boot. That one." Heath pointed to the sodden cordovan-colored boot standing solitary watch on the cold hearth.

"E, would you please make Anna a cup of tea, real warm but not hot, lots of sugar," Gwen said.

"No sugar," Anna said as E turned to go.

Gwen tilted her chin at her great-niece. Anna would be getting sugar.

"Do you remember anything?" Heath asked.

Anna thought. Heath waited, her fingers drumming lightly against the face of her phone, itching to call for help. "May I call Superintendent Barnes now?" Heath asked.

"Not yet. I . . ." Anna's voice faded out. Her train of thought had evidently derailed. "Let me figure out what happed first," she said, finding her way back.

Had Anna not been showing signs of returning life—if not sanity—and Gwen not been a doctor, Heath would have made the call regardless of Anna's protestations. As it was, Anna seemed to be out of danger.

Danger of what, evidently not even Anna knew.

THIRTY-SIX

Anna was awake. A dozen times before, she'd thought she was awake, only to slip back into nightmares until she could no longer tell what was real, what had happened, and what was only a dream.

Only a dream.

There was no "only" about the dreams that pulled her down. They were a force as powerful as any she had encountered. They followed her into the waking world and threatened to drag her back.

"I am awake," she said. Her voice creaked. Her tongue was as stiff and dry as weathered wood. If taste was any indication, weathered wood from the bottom rail of an old pigsty.

"You're awake," a kind voice agreed. "And alive."

Anna rolled her eyes, eyeballs scratching against lids that felt packed with sand. "We'll see," she rasped. Heath was bent over her, a huge annoying smile on her face. "I feel like shit. My face hurts."

"You're hungover," Heath said, still grinning like a fool. "Your head got a hard whack, but it isn't broken, according to Aunt Gwen."

Anna reached up with shaking fingers and felt above her eye. There was a lump the size of a walnut, and tender to the touch. Not broken; that was good news. At least not broken on the outside. The gray matter inside of her skull felt as if it had been scrambled like eggs. Lying down was disorienting, and she struggled to sit up. The room spun. Her stomach lurched into her throat. A hammer wielded by an invisible hand slammed into her left temple.

"Do you want to sit up?" Heath asked.

"Of course I want to sit up!" Anna grumbled. "Do you think I'm flopping around because I like looking like a landed fish?"

"Somebody got up on the wrong side of the ocean today."

Elizabeth was perched on the end of the couch where Anna lay. Anna tried to glare at her, as Heath, more trouble than help, worked to get her into a seated position without falling out of her wheelchair.

"E!" Heath said. Rising smoothly, Elizabeth trotted around the back of the sofa. Between the two of them, Anna was shoved and shored up into a sitting position.

"Damn, but I feel like shit," Anna said as bile rose up her gorge. "I'm going to be sick." Heath bobbed out of her line of sight, then bobbed back up again, a bowl in her hand.

"Gwen said you might be," she said, putting the bowl between Anna's hands.

Anna retched into the bowl, spewing up thin acid and stinking chunks.

"Done?" Heath asked gently.

"Don't be so nice," Anna said. Nice made tears threaten, and Anna was too sick to cry.

Heath smiled. "Take this, would you, E?"

"Eeeeew," Elizabeth grimaced as she removed the mess from Anna's lap.

"How long was I asleep?" Anna asked.

"Half the day," Heath said. "Gwen thought rest was the best thing for you. She gave you an antibiotic, but we didn't try and clean or dress your wounds."

"I have wounds?" Anna asked, surprised. When every inch of one's body hurt, it was hard to tell.

Elizabeth was back on her perch. "One of your heels is all scraped up, and your bottom has major road rash."

An image of her booted toes, seen down the length of her naked body, bouncing along black asphalt flashed through Anna's mind.

"I was dragged," she said, more to herself than them.

A cackle of questions battered in stereo. "By who? Where? Why? Do you remember? Dragged?"

Anna ignored them. Her skin was too tight, her hair stiff and matted; thinking was difficult. Poison pervaded her being. She was sick unto her bones.

"I need a shower," she said softly. Then, raising her head, she looked into Heath's concerned face. "A shower."

Heath and Elizabeth exchanged glances. Anna glowered. "Help her with a shower, E," Heath said finally.

"I don't need any help." Anna stood up, tottered, then fell back on the couch. For a moment she sat blinking stupidly as resistance drained away. "That would be good, E," she said with moderate civility. "Thank you."

Leaning against the tile wall for support, hot water pouring through her salt-encrusted hair, Anna began to feel slightly more human. Most of the night and the day before were a blur. She remembered going to bed. She remembered seeing the toes of her boots. She remembered plastic sticking to her face. She remembered someone saying she was a lobster.

Four memories that didn't add up to anything. Caked in salt, contusions on her butt and heel, a knot on her forehead, a small hole that ached in her left arm, up by the shoulder, probably a needle stick: drugged, dragged, and dumped into saltwater. Without the aid of memory, logic dictated that much. Since she was not dead, one could assume she had subsequently been fished out of the saltwater. Heath and Wily had found her naked, tied to the cargo ring on the lift, shortly before sunrise.

Again, since she wasn't dead, logic suggested she was put there by the fisher-of-out, either so she would receive help or as a warning to the island's residents. E, as a stalkee, being the most obvious.

Both theories were absurd.

That didn't make them untrue.

"Are you still alive?" Elizabeth asked from the other side of the shower curtain.

"Getting there," Anna said. She could see the girl's shadow where she sat on the commode, standing by in case Anna fell or drowned.

"Let me know when you're ready to do your back," E said.

Elizabeth's comfort with her own and other people's bodies was a wonder to Anna. Nudity, injury, snot, puke, washing hair, clipping toenails—E did these things for other people as casually as she did them for herself. Maybe loving someone who occasionally required personal assistance had given her these skills. More likely she was born with them, and loving Heath had brought them to flower.

John Donne said no man was an island. He didn't say anything about women. Anna keenly felt her physical isolation from the rest of the human race, with the exception of her husband, Paul, an isolation she preferred. Every woman in her own skin, every mind in its own cranium.

Until she couldn't take care of her own skin or trust her own mind.

"I'm ready," Anna said.

"Incoming," Elizabeth replied cheerfully as she opened the shower curtain. Anna braced both hands against the opposite wall, holding herself up, while Elizabeth carefully washed the scrapes on her buttocks.

"Not as bad as we thought," E said. "Sort of like a skinned knee, but all over. Not so much bleeding as oozing. Some bleeding on your bottom, but nothing as bad as your heel. Aunt Gwen did that up while you were out cold. Now that the bandage is wet, she'll have to redress it. She said your heel is pretty much like hamburger. Nothing broken, though. She didn't want to mess with your back until you'd slept. We took a look at it. Heath and I thought we should put you out of your misery, but Aunt Gwen said it wasn't too bad, and it isn't."

Whoever had dragged her across the pavement must not have dragged her far, Anna decided. A protracted trip would have left her skinned alive.

"Where is Gwen?" Anna asked, mostly to keep Elizabeth chattering. Unlike the prattle of other people, the prattle of her goddaughter was soothing, like rain on a tin roof. Usually Anna listened for clues of what was happening in E's world, and heart, and mind. Sometimes, like now, she just rode the flow of words, enjoying the murmur of a happy life burbling past her ears, a sweet cacophony more soothing to the soul than silence.

"Aunt Gwen is in Bar Harbor meeting Dez Hammond—one of the old ladies who lived here—for coffee. Aunt Gwen felt guilty about abandoning you, but she said it was very important. An errand for Chris Zuckerberg, the other lady, the one that's sick. Some sort of meeting Ms. Zuckerberg was too sick to go to.

"Aunt Gwen took her medical bag. She said she was going to get a DNA sample or something. She had a glass tube and Q-tips and everything. Very *CSI*. Of course she wouldn't tell us what it's about since it's a doctor thing."

Anna's knees were growing weak. Her arms, bracing her against the shower wall, were tiring. "Are you about done?" she asked.

"Done," E said. Anna felt a towel being draped over her shoulders. Pulling her aching arms away from the wall, she noticed a red mark on the inside of her arm at the elbow. "Another needle stick," she said, turning to show Elizabeth the way a little girl might show her mother a splinter.

"That was Aunt Gwen. She took blood while you slept. You didn't even move an eyelid," Elizabeth said with obvious pride in her aunt's needlework.

"Took blood?" Anna echoed stupidly.

"*CSI* on every channel today. She's getting it tested for drugs," E said matter-of-factly.

"She's not in law enforcement," Anna said.

"She's a doctor. They do all that blood stuff."

Of course. "I'm not thinking straight," Anna admitted.

"Duh," E said, holding out a second towel for Anna's hair. "Sit."

Obediently, Anna sat on the lid of the commode and let Elizabeth towel-dry her hair. Gray splotches floated in the corners of her eyes, as amorphous and will-o'-the-wisp as her recollections of the previous night. The shower had washed away the salt, the blood, and the last of the anger she'd brought with her from the other side. Without the anger, her brain was a cold and sluggish thing, thoughts being forced out like the last of the toothpaste from the tube.

"Was I raped?" she asked, before her brain had time to mention that might not be an appropriate question to ask a sixteen-year-old girl, and one's goddaughter at that.

"Nope," E said as if it were the most obvious question in the world— and it was. "Aunt Gwen said there was no evidence to indicate any kind of sexual trauma. She did a rape kit anyway. Don't worry. The rest of us, even Wily, were banished from the entire house while she did her exam."

Anna was absurdly relieved. Bad enough if E and Heath had seen that sort of thing, but if Wily had, she'd have had to resign from the pack in shame.

Three taps sounded on the door. "Are you guys about done?" Heath asked. "E, your visitor has finally seen fit to come, so make sure Anna has something decent on."

Both caught the sour emphasis Heath put on the word "visitor." Anna raised an eyebrow.

Turning to take a terrycloth robe from a hook on the back of the bathroom door, Elizabeth said, "It's my friend."

"The one with the boat," Anna said.

"Yes."

"What made you decide to blow Boat Boy's cover?" Anna asked.

"Before, he needed you not to know more than you needed to know. It's the other way around now," Elizabeth said as she held out a thick yellow chenille bathrobe.

Anna snorted. Now she was on a need-to-know basis with her goddaughter. Elizabeth had grown from a skinny little kid into an entire human being, and Anna had seen every bit of it, a terrifying miracle.

"Are you going to arrest him?" Elizabeth asked.

Anna stood and let her goddaughter help her into the robe.

"I sure as hell feel like arresting somebody," she said.

THIRTY-SEVEN

The shower worked wonders. Anna was fairly steady on her feet. Her mind was clear enough for minor calculations. The mirror proved unkind. There was a nasty bruise on her forehead, her skin was pasty, and her eyes had dark circles beneath and red rims around. No beauty contests would be won today.

As she walked from the bath into the room around the tower, the lift bell rang.

"That will be Aunt Gwen," E said, hovering behind Anna's right shoulder. "She wanted to be in on this, and her meeting with Mrs. Hammond was over."

Elizabeth settled Anna on the sofa with so little fuss, Anna didn't even mind. Heath rolled in from the kitchen to hand Anna a mug of steaming cream of tomato soup. Tears stung the corners of Anna's eyes. Tomato soup was just the thing, the only thing, her stomach wanted. When she was growing up it was the food for ailing children. Dotted with chicken pox, she and Molly had sat across from each other at the scarred old kitchen table spooning soup with oyster crackers. Later it had been mumps and tomato soup and ginger ale. Then measles. Because of tomato soup, she and her sister had lived to adulthood.

She sipped, sighed, and silently blessed Heath with a smile. "Where's Boat Boy?" she asked.

"He went to meet the lift," Heath said, rolling over to one of the wide windows. "Seems Gwen decided John Whitman should be here."

Despite the healing magic of soup, Anna wasn't up for a party. "Why?"

"Boat Boy is named Walter. Walter is John's grandson," Elizabeth said.

"Curiouser and curiouser," Anna said. Then, "Walter Whitman? As in *Leaves of Grass*? A poet, no less?"

Evidently E hadn't heard of Walt Whitman. Anna would fix that another day. She took another fortifying slurp of soup.

Gwen, John, and Walter Whitman came in from the patio.

Boat Boy was so handsome Anna scowled. Light brown hair waved back off a square brow in what had been called a surfer cut when she was in college. Shoulders were broad and arms muscled—from rowing boats with muffled oars, no doubt. Lips were chiseled, eyes wide set and a deep rich hazel. The plaid shirt straining across his chest was almost a cliché in its woodsy perfection.

Unless John had more than one son, Boat Boy Walter was the son of the lobsterman shot for poaching, the boy accused of being an accomplice.

Gorgeous, an orphan, and a fugitive.

Anna had to admit, had she been sixteen and marooned on an island with annoying adults, she would have jumped ship with this boy in a heartbeat.

"This is my grandson Walter," John said.

Anna opened her mouth to introduce herself. What came out was "I'm not a lobster." Clapping her mouth shut, she frowned. Kaleidoscope fashion, parts of her lost night were spinning through her gray matter.

"A lobster trap," Walter said apologetically. "I thought you were a lobster trap. It was wicked hard gettin' you out of the drink."

"Lobster" was pronounced *lobstah;* "hard" was *hahd.* Coming from the Apollo-meets-Ralph-Lauren vision, the hard New England accent sounded out of place, yet it, too, was charming. Anna reminded herself that often as not, Prince Charming turned out to be just another clown.

"Let's all sit," Gwen said sensibly. "This may take a while."

Walter and his grandfather sat on the outer edge of the chairs, elbows on knees, hands clasped, the way Anna remembered the hired hands sitting when she was a kid. Comfortable, assured, but not wanting to be seen to be taking the boss's hospitality for granted.

"You saved my life," Anna said to Walter. "Let's start there and work our way back. That way I'll be in a more forgiving mood when we get to the kidnapping of my goddaughter."

Anna had been shooting for a spot of humor, a little levity to ease the proceedings. Through a furry brain and a swollen lip, the words came out more like a threat. John started a low grumble in his throat. Wily echoed it from the cold hearth, where he lay watching the proceedings with interest.

"Her bark is worse than her bite," she heard E whisper.

"She bites?" Walter whispered back, then caught Anna's eye and grinned sheepishly. "No disrespect meant," he apologized.

"I do bite," Anna admitted with a sigh. "But I'm not rabid, so, if it happens, you'll survive."

"Tell the woman your story," John said, jutting his chin in Anna's direction.

"You'll know by now, it was my dad was shot by Billy Gomer. Killed for poaching," Walter began uncertainly.

"I didn't know the shooter's name, but I'd heard," Anna said. It had been two, maybe three weeks since this boy's father was murdered. Walter's words—and, to give him credit, tone of voice—were matter-of-fact.

The eyes and the small muscles around his mouth told Anna of the grief and strain. "You were accused of doing the same," she said before sympathy could get the better of her.

"That's right. But we were no poachers. Neither my dad nor me. It was about a patch of good fishing that was being fought over and we won. We were taking forty to fifty percent more lobsters out than Gomer ever did, so he starts saying we were taking from his line. He and my dad got into it, and Gomer shot Dad. Killed him right there." Walter clamped his lips together and stared at the floor. These were not men who wore their hearts on their sleeves. Pain was not for public consumption.

"Is this Gomer fellow in jail?" Anna asked.

Walter's grandfather barked a bitter laugh. "Billy is goin' on eighty. Twelve kids, nine of them boys, and all got a patch and a vote. There won't be any goin' to jail for Billy Gomer."

"Mr. Gomer is mean to the soles of his boots," Walter said, shaking his head. "But he's known to be honest. I think he believed me and Dad were poaching because he couldn't believe the truth, which is we're better fisherman than he ever was."

"I'd say that's about right," John added. "I'd say old Gomer believes himself. Since he's sworn he'll shoot Walter if he gets a chance, I don't much care what he believes or doesn't believe." The older man's jaw set in a concrete square. Anna would not want John Whitman as an enemy.

"I don't think he will," Walter said. "The fight was always between him and Dad. Much as I'd like to see it, I don't think there's any good to be had by lockin' Mr. Gomer up. He's sure to die in a few years anyway."

Another day Anna might have been fascinated with the ins and outs of lobster fishing in Maine. At present her head was heavy and her face hurt her, and undoubtedly hurt them to look at. "I'm sorry about your dad," she said as kindly as she could manage. The soup had helped. She almost liked herself.

Her well-meant words started to eat away at Walter's stoicism, so she went on. "But how does this relate to saving my life and kidnapping my goddaughter?"

John Whitman stood abruptly. "There was no kidnapping." His scarred hands were balled into fists. Suddenly he wasn't quaint or colorful.

"It's okay, John," Gwen said quickly. "Ranger humor."

"I don't have much use for park rangers," John grumbled.

"They grow on you eventually," Heath said dryly.

Slowly, John lowered himself back onto the edge of the chair, his hands again folded between his knees.

Walter took his time, looking first to his grandfather, then to Elizabeth. He must have found what he was searching for, because he went on. "Mr. Gomer's talk got my fishing license suspended, pending investigation."

"An investigation that isn't going to happen," John said grimly.

"Probably not," Walter agreed. "People forget others' troubles pretty quick. The lines Mr. Gomer shot Dad over are right here off the island, between Boar and Mount Desert. Rich beds. I figured if I could find out who was stealing from the traps, I could clear Dad's name and get my license back."

"So you went into hiding, and have been watching the area?" Anna asked.

"That I have. I'd been camping out in the old wing of the house, the one seaside."

"Walter was our ghost, remember, Mom?" Elizabeth asked.

Heath nodded. A story Anna would have to hear later. Clearing his father's name, and his own, to get his fishing license back might have struck Anna as a silly piece of teenage posturing in another place. In Maine, once the Whitmans' licenses were suspended, their trap line would have been farmed out to another fisherman.

Chances were good Walter had worked with his dad and granddad since he was old enough to mend traps. He'd probably apprenticed for two years under his father to get a license. Lobster fishing might very well be all he knew and all he wanted to know.

"You've been living on Boar and watching the water at night?" Anna clarified.

"That's about it," Walter said.

"You were watching last night," Anna said.

"I was. I saw a boat I've seen before. A small dark-colored outboard. Both times before, I lost it. Weather once, and once it was just plain too dark to see where it went. It has no running lights. There are three green LED lights near the bow, but they're no bigger than that." With his thumb, Walter indicated the tip of his little finger. "And they aren't bright. Decoration maybe. Whoever owns the boat dives at night. Robbing traps is my guess. Last night, there was some light and the seas were calm. I saw that same boat coming onto the line of traps, so I rowed out as close as I could without them noticing me."

"Muffled oars," Anna said.

"That's right, and their engine noise to cover for me."

"More than one?" Anna asked.

"This time there were two in the boat. Last two times just the one. I saw them throw something over the side. I figured they were up to something, so I pulled out what they'd tossed in."

"My exceeding good luck," Anna said. "Which way did they go?"

"They came from the north up by Schoodic, and headed down toward Somes Sound when they left."

"And you were stuck with a very strange catch," Gwen said.

"Odd things get thrown in the ocean," John said.

"Anna is an odd thing," E said.

"You put me on the lift?" Anna asked.

"I knew the bell would wake up Elizabeth, and I knew her great-aunt was a doctor," Walter said. "I suppose I could have stayed, but I couldn't see what use it would be to anybody."

Anna thought about that for a moment. There was really no point in his staying. Her desire to dislike young Walter was slowly being overwhelmed by warm cozy feelings.

"Why did you tie me down to the cargo ring?" she asked in a last attempt to find fault with the boy who stole Elizabeth's heart—and kidnapped Wily.

"So you wouldn't fall off," he said simply.

The tail end of Anna's dislike vanished like a snake down a hole. All in all, she was glad to see it go. Disliking people was labor intensive at the best of times, and today wasn't the best of times.

THIRTY-EIGHT

There had been little more either John or his grandson could tell them. Anna had been wrapped in black plastic—either a bag or a sheet. Walter had torn it open. The plastic had been lost at sea. If there was anything in the bag with her, he hadn't noticed. Nor could he tell them any more about the mystery boat than he already had.

The Whitmans left for Bar Harbor, promising to look for the dark boat on their way into town. Walter promised he'd call E in the morning.

Elizabeth was positively wriggling with delight at having her beau outed and approved. Walter seemed as pleased as she to be out of the shadows. Another point for him.

Anna held out no hope the Whitmans would find the runabout that had nearly served as her hearse. Not only had it been headed in the opposite direction—Somes instead of Bar Harbor—but there were coves and jetties, private boats and commercial, in a thousand places in the waters around Acadia. Small, dark-colored, outboard—didn't narrow it down much.

The lift bell had barely rung, lowering the Whitmans to the jetty, when Gwen had a blood pressure cuff around Anna's upper arm. "A friend of a friend, a doctor at Mount Desert Hospital, was more than kind. She ran the tox screen on your blood. A heavy dose of Rohypnol and a muscle relaxant. You should be feeling better by tomorrow, almost your old self," she told Anna.

That was good news. Anna had been doped once, and once slipped LSD. By good fortune she'd never been given anything highly addictive or—so far—fatal.

"I wish rufies were harder to come by," Heath said. "If you pay attention to the news, it seems there are more date rape drugs than sex ed classes in most school districts."

"I'd hate to have a daughter in this day and age," Anna said.

"Ah, but you do," Gwen murmured.

That was another drawback when it came to children. One got fond of them, and then they went speeding away in a convertible with a bottle of Jack Daniel's and no seat belt.

"Have you yet seen fit to share with Heath why you didn't want the medical establishment or law enforcement called?" Gwen asked as she pumped the rubber bulb tightening the cuff.

"She did," Heath said. Heath was sitting in Robo-butt near the cold hearth, one hand idly playing with Wily's right ear, the other holding a glass half full of bourbon-and-water.

"Murdering me doesn't make sense," Anna said, feeling the slight claustrophobia the tightening of a blood pressure cuff always gave her. "I've been trying to work it in with the cyberstalker and/or the Duffy murder—not because either makes sense, but because they are the only items of interest I've been involved in since coming to Maine. I think I might have a better shot at getting to the bottom of it if I remain dead for a while."

"A hundred twenty over seventy. Better than most twenty-year-olds," Gwen said, deflating the blood pressure cuff. "I can see wanting to stay dead—no one pesters the dead. But won't the Acadia people wonder where you are? Aren't you acting chief ranger?"

"I called in sick, told Peter what I was up to. We argued. I won," Anna explained succinctly.

A cell phone played a few bars of "Yankee Doodle Dandy." "That's mine," Gwen said. "Would you get it, E?"

Elizabeth picked up the phone. "It's Mrs. Hammond," she said, passing the phone to Gwen, who sat on a stool at Anna's side.

"Dez," Gwen said into the phone. Her face went tight and tired. Without the burning energy within, her flesh pulled down. Pouches showed beneath her eyes. Shadows hollowed her cheeks.

Shangri-La, Anna thought as she watched her friend aging in front of her.

"Okay," Gwen said. "Okay. Let me know if I can do anything. Soon as it comes in, I promise. No, I don't doubt it either. It's a crying shame, that's what it is. Call me tomorrow?" Gwen pushed the OFF button but continued to stare down at the phone.

"What is it?" E asked.

Anna knew it was death. Death masks weren't just for the dead. Many times she'd seen them slipped onto the faces of survivors. Gwen wore one now.

"Chris died today, while Dez and I were in Bar Harbor," Gwen said.

Heath rolled over and put her arm around her aunt. E knelt on Gwen's other side and laid her head in her lap. Gathering of warmth and strength, being enfolded in the arms of loved ones, Anna knew, was beneficial for most people, so she watched in respectful silence. Wily, probably feeling sorry for her because she was not exactly of the human race, jumped up beside her on the sofa. A pain-filled whine let her know what the thoughtful gesture had cost his old injuries.

Gwen sniffed and rubbed her eyes. "It's not as if Chris and I were close. For the past twenty years it's been mostly Christmas and birthday cards, maybe a call now and then," she said after blowing her nose. "It's not a surprise. Chris—and Dez and I—knew she wasn't going to live to a ripe old age. It's just that the timing couldn't be more tragic."

"Because she was so young?" Heath asked. To Anna she said, "She wasn't even sixty."

"Fifty-seven," Gwen said. "Had her first heart attack at fifty-four."

"Is that usual?" Anna asked.

"More so now than it used to be, what with obesity, blood pressure drugs, and so on. Chris wasn't obese. She had a weakening of the vessel walls in her heart muscles. Every doctor has a theory, but none of us agree—not that I know much about hearts over the age of ten."

"Is that what you and Dez met about? Ms. Zuckerberg's health?" E asked. As for Anna, Chris was just a name to Elizabeth.

"No. Worse in a way. Because we were out, Dez wasn't with Chris when she died. That will be hard on her. They've been together over fifteen years," Gwen said. Sighing, she moved from the stool to a comfortable armchair. "I could do with what you're having, Heath."

"Anna?" Heath asked as she rolled toward the kitchen where the bourbon bottle lived.

"No more drugs for me in this lifetime," Anna said.

"Lesbians?" E asked.

"Why does everybody have to be a lesbian!" Gwen snapped. "They became friends when they were girls. Dez was the maid here when the babies were born. After Dez's husband died, and Chris's health started to go, she came to live here with Chris. Lesbians! For heaven's sake. Can't anybody just be friends with anybody anymore?" Gwen grumbled.

Heath rolled back in with an obviously much-needed bourbon. Anna had never seen Gwen irritable. The pediatrician's mood was always so bubbly Anna occasionally wondered if she prescribed a little something for herself.

"This baby thing is new," Heath said. "Until we got to Boar, I didn't know Chris had children. I didn't know she'd ever been married."

"You said she didn't have kids," E said accusingly.

"So I did," Gwen admitted. "That was an attempt to keep you out of more misery and keep Chris's secret. I failed at both. It's been a long day. Now that Chris is gone, I guess her old secrets can't hurt her. Chris never married, but she did have children. Forty years ago—forty-two now, I guess—when Chris was fourteen, she gave birth to twin girls. Here on Boar Island. I was the doctor. It was my first paying job out of medical school. Her mother—a witch spelled with a *b*—didn't want anyone to know her daughter had gotten pregnant. Because Chris was a minor, the witch didn't need her consent to give the babies up for adoption—or so she said. There was enough family money to make her right, no doubt.

"A few years ago a couple of things happened. First, Chris's mother finally had the decency to kick the bucket—Chris had never gotten free of her, not really—and Chris had her first heart attack. That was when she decided to find her daughters if she could."

"Nearly sixty and still afraid to admit she'd had twins when she was fourteen?" Elizabeth asked. "People now would be going on talk shows and writing books about it."

"Not Chris. From age eleven to age thirteen, Chris was molested by their rabbi. When she became pregnant, she told her mother. Her father tried to beat the truth of who the real father was out of her. Her mother packed her off to Boar Island with only herself and a maid—Dez, all of twelve years old—for company," Gwen explained.

"Her own mother didn't believe about the rabbi?" Elizabeth asked. "What a rat."

"Worse," Gwen said. "Her father didn't believe her, but her mother knew she was telling the truth. The rabbi was beloved and rich and the witch didn't want to damage her own social standing by crying 'Pervert!' "

"Did she find her daughters?" Heath asked.

"Three or so years ago she put an ad in the papers, you know the sort of thing—seeking identical twins separated at birth, would now be thirty-something, legacy involved," Gwen said. She took a swig of bourbon and held it in her mouth for a moment before she swallowed. Anna took over the task of fiddling with Wily's ears.

"She didn't get an answer to that ad, or the next one, or the one after that. Assuming the girls would have been adopted out locally, and quietly, and without any paper trail, Chris only put ads in papers around this area," Gwen told them. "All of a sudden, last week, somebody answered an ad from a while ago. Chris was so excited. Not a good thing when your blood vessel walls are disintegrating. She insisted that Dez and I go meet with the woman—Dez to question her, me to get a DNA sample if the woman was willing."

"You'd have to," Anna said. "The word 'legacy' should have brought out every greedy woman for miles. I'm surprised there were no responses to the first ads."

"Mainers are a decent people," Gwen said.

"When they're not shooting each other for poaching," Anna whispered to E, who'd joined her and Wily on the sofa.

"I took the sample, a cheek swab, but Dez and I think she's legitimate—"

"Not literally," Heath said.

Gwen frowned at her, then went on. "Other than the bleached-out hair, she is the spitting image of Chris when she was in her early forties: same color eyes, same overlapping front incisors, same oval face and straight eyebrows."

The description tugged at Anna, but she let it pass. After being drugged, bagged, and dumped, a little paranoia was surely normal.

"How did she know she was a twin?" E asked. "I mean if they were separated at birth and all that, you wouldn't know, would you?"

"That was the only fishy part," Gwen said. "We asked her that same question—though believe it or not, neither one of us thought of it at first. She said she had recently found her sister, but she wouldn't tell us who it was, or if the sister knew about our meeting—nothing. Though she seemed like a good woman, if on the naïve side, I couldn't help but wonder if she planned on sharing the legacy with her twin, and of course she has to. Chris needs to give them both the news. Needed to."

The sun was low over Mount Desert, knifing into the room in a wedge of rich coppery light. Gwen squinted into the shaft of dancing motes for a moment. "Chris died. Damn. She will never get to see her daughters—not even one of them. It just makes my heart ache."

"What's the legacy?" E asked. Anna had been wondering the same thing but had become too civilized to blurt it out at the graveside, so to speak.

"Boar Island, this house," Gwen said. "There isn't much left in investments, but I imagine one could get a pretty penny for a private island off the coast of Acadia National Park. The historic value of the lighthouse would be worth something, I would think."

"Jeeze, yuh think?" Heath mocked gently. "I bet this rock would be worth millions of dollars to some rich New Yorker who wants a six-thousand-square-foot summer cottage to use for a couple of weeks each year. Not a bad legacy. Juicy enough to want to steal it from your sister."

"That's the good news part of the legacy," Gwen said, then sighed again, more deeply this time. "The bad news is that their biological father—"

"The child molester the witch was so into protecting," Heath butted in.

"Died of Huntington's disease," Gwen finished.

"Shit," Heath breathed. Gwen shot her a reproachful glance.

Elizabeth stared at her mother, then turned to Anna. "What's the big deal? He was a pervert. Who cares if he died? It's not like they'd want to look up dear old Dad for the holidays. I sure wouldn't."

"Huntington's is hereditary," Anna said. "There's a fifty-fifty chance the child will have the disease if one parent carries it."

"It is a terrible disease," Gwen said. "Pitiless. It's a neurodegenerative genetic disorder, which means the nerve cells in the brain break down. There's a whole host of symptoms ranging from loss of motor control to severe psychiatric disorders and dementia."

"Gosh," Elizabeth said. "You'd think they'd know they had it already."

"Most people start showing symptoms in their late thirties and early forties. Sometimes it manifests earlier or later, but if you didn't know your family history, you might not know what was happening to you," Gwen told E. "That's what Chris was worried about, that they wouldn't get medical care if they had it, or that, without the money from the sale of Boar, they couldn't afford it. A person with Huntington's can live twenty or more years after the first onset of symptoms, getting progressively worse and worse."

"Is there anything you can do about it?" Heath asked.

"Not much," Gwen said.

"Then who'd want to know they had it till they had it?" E asked.

Anna suspected she wasn't so much asking anybody in particular as demanding answers of the universe. Why would anyone want to get tested? A fifty percent chance of no longer worrying about it. Why would anyone who wasn't worrying about it want to know?

Gwen answered E's question. "There are some drugs that show promise. There's also the issue of safety to self and others."

"Driving," E said.

"Gas stoves, matches, babysitting, getting lost, knocking over hot coffee, the whole gamut of dangers, and we haven't even gotten to psychiatric issues," Gwen said. "At some point it becomes unsafe not to seek medical care."

"My biological father is dead and I don't know his medical history," E said. "Could I have it?"

"You could," Gwen answered slowly. "But you're more likely to get cancer or pneumonia or hydrophobia. Huntington's is rare. If you're going to dwell on it, I'll get you tested."

"You don't have the gene," Heath said. "Your father died in a motorcycle accident when he was fifty-five, remember?"

"Right," E said, sounding relieved rather than sad. Anna was unsurprised. E's father had been absent since she was eighteen months old. "Did you tell her—the daughter?"

"We didn't. Chris wanted to do that," Gwen said. "Now Chris is gone. I'm afraid the twins do have the gene. This poor woman seemed to have some cognitive dysfunction. We had to repeat ourselves. Sometimes she appeared confused, unnaturally docile."

"Maybe she just isn't very bright," Heath offered.

"She also showed chorea. Involuntary movement in her hands." Gwen flicked her wrist.

Suddenly, what had niggled in Anna's brain snapped into place: bleached blonde, overlapping front teeth, cigarettes being flipped out on the ground.

"Paulette Duffy?" she asked.

THIRTY-NINE

Once again Anna was sitting at Peter Barnes's kitchen table. As superintendent, he could keep a nine-to-five, Monday-through-Friday schedule if he wanted. Since the baby had been born, he did. Lily was watching television in the front room; Olivia, in a soft pink Onesie, was curled up on the couch beside her, making tiny grunting sounds like a piglet.

Anna set her teacup down and gazed past Peter at the charming picture on the couch. Mother and daughter, happy, safe, beautiful. Would that it would always be so.

"Elizabeth's cyberstalker has sent an ultimatum," she said more abruptly than she'd intended. "E's supposed to show up alone, in person, at a time and place to be determined. Or else."

"Preying on children! God, but it makes my stomach turn! Throw in sexual perversion and I'm ready to change my stance on the death penalty," Peter said. He didn't glance at his baby girl, but Anna noticed his head jerk as if he'd been going to and stopped himself. Attitudes changed when one had skin in the game. Taking a hit while fighting for the principle of a thing was fine, but when the good fight began to cause collateral damage to innocents, how to be a hero became more complex.

"Heath would be too conspicuous in her wheelchair, and logically, the stalker is someone who knows Elizabeth; ergo, he might know Heath or me or even Gwen. I was hoping to borrow an unknown face so it won't be only me and Gwen. Though smart and fierce, Gwen is small and somewhere north of seventy-five."

"There's always the Bar Harbor police, the Maine State Troopers, the sheriff's department," Peter said drily. "All perfectly legitimate and, from what I've experienced, competent options. Not as reassuring as an elderly pediatrician, I'm sure, but they do their best."

"I have great respect for small-town police and sheriff's departments," Anna said. "They see a little of everything and have to deal with it by themselves. They tend to be generalists, the way rangers were in the good old days, before we carried guns. It's the time-frame and subject matter that make me want to keep it personal."

"How so?" Peter asked.

"With cyberbullying, police don't yet know what to do, where they stand, what the procedure is; nobody really does. The police back home more or less blew Elizabeth off. Not out of malice, more out of this-isn't-my-jurisdiction.

"The or-else meeting is tomorrow. That's not much time to coordinate with officers who may not deal well with a girl from Boulder, Colorado, hiding out in Maine, who says she's meeting a stalker who posts dirty things about her on the Internet. I doubt we'd get things sorted out in less than the twenty-odd hours we've got."

"Put the guy off. Tell him you'll meet day after tomorrow, or next week," Peter suggested. "That might give you time to get things set up with local law enforcement."

"It might. It also might scare him back into the cyber woods. Then E will have to live not knowing when the bastard is going to pop out again."

"I wouldn't wish that on anybody, especially not a teenaged girl," Peter said.

"Marriage and fatherhood have made you downright sensitive," Anna joked.

"Estrogen seems to have a civilizing effect on me," he admitted. "I can't give you anybody. I shouldn't have let you and Denise go on NPS time. Bad judgment on my part, and let's hope it stays our little secret, at least until I'm retired. What I can do is give Artie the day off—you're on sick leave—and if you and Artie choose to spend the day hanging out with septuagenarian aunts and underage girls, that's your business."

Anna's eyes were blurring. Drug residue. She blinked rapidly to clear them.

"You look like shit," Peter told her kindly. "You should have let me come out to Boar."

"I had cabin fever," Anna said. Talking hurt—her upper lip was bruised—but nothing like the pain in her left heel or her butt. Gwen had bandaged her various scrapes. Anna felt like she was wearing diapers under her jeans. "I needed to get off the island. I'll be back in Schoodic tonight."

"Hoping for another attack?" Peter asked. He took a sip of hot tea, raising his eyebrows over the rim of the cup at her.

"No. I'm dead, don't forget," she said.

"Right. How's that supposed to work for us?" he asked.

Anna rubbed her face. "I must admit I wasn't thinking too clearly when I wanted to stay dead. I had a sort of half-baked notion that I could appear like the ghost of Hamlet's father, and the guilty parties would fall down and confess, or at least look much amazed. Trouble is, this ghost doesn't know to whom it would be profitable to appear. Now I think I'd like to stay dead until we get this business with the stalker over with. If I'm dead, nobody will be taking potshots at me."

"Artie and I made a quiet visit to Schoodic today and had a look around," Peter said. "We found a broken needle—the kind that fits in a plastic syringe—in front of the Rockefeller building. It's been bagged and will be tested."

"Gwen went through the Mount Desert lab," Anna told him. "Rohypnol and muscle relaxants were in my blood."

"Good to have friends in high places," Peter said. Being superintendent of a major national park couldn't get evidence tested in a four-hour time frame: lack of funds and facilities, the need to stand in line behind other law enforcement organization at shared labs. "We found your other boot," he went on. "Once it's been through the system, you can have it back. It was about halfway between the Rockefeller building and Schoodic Point. Schoodic was probably where the boat was beached. Nothing interesting in your apartment or on the stairs."

"No *CSI Acadia*?" Anna asked with a smile. "No tiny thread or droplet to lead us to the bad guys?"

"Sorry," Peter said. "Have you remembered anything new?"

"I don't know," Anna said honestly. "The Rohypnol has an amnesiac built in. It's not total, but everything is stretched and warped, like the memory of a dream. Walter said there were two people in the boat, and I sort of remember two people in my apartment—or the parking lot or somewhere. I haven't any idea whether I really remember two or, because I was told there were two, I think I remember. Most of the day I've been poking at my poor raddled brain. I think I might think the two were small. I think I might think they were dressed like ninjas, all in black. I think I might think they wore white gloves like Mickey Mouse. I don't trust my own memories. Before I can believe myself I need corroboration from people that weren't stoned out of their minds."

"We talked to the sculptors," Peter said. "Nobody saw anything or heard anything. We talked to your boyfriend—Walter Whitman—"

"Don't speak ill of my savior," Anna said. She sipped her tea. Earl Grey. Right up there with tomato soup for curing what ails.

"Seems like a good kid. A little monomaniacal about clearing his dad's name, but I can understand that."

"Good thing he is, or I'd be sleeping with the fishes," Anna said.

"He gave us a statement about the boat that dumped you, and precisely when and where that dumping occurred. We put out an APB to the Coast Guard and local marinas. Today I'd hoped to get a diver down where you went in. Something might have fallen from the bag you were in, or their boat. Problem is, Denise Castle, the ranger who drove you around, is our only certified diver, and she just retired."

"She went through with it?" Anna was surprised at that. Denise didn't strike her as a woman who had anyplace else to go. It wasn't anything the woman had said or done, it was the starkness of her apartment: nothing personal, no pictures with people in them, family, friends, or even co-workers. Just that one bedside photo from which Peter Barnes had been amputated.

"She did. I think she was as shocked as everybody else."

"Struck me that way, too. She'd not talked about it before?" Anna asked.

Peter looked into the other room, where his wife and child nestled in the flickering light from the television. "Why do you ask?"

"Not sure," Anna said.

Peter sighed and rubbed his jaw like a bad actor trying to indicate he's thinking. "Yes and no," he said finally. "She seemed to be happy here, but—you know Denise and I lived together for eleven years?"

"I remember, vaguely," Anna said.

"After the first shit was done hitting the fan, Denise seemed okay. Then Lily came and the baby. Denise seemed fine with that, seemed totally over the split. She brought Olivia a really beautiful coming-home gift—an angel figurine from Lenox, not cheap—and has been nice to Lily. I happen to know Denise has no family and no real friends, so on the one hand, I was surprised she just up and retired without any notice. On the other hand, there have been a few times I've caught her looking at Lily or me, or seen her face go kind of odd when somebody mentions our house, that makes me think she might not be as much over the split as she acts. So I wasn't surprised she up and retired. Does that make sense?"

"Why now?" Anna asked. The timing of an incident could tell one a great deal. That was the moment when something changed. "After hanging on through the split, the marriage to Lily, the birth of Olivia, why did Denise choose now to retire?"

"Who knows," Peter said wearily. "I haven't a clue as to why Denise does anything. We got Walter Whitman squared away with the local police," he said, changing the subject. "There wasn't an arrest warrant out for him. Town police try and stay out of lobster wars. If there's any danger to Walt, it'll come from other lobstermen. John Whitman thinks blood has cooled enough the kid could come out of hiding, but that won't get him his line back. Without fishing rights, he hasn't got a future. At least not around here. I told him to talk with Gwen. If he's going to be squatting on Boar to do his spying, it should be with the owner's permission."

"The owner is dead," Anna said. "Chris Zuckerberg bought the farm this afternoon."

Peter sat back in his chair. Inwardly, Anna flinched. Wrapped up in her own troubles, she'd forgotten that Peter probably knew Ms. Zuckerberg. Not only was Acadia a small world during the winters, and people got to know one another, but any self-respecting superintendent would want to have some kind of relationship with his rich, private-land-owning neighbors.

"Sorry," Anna murmured as she hid her nose in her teacup. "Did you know Chris had kids?"

"I didn't," Peter said.

"Twins, girls, adopted out at birth. Chris was trying to find them when she died. Actually had found one—or thought she had. Paulette Duffy."

"Mrs. Kurt Duffy?" Peter asked.

"That's the one," Anna said. "Odd, isn't it, how one day you've never heard of Paulette Duffy, then she's popping up everywhere?"

"Not so odd. Every time I learn a word I've never heard before, guaranteed I'll hear it three times before the week is out."

"There was a legacy, enough to make murdering a husband worthwhile if one didn't wish to share. Though, from what I hear, most women would have murdered Kurt Duffy for free," Anna said.

"Iron-clad alibi," Peter said. "Half a dozen acquaintances and strangers can attest that she was in the Acadian at the time of the murder."

"But if Paulette is Chris Zuckerberg's long-lost child, she has an identical twin sister," Anna said.

Peter digested that for a minute. "Damn," he said finally. "So mysterious twin sits at the Acadian while Paulette kills her husband?"

"Maybe," Anna said. "Or maybe the other way around. Or maybe they're both innocent."

"Speaking of innocents."

Lily was standing in the kitchen door, Olivia in her arms. "It's Livvy's bedtime."

Peter leapt up like a terrier offered a treat. "Come on," he said to Anna. "You can be an aunt."

Because they clearly thought she would like nothing better than to watch them tucking their baby into its bed for the night, Anna obligingly rose and followed the familial parade up the stairs.

As she would have expected, the nursery was a froth of girly pink, but well done and spotlessly clean. An old-fashioned white antiqued-wood dressing table, with a large looking glass in a matching frame, mirrored the bassinette with its rows of white lace, a mobile of pink and blue and yellow ducklings hanging from the hood.

Peter and Lily cooed and prattled. Anna looked at the guardian angel. It was a lovely thing, not the usual flowing skirts and tiny feet, but a bell-shaped dress with many colors and sturdy handsome wings. On its arm was a basket of flowers.

Anna picked it up.

"Denise gave Livvy that," Lily said. "Wasn't that sweet of her?"

Anna turned it over.

"Sweet," she said, but either it wasn't a Lenox or it had been broken and repaired. The bottom was patched with plaster of paris.

FORTY

It was late when Denise finally staggered into the foyer of her apartment building. Her mailbox was empty. She'd half expected a note from Paulette reporting on her latest betrayal.

There was nothing. Good, she guessed. Maybe.

Using the handrail as if she were a woman twice her age, Denise dragged herself up the stairs to her apartment, fumbled the key into the lock, and nearly fell into the front room.

This had been one of the longest days of her life, and it had come at the end of one of the longest nights. Exhaustion swelled like a balloon in her chest. Her head throbbed. Her hands jumped with nerves. Exhausted, but not sleepy, not the least little bit. High-pitched, sharp-edged nervous energy sang through her veins, sawed through her bones, and squirted acid into her belly until her throat burned nearly to her back teeth.

The Miata, her pathetic attempt at joie de vivre after Peter had summarily tossed her out, was gone. She wouldn't miss it. In its place, paid for in cash—it took as long to pay the idiot salesman in cash as it would have to get a loan and buy it on time—was a midsized Volvo XC90. Safe.

That was what she wanted in a car now, safe and family-friendly. The car had cost a good chunk of her savings, but there was no choice. A family couldn't drive around in an accident waiting to happen.

For color, she'd chosen white. There were a zillion white sort-of SUVs with mommies and kiddies in them on every road in America. The Volvo would blend in.

Dropping keys and purse onto the coffee table, Denise let gravity suck her butt down onto the sofa. Her apartment. Sterile and neat and utterly hers. Nothing where it shouldn't be. Everything where it should. This was gone, too. Or as good as. She'd turned in her two-week notice to the landlord. In winter, she would have been stuck with six weeks' rent money. In summer, apartments were at a premium, so she'd only had to flush two weeks' worth of rent down the rat hole.

Rat.

Paulette.

"No, no, no," Denise muttered, banging her head against the soft back of the couch with each word.

Denise had quit her job, bought the most expensive car she'd probably ever own, given up her apartment, and killed two people, for Paulette. Not to mention the hundreds of dollars she'd dumped at Walmart that afternoon. All the while she was hacking off chunks of her life so that their new life together might have a chance at success, Paulette was betraying her.

It was because of the Walmart shopping spree that Denise knew this. Thinking it would look odd for a retired ranger, who had given two weeks' notice to her landlord and was supposed to be moving out, to be carting armloads of goods upstairs to her apartment, Denise had taken the risk of driving the lot of it to Paulette's house in broad daylight. In a new Volvo, she figured if any rangers saw her, they'd never think it was her. Fancy Volvos and GS-9s didn't exactly go together.

Paulette hadn't been home. At first, Denise was relieved. This wasn't the time to be arguing about what she'd bought and why and where it should be kept.

Denise had driven behind the house to unload her purchases into the nursery. Paulette wasn't in the nursery. Where was Paulette if she wasn't at work and she wasn't at home?

Denise trotted through the trees to the house. Forcing the kitchen door didn't take much brute strength. A firm shove of her shoulder overwhelmed Paulette's flimsy attempt at security. Since they were family, Denise didn't consider it breaking and entering, more like she'd forgotten her key. Paulette should have been home. Denise needed to reassure herself that nothing had happened to her sister; that she hadn't panicked or gotten sick.

Denise needed to know where Paulette was.

The old ads for twins separated at birth, along with the postcard with the cell number on it, were on the kitchen table amid the coffee rings. That was all Denise had to see. She knew what Paulette had done. She'd called the person to ask about the legacy. While Denise was buying and selling and giving notice, Paulette was meeting with their *mother,* or some lawyer or con woman. Undoubtedly Paulette was drinking up whatever bullshit this individual was pouring out. Undoubtedly Paulette was babbling out their secrets with girlish gusto, hoping for a big fat legacy or, worse, the loving arms of the bitch that had whelped them.

Denise groaned. Sitting forward, she held her head between her hands, pushing hard on her temples with her palms. Her disposable cell phone had fallen from her bag and lay on the coffee table. She could call Paulette, let her know this shit wasn't going to fly.

A hand detached itself from Denise's head, floating into her field of vision. Not like it was her hand reaching for her phone, more like it was a detached hand, like a balloon-hand in the Macy's Thanksgiving Day parade, floating on wires high above the crowd, then settling down toward the tiny phone on the table.

Denise reached out with her other hand, caught the one floating, and shoved both of them between her knees. "Poison thoughts," Denise whispered. "If you think poison thoughts you'll die."

Instead of taking up the phone, she opened her laptop. A glance at the time told her Olivia would be in her crib. If she was lucky, Peter and Lily would have finished their bullshit cooing and baby-talking, and cleared out of the room. Seeing a baby, a new life, free of the crap that was dripped into every human's veins over time until the whole person was a toxic waste dump, would settle her, calm her mind. Keep the poison thoughts from killing her. At least for a while.

She tapped on the mouse pad, opening the live feed to the camera in Olivia's nursery. Peter and lovely little Lily bent over the bassinette making faces they thought were amusing but, in truth, were scary and ugly. Then the world spun, the camera showed the wall, the ceiling, then . . .

"Shit!" Denise screamed, throwing herself back against the couch cushions, covering her eyes. When she uncovered them, all was as it had been, Peter and Lily cooing, the world right way up, Olivia in her bed.

For an instant Denise could have sworn she had seen a face. The face of a dead woman. Anna Pigeon's face. The video wasn't recorded; she couldn't go back. Had she been able to, there would have been no point. She had seen Anna Pigeon's body in a black plastic sack sinking beneath the waves of the Atlantic.

The fear and paranoia burning like acid in her gut were from fatigue, not because of anything real. She'd not slept for over forty hours. Too tired and thoughts got crazy. Way too tired and one could even hallucinate.

Anna Pigeon was dead.

Paulette was her soul, her gentle self, her family.

Obstacle removed; identical twin good and right and safe.

There was no Anna.

Paulette might have gone to meet somebody, but she wouldn't break trust with her sister, her identical twin sister. The legacy was for them, for their family. Denise herself had told Paulette to pursue it. Paulette might even be meeting with a Realtor. Could be Denise was wrong about the meeting with the legacy person.

But Denise wasn't wrong. She could hear how right she was barking down among the chunks of disappointment and misery in her brain's junkyard.

"Doesn't matter," she said aloud.

The day—and the night before—had been good, she told herself. Better than good. Denise took out the slip of paper she'd been carrying in her front pants pocket so long it was growing soft. From her bag she got a pen, one with red ink.

Kill Kurt (Denise)

"Check," Denise said, and put a neat red check mark next to it.

Sell Land (Paulette)

"Better be soon," she muttered as she passed that one over.

Remove Obstacle (D&P)

Denise paused. The dead pigeon's upside-down face blinked like a strobe light, setting parts of her mind afire. "Check," she hissed, and scribbled out the words with such force that the pen tore through the paper.

"Stop it," Denise said aloud. Her hand flicked. The pen flew from her fingers, fell to the white sofa, and rolled, leaving a thin red trail. Denise forced herself to look away from the bloody little snake-track on the perfect white of the fabric. "Calm. Slow and steady wins the race. Nerves. Fatigue. Finish and rest. That's a girl," she crooned to herself. When she felt the spate of rage diminish, she went back to the list, carefully avoiding glancing at the ink stain.

Quit NPS (retirement pension) (D)

"Check!" Denise said as she marked it.

Find out about "Legacy" (if it exists) (P)

Denise was sorely tempted to check that off, as a sign that she believed in her sister. That her sister believed in them. If she didn't know for sure, though, she couldn't do it. She never broke her own rules. Well, hardly ever.

In a spirit of compromise, she set aside the pen, fished a pencil from her purse, and put a pencil mark next to that item on the list, a faint gray check mark. For now that would have to do.

Car, shopping, etc.

"Check!" and check.

Give landlord notice

"Check!" and check.

Family—Mt. Desert Hospital (D&P)

The injection into the four-ounce, hermetically sealed waxy box, the seventh of those in Lily's cupboard, would be used by lovely little Lily late in the afternoon tomorrow. Lily used sixteen ounces each day.

That wasn't enough to check it off the list.

After nearly two days without rest, the pen that had so recently flown from her hand of its own accord became too heavy to lift. The list blurred. Denise leaned back on the couch cushion and rubbed her burning eyes, wishing she hadn't sacrificed the last of her Valium to the obstacle issue. Tomorrow *Family* would get checked off, then, one by one, the rest of the list. She would do it tomorrow. After all, tomorrow was another day.

Scarlett O'Hara had said that.

But then, Scarlett O'Hara was one crazy bitch.

FORTY-ONE

Denise's scalp stung, her eyes stung, her nose stung. In law enforcement training at FLETC, the students had been pepper-sprayed—"to know what it feels like." Sadistic bastards; they just liked tormenting the new kids. Right now, right here in Paulette's kitchen, she felt the same sensations. Besides that, her neck was going to snap.

"What's next? Waterboarding? Do you do this once a month?" she asked.

"Every six weeks. You get used to it," Paulette said as she finished rinsing the bleach from Denise's hair. "Done. You can get your head out of the sink."

Lifting her head with the care she'd use lifting a bowling ball with a soda straw, Denise straightened in the chair while Paulette wrapped a towel around her head.

"You're going to be beautiful as a blonde," she said, disappearing into the bedroom.

Denise wasn't sure about that. There were other reasons she'd decided to bleach her hair tonight, reasons she chose not to share with Paulette—at least not yet.

Paulette reappeared brandishing a blow-dryer.

"As beautiful as you?" Denise teased.

"Just exactly as beautiful," Paulette said with a laugh.

"Identical," Denise said with an answering smile. She was teasing her twin sister, in fun. If the painful process of stripping the color from her hair had no other use, Denise still would have done it. Playing beautician, Paulette was relaxed, smiled more, even laughed. For a while she seemed to have forgotten the dark web they were weaving, some strands already destroyed forever, some yet to be spun. Denise felt the glow of awe she had experienced that first night as they sat in front of the mirror in the bedroom looking at themselves, at each other, at *theirself.*

This was what it would be like all the time. Once they had a place of their own, safe in a warm part of the world, every night they would laugh and tease, watch movies and eat popcorn. That wasn't part of Denise's childhood, yet she'd done that sort of thing with Peter. At the time it must have been nice, but that recollection had been rotted and discolored by the times between then and now. As a memory, it was a corpse, and that corpse stank like carrion.

Paulette plugged the blow-dryer into an outlet on the counter. Hot air blew over Denise's neck, breathed past her right cheek and ear. She closed her eyes. Her sister was fixing her hair. Right out of one of those books she used to vandalize at the library when she was a kid. The happy family bullshit that infuriated her. Maybe it wasn't fiction after all. Maybe all those Dick-and-Jane children's authors weren't lying through their teeth.

The new Volvo was parked behind the shack. The back porch light was off. Still, it was a risk for Denise and Paulette to be together. The closer they got to endgame, the more dangerous it was to be seen in one another's proximity. People didn't remember much about random days.

They remembered where they were when Kennedy was shot, what they were wearing when the World Trade Center towers came down, what they had for dinner before they'd gone to see *The Dark Knight Rises* in a movie theater in Aurora, Colorado. Denise didn't want anyone popping out of the woodwork and saying, "Yeah. I saw Denise Castle and Paulette Duffy together right before the shit hit the fan. You know, they were real chummy. They even kind of looked alike."

Denise wanted to leave Maine unremarked and unremembered. She wanted Paulette to drift out of the minds of the people who knew her the way perfume drifts out of a bottle. The best way to get away with murder is never to be suspected in the first place. Once law enforcement decides on a person of interest, they keep sticking their noses up that person's ass if for no other reason than it makes it look like they're doing something when they don't know what the hell to do.

Unfortunately, they had to be in the house; the bleach job required running water. That turned out to be a perk. Denise didn't want Paulette going out past the Volvo and seeing all the things she had bought. Later, Paulette would be glad, grateful even, but it might be hard for her to understand at the moment. Besides, they were having fun! Good, clean family fun. Like a couple of Mormons, Denise thought, and was taken aback at her sourness.

Having fun must be like a lot of things in life. To do it right required practice and training.

Denise's hair was dried. Paulette had set the electric rollers next to the sink and plugged them in. She insisted Denise wasn't to look in a mirror until the process—she called it a "transformation"—was complete. After the transformation would be the "reveal."

Though she'd lost the thread of why they were happy, while the curlers heated, Denise went on pretending she was. Paulette rolled her hair as the television played a reality show where people made assholes of themselves and a laugh track, like Denise, pretended it was funny.

Paulette combed out her hair and insisted on putting makeup on her. Feeling like a clown, Denise went on pretending. Maybe fun was like faith for alcoholics, fake it till you make it.

Eyes closed, promising not to peek, she let Paulette lead her through the bedroom and into the bathroom.

"The mirror's smaller than the one on the bureau, but the light's better," Paulette said, excitement bubbling in her voice. "You can look now."

Denise opened her eyes, expecting to see hair like Paulette had, broken and dried out like an overused broom. Regardless of her decaying attitude, Denise was impressed by the reveal. In the mirror was a beautiful woman. Smooth, blond, gleaming hair waved down past her chin. Soft rose colored her cheeks. A darker hue made her lips look fuller, younger. Mascara rimmed her eyes, turning the muddy hazel to dark green.

For a long, long moment Denise didn't know who she was looking at. She knew she was in the body of the person reflected in the mirror, but that face, that hair, those lips had no connection whatsoever with Denise Castle, dour and green and gray to the shattered remnants of her soul.

"Do you like it?" Paulette asked anxiously.

Denise nodded. The beautiful blonde in the mirror nodded.

If she'd had Paulette five years ago, if she'd gone blond, curled her hair, worn makeup, would Peter have needed space? Would he have chucked her out? Fallen in love with Lily?

"Doesn't matter," Denise snarled, and the plump pink lips in the mirror snarled with her.

"You hate it!" Paulette cried. Over her shoulder, reflected in the glass, Denise saw her sister's eyes fill with tears, her open happy-face curl into a pained wad.

"No. I love it. I was thinking of something else." Denise tried to undo the damage, but the moment had gone.

Though she primped and complimented her own reflection over and over, Paulette wouldn't cheer up. Denise was never so glad to see the back of anyone as she was to see the last of the pink scrubs disappear out the front door when Paulette left for work at seven forty-five.

"I'll lock up," Denise promised from where she sat on the sagging dirty couch. "I just want to finish this episode of . . ." Denise had no idea which show was on. Assholes. That was what was on. Fortunately, Paulette was more intent on leaving the dudgeon than she was on what Denise was saying.

The moment Denise could no longer hear the burr of the Duffys' pickup truck on the asphalt, she leapt to her feet.

She worked quickly, not because she was afraid Paulette might come back for some reason but because she wanted to get out of that house, out of the room where she'd killed Kurt, and away from the ammonia fumes of her new persona.

Under the bed, she found a suitcase. Rummaging through drawers with the insensitivity of a hardened burglar, she grabbed what she thought Paulette would need. One suitcase would have to be enough. What Paulette had was cheap and tired. They would both buy new wardrobes once they were settled. Cosmetics, shampoo—all the gooey stuff—they could pick up on the road.

Suitcase slammed shut and zipped, Denise snatched a set of scrubs and a pair of Crocs out of the closet. Stopping, she looked around the room. This was the last time she would see it. If things went as planned, Paulette would never see it again.

On the back porch, suitcase in hand, scrubs over her shoulder, Denise stopped again. Turning back, she stared at the weathered wood on the side of the house, the torn screen door, the peeling paint of the trim. Too bad a fire would call attention to the place. But for that, she might have thrown a match into the tinderbox.

Given her mood, if she could have, she might have burned down the world.

FORTY-TWO

Cybercreep had mandated a night meeting. Because it was the height of the season, bars, cafés, and many shops were open until eight or later. Cecelia's Coffee Shop was open until nine thirty. The cybercreep said they needed to be there at nine.

Everything about the time bothered Heath.

Poor little creep probably was hoping for darkness, she thought. Too bad the sun wouldn't set until nearly ten o'clock. That failed to comfort her. Dusk was probably worse. Often it was harder to see at dusk than it was in the middle of the night. Dusk was like a gray fog; normal shapes fooled the eye, strange shapes appeared familiar.

Of course, Bar Harbor would be lit up for the tourists.

Light was probably worse than dusk. Light meant shadows. Black shadows under docks, between boats floating in black water.

Everything about the place bothered Heath.

Why not midnight in a haunted house, or in the deep dark of the forests? Anna said the lonelier the place, the easier it was to spot the bad guy coming, to see where he parked, to hide in place until the appointed hour. In towns there were crowds; plenty of people that wouldn't be him, and only one son of a bitch who would. Hard to tell the good guys from the bad guy.

Meeting in town probably meant that he wasn't planning on kidnapping E. That, too, bothered Heath. Since it was almost a guarantee he meant Elizabeth no good, if he didn't intend to take her, then he must intend to harm her. An attack in town would be sudden, like a lightning bolt from a cloud of tourists, all but one of whom were innocent. A gunshot? A head shot? Heath shuddered at the image and gasped.

"You okay, Mom?" E asked. They were just rounding Bald Porcupine Island. E was seated beside Heath in the stern of John's boat as it turned toward the dock at Bar Harbor. They were holding each other's hands, leaning close to be heard over the noise of the engine. Gwen was at the console with John.

"Never better," Heath muttered. "Never better."

"Would it cheer you up if I told you that you look like a whale that got spray-painted at a 'Back to the Sixties' party?" " Elizabeth asked.

Heath stared down at her lap. She was wearing Dem Bones beneath a riotously colored maxiskirt. Over that was a long fuchsia tunic with turquoise embroidery down the front that Anna had picked up at the thrift store where she bought the skirt. Heath's punishment for insisting on being part of the festivities. Sunglasses were out since Cybercreep had opted for night ops, but she wore a moderately battered purple sun hat with a wide brim. All in all she was, if not a perfect picture, at least a pretty good likeness of an overweight tourist with a good heart and bad taste.

If the pervert did recognize her, she would never forgive him.

He won't, she told herself, as she had insisted to Anna. For the past seven years—all of her life with Elizabeth—anyone who knew her knew her in a wheelchair. Many never saw past the wheelchair. Upright, walking, even with canes, was the ultimate disguise. Heath Jarrod was "the lady in the wheelchair," not "the fat lady hobbling down the sidewalk."

"And you look like a fourteen-year-old boy," Heath teased her daughter.

Elizabeth smoothed her palm down the flat front of her shirt, her breasts squashed beneath the Kevlar. "This thing is more uncomfortable than a bra. I'm surprised Anna wears one."

"I don't think Anna's worn a bra since she burned her last one in 1971," Heath said.

"The bulletproof vest," E said with exaggerated patience. Heath had known what she meant; she'd just wanted to make herself think things were a joking matter when they weren't.

"Regulations," Heath said. "Otherwise, I expect she wouldn't."

"Will she have somebody else's tonight?" E asked. "I hadn't thought about that. If I have hers, will she be, like, vulnerable and stuff?"

"Anna can take care of herself," Heath said. As the words came out of her mouth she remembered Anna tied to the lift, naked, unconscious, and covered in blood.

As if her mind were running along the same channels, Elizabeth said, "Anna isn't getting any younger."

"Older is tougher, like beef and redwoods," Heath said.

"Do you know where she'll be?"

"No. Not exactly. She's sort of wandering the general area. But she'll be close."

Cybercreep had insisted Elizabeth come alone. Unless he was a total idiot, he had to know that there would be watchers, that this was a trap as much for him as for E. He must be gambling that no one would dare be too close, that he would have space to do whatever it was he wanted to do, then get away before they could catch him.

"Maybe he just wants to talk," Elizabeth said.

"Let's hope so," Heath replied grimly. "We're here."

John had cut power. Under his experienced hands the boat was gliding effortlessly alongside a dock below a large parking lot that served the picturesque downtown area of Bar Harbor. Nimble as his own grandson, John Whitman leapt over the gunwale to snick two yellow lines fast, one at the bow and one near the stern.

Walt had wanted to be a member of the party. Anna had nixed that. Heath had no doubt the nixing was a waste of breath. What red-blooded young hero wouldn't want to save the damsel if he got the chance? Walt would be lurking somewhere around the town square. Since he had been unknown—even to her—until the previous day, Heath wasn't worried his appearance would scare the cybercreep into hiding or precipitous action. In fact, Heath hoped he would disobey Anna. If Heath had her way, the town would be full of young, strong, kind, brave boys in love with her daughter.

Young, strong, kind, brave, *sane* boys.

Were boys who bullied, took sexual advantage, loved pornography, and the shame and subjugation of women, technically insane? Given that society at large behaved in much the same manner, didn't that make the nasty boys the norm? Was virtue, once its own reward, now a symptom of a mental disease?

Physical demands chased away the bitter thoughts as, with the help of John and Elizabeth, Heath disembarked and got herself squared away on the pier: hat firmly on head, crutches in hand, tunic over thick waist and legs, feet pointed toward the landing ramp.

From the low dock, Heath could see that the town was lit up and the parking lot was full, but little else. It wasn't more than a couple hundred yards—and two ramps—to where she had chosen to plant herself for the duration. Over the past couple of weeks, she'd gotten good with Dem Bones. Two canes were still needed for balance, but her gait was relatively smooth and her endurance far greater than it had been at the start. Still, she didn't want to use up her strength getting up to city level and through the parking lot, so she waited while John unloaded Robo-butt and Gwen unfolded it.

Gwen stayed with the boat while John rolled Heath up to the pavement, then halfway down the long parking area. There, he took the wheelchair and left her and Elizabeth standing in the shadow of a Chevy Suburban. He and Gwen would wait with the boat, ready to leave if leaving suddenly became necessary.

The time was eight fifteen; the sun was low in the west, veiled with clouds, the sky a deep lavender. Heath's eyes took a moment to adjust to the bright lights and big city. They had expected some foot traffic at this hour, but the square was packed with bodies. "What in hell . . ."

"People are wearing their pajamas!" Elizabeth exclaimed.

"And bathrobes and slippers," Heath said. "And I thought I looked silly."

For a minute or more they stared at what looked like a combination sleepover and shop-a-thon. "Lookie," Elizabeth said, pointing east of the parking lot where a lush lawn stretched in a smooth green apron down to the Atlantic. A vinyl sign, hung between two poles, read SEASIDE CINEMA! TONIGHT SHOWING *THE PAJAMA GAME*. Though it was not yet dark enough to start the movie, blankets were already spread, and pajama- and nightgown-clad moviegoers were lined up buying popcorn and sodas at a snack bar made to look like an old horse-drawn wagon.

Around the grassy area, the shops had doors open and lights on. Handwritten signs advertising Night Owl Specials, Midnight Snacks, and Pajama Party Sales were stuck on sandwich boards on the sidewalks and taped in windows.

"Holy shit," Heath breathed. "Talk about the unexpected."

"I bet this is why Creep-O wanted to meet 'day after tomorrow.' I wondered about that, but just thought he had a dentist appointment, or date, and wasn't free to torture people yesterday. I bet he was waiting because there'd be this big crowd today."

Heath bet her daughter was right. She bet she wanted to call this whole thing off, run—or walk mechanically—back to the boat, escape to Boar

Island, disable the lift so nobody could call it down, and barricade her daughter in the tower.

Anna was here, she reminded herself, and a beefy ranger named Artie. Walter was surely here somewhere. Elizabeth was wearing a bulletproof vest. She knew not to eat or drink anything given to her by anybody, including waitstaff. She would never be out of Heath's sight or Anna's.

Damn, but Heath wished she knew where Anna was. It took an effort of will not to try to find her in the flannel-and-fleece crowd.

"Are we ready?" Elizabeth asked. "I feel overdressed."

To Heath's eyes Elizabeth looked beautiful, and as fragile as a butterfly fresh from the cocoon. She wore skinny jeans, tennis shoes—for running, Anna had insisted—and a loose boy's plaid shirt Walter lent her to disguise the thickening of the vest. Heath gazed at her daughter so long that Elizabeth started to roll her eyes. "Sorry," Heath said. "You look fine."

"Fat," E said. "Somebody should tell Anna that Kevlar makes you look fat."

"Go," Heath made herself say.

E walked farther down the parking lot. A few rows before the street, she stopped and hid in the shadow of a pickup truck, the kind that look like they're on steroids and have never hauled anything heavier than the ego of their owner. Both E and Heath would stay out of sight until twenty minutes of nine. At that time, Heath would make her way across the grassy square and pretend to window-shop in the stores to either side of Cecelia's Coffee Shop. At ten minutes of nine, Elizabeth would enter the square from the parking lot, walk straight across the center of the lawn where the most light and people were, and take a seat at one of Cecelia's outdoor tables. If no tables were free, she would stand with her back against the wall of the coffee shop, watching the square, until she was contacted. Artie, the only person other than Walt that they were sure would be a stranger to the cybercreep, would already be in place, seated at an outdoor table absorbed in the American obsession of drinking caffeinated beverages while staring at electronic devices.

If the creep did contact Elizabeth, and did not attempt anything hostile, both Heath and Artie would photograph him with their devices. Artie and Anna would tail him when he left. No attempt to capture him would be made near Elizabeth. Less dangerous that way.

If the creep made hostile motions, Artie would take him down.

Heath ran through this in her mind as her legs were propelled off of the concrete and, with scarcely a hitch, onto the lawn. Canes were a great help. People tended to make way for a wheelchair, not so much for canes, but some. When they didn't, she batted them gently with the end of the cane, and apologized. Dem Bones was miraculous, but running obstacle courses and doing ballet had yet to be programmed into it.

Crowds. Dense crowds.

This bothered Heath more than the time and the place.

Artie was armed, and licensed to carry concealed weapons when off duty, as was Anna. The density of the crowd made that problematic. A bullet could easily pass through the villain and into two or three innocents before it came to a stop. At the moment, Heath didn't care if it mowed down all of Pajama Land, as long as E was safe.

Anna would care, as, Heath presumed, might Artie. Better no guns, she told herself as she maneuvered around a big man with a bushy beard wearing blue footy pajamas and a Red Sox baseball cap. E would be too close to the action; it would be too easy for a bullet to go astray. If the cybercreep had a gun—

No, Heath told herself firmly. That was not a thought she had allowed herself to entertain for the past forty-eight hours, and she wasn't going to entertain it now. If the bastard had a gun he wouldn't need all this meeting business. He could wait outside their house, or E's school in Boulder, and just blow her away at his convenience: no waiting, no air travel, no coffee date.

Sweating so profusely her hands were slick on the rubberized handles of the canes, Heath reached the far side of the square where Cecelia's was located. Twelve o'clock—that was what had been decided so they could tell one another where to look: The green was a clock face, Cecelia's was twelve o'clock, the grassy point—now the cinema—was at nine o'clock, the parking lot where she and E entered six o'clock, and the west part of town three o'clock.

Heath was across the narrow street from the coffee shop at twelve o'clock, the outdoor movie theater at nine o'clock on her left. For a minute or two she stood still, breathing, trying not to sweat, to fit in as a general-issue tourist at a pajamarama. If such a thing existed.

After a moment she spotted Anna. Had she not seen her in costume before she left Boar, she wouldn't have recognized her. Munching popcorn, Anna was leaning against a tree at about ten o'clock, ankles crossed. Her long braid was concealed beneath a loose flowing shirt over wide-legged soft palazzo pants. A Greek fisherman's cap, the cheap kind available in most of the souvenir shops, was pulled low on her forehead. The greatest disguise was the makeup. Anna Pigeon wore red lipstick, smoky eye shadow, and mascara. Beautiful and urban on someone else, it was oddly disturbing on the ranger, rather like seeing false eyelashes on a young Clint Eastwood.

Anna had to have seen her; Heath looked like the *Mayflower*, as envisioned by Peter Max, under full sail, but her gaze wandered past and through without a flicker of recognition.

Encouraged by the sight of her friend, Heath managed the step off the curb and crossed the street to the shops. Artie looked up as she passed. He didn't recognize her. Heath felt a mild lift of her spirits.

Facing a children's bookstore as if she were shopping, she watched the reflection of the front row of cars in the big parking lot at six o'clock appear and disappear as waves of people ebbed and flowed over the green space. She didn't see Elizabeth until she was halfway across the square, seeming very small in the big shirt and dark, tight jeans. Shoulders slightly hunched, she looked around as she walked, peering into the faces of the people she passed.

That was okay. Cybercreep would expect Elizabeth to appear frightened. After all, he'd spent weeks carefully fraying every single one of the girl's nerves. One of these happy people in bunny slippers was feeding on E's fear at that very moment. Anger, so intense it dimmed her vision, flooded Heath's entire being.

Her vision didn't clear. The world was viewed through a glass dimly. Heath's head swam; her balance faltered.

Lights had gone from the windows. Gone from the square.

Her tenuous vision of her daughter's reflection had vanished.

FORTY-THREE

First the streetlights around the green went dark, then the lights on the storefronts. The sky had faded from lavender to deep blue. The pajama-clad throng melted into amorphous shuffling grays and blacks, an occasional spark of red or green as beams of flashlights startled color from a sleeve or back.

Sharp pieces of the previous night flickered through Anna's brain: shadows shifting into ninjas, gun falling from her hand, darkness sucking her down. Dizziness overtook her. Blindly, she reached out for the tree trunk. Coarse bark brought her back to her body; the ancient strength of the tree steadied her.

Slowly, Anna squatted, carefully set her box of popcorn on the ground, then rose, stepping away from the tree.

Music began, a loudspeaker playing the Broadway overture to *The Pajama Game*.

Specters that had been born on the residue of Rohypnol faded. This was not a flashback, not a vast conspiracy to throw Elizabeth into the dark. The movie was about to start. Simple, prosaic, *Pajama Game* in pajamas, quaint, colorful, charming, and a huge pain in the ass.

Irritation burned in the pit of Anna's stomach. She had not foreseen this. A blind woman should have known that when the movie started the lights would go down. Cybercreep had known it. The people in the square had known it. Anna was the fool. Had she time, she would have cursed herself. Taken by surprise, none of them might have time, especially Elizabeth.

A chill of hypervigilance shivered through Anna. Cold tingled in her feet and hands and the top of her scalp. Whatever was going to happen would happen now, while people were on the move, while the lights were down and the area still crowded.

Counting on the invisibility cloak created by her shade tree and the lowered lights, Anna leapt onto a park bench. Her skinned left heel cursed her with a stab of pain. She ignored it. From the higher vantage point, she could see over the milling crowd. Most were drifting toward the lawn in front of the movie screen. A few continued to shop, eat, and talk in the shadows beneath awnings of stores and branches of the maples in the park. Blankets were being shaken and spread. Last purchases were being made at the snack bar.

Soft, fleecy, plaid stuffed animals in the arms of children and some adults, pillows and blankets in baskets: This was not the stuff of creepiness. Who looked like a sexually perverted bully in footy pajamas? Fuzzy slippers and terry robes could disguise a lot of sinister intent.

Despite the sudden change in atmosphere, Elizabeth was staying on track, walking a little slower than before but still heading straight—or as straight as she could through the pajama swamp—for Cecelia's.

Good girl, Anna thought.

Keeping E in her peripheral vision, she began searching in ever wider concentric circles out from her goddaughter, automatically discarding the very young, the very old, and families holding hands as parents walked children toward the cinema. A young man, rising and walking in the opposite direction of the crowd, his stride that of a man on a mission, caught her attention. Walter Whitman. He had been sitting on a low stone wall between the grassy movie space and the sea. As she could have predicted, he was making a beeline for Elizabeth. Clearly he, too, had been watching her.

Heath was in front of the children's book store beside the coffee shop, her back to the windows. By the panicked way her head bobbed and craned, she had lost sight of her daughter.

On the west side of the grass, at about two o'clock on their imaginary clock face, a single man wearing khakis, a short-sleeved blue shirt, and sandals with socks stood on the sidewalk. In the dim light, age was hard to guess, but he had a full head of dark hair and stood, hands in pockets, with the slouch of a man in his twenties or thirties.

Anna punched WM2 into the text line on her cell phone, then hit SEND. Artie, attention torn from his laptop by the change in illumination, turned back to it. Heath took her cell phone from a pocket in her smock and looked down into the pale blue square of light. Then both looked for the white male at two o'clock.

A shake of the head let Anna know Heath didn't recognize him, but then she wouldn't necessarily.

Artie stayed with WM2. Anna continued her scan. Elizabeth was nearly across the grassy area, about fifty feet from the coffee shop. Two of the tables had been vacated by moviegoers. Once E was seated, she could take out her cell phone, put it on the table, and see the texts. Anna had wanted her to keep her hands free at all times and, when approaching the meeting place, to do nothing that might scare Cybercreep away.

Three doors down from Cecelia's, a dumpy woman emerged from an ice cream shop, her head a puff of pink lace in a many-tiered curler cap, her robe a tatty old blue-and-white-striped cotton. Plump doughy hands clutched a large satchel to her chest. By the contours of her figure, Anna guessed it must be filled with Red Hots, Jujubes, Goobers, and other treats one only ate at the movies.

A stride or two behind Elizabeth, and five yards to her right, a man paralleled E's path. Paunchy, hair thinning, stoop-shouldered: Anna put him in his early forties. He wore red-and-blue plaid flannel pajama bottoms and a pale blue, zip-front, lightweight jacket. On his feet were hiking boots. His face was unremarkable except for a simian brow that didn't match the ordinariness of his other features.

WM//E3, Anna texted. She knew they would understand the white male at three o'clock and hoped they would understand the parallel mark.

Artie glanced in WM3's general direction. Sitting, he wouldn't be able to see the man. Heath was having trouble spotting the guy as well, her head moving back and forth and looking suspicious as hell.

BCOOL, Anna typed. Shrinking in on herself, Heath settled. Then the shrinking ceased. Heath regained her stature the way a resurrection fern will after a good rain. Heath had seen Elizabeth.

E had reached the road that separated the shops from the grassy space. Walter, Anna noted, was making his way toward Cecelia's using the sidewalk. A clever boy. Anna was sorry she'd nixed his coming.

No one else stood out from the thinning crowd. No beady-eyed perverts slinking around in their pj's. Had the cybercreep seen Heath or Anna and disappeared back into whatever hole he lived in? Was he standing them up to throw them off guard the next time he called for E to meet with him, or the time after that, so he could strike when they were no longer alert?

The crowd on the green had thinned to twenty or so stragglers. Stores were still doing a desultory business. The man in sandals went into the ice cream shop. Paunchy ceased to parallel E's path and veered onto an intersecting course. The woman in the curler cap stumped stolidly down the sidewalk, evidently bent on getting a Frappuccino to wash down the candy.

Elizabeth reached the coffee shop. She slid into a chair at one of the abandoned tables, took out her cell phone, and began fiddling with it.

The man with the paunch stopped fifteen feet shy of Cecelia's. Standing on the curb before the narrow street, he squinted as he stared across the road to where E was sitting. Artie moved his laptop so he could watch him without seeming to take his eyes off the screen.

Paunchy shoved both hands into the pockets of his windbreaker, his protruding brow shadowing his face.

Anna's brain, still tainted with the Rohypnol, reeled: the doughy hands, the oversized bag clutched to the woman's breast. This was important, this was trying to take her mind from its set track.

The man on the curb pulled a black rod from his pocket. Anna couldn't make out what it was, but it wasn't flat; it wasn't a cell phone. Pink Curler Cap was almost to Heath, her small sneakered feet marching determinedly along the dull gray concrete of the sidewalk.

Anna's brain locked between the dumpy little woman in the old housecoat and the man with the black rod. Walter bolted through the fog swaddling her mind to smash into the man on the curb. The boy didn't hit him with a football tackle or a fist; he plowed into him like a ship at ramming speed, the entirety of his strong young body smashing into the smaller man, knocking him ten feet onto the green.

"Get off me! Get off me!" the man screamed as Walter followed him down and pinned him to the turf with his weight. "Help! Help!" the man cried. No one moved to help. Anna had worked in tourist destinations most of her life. Tourists had no connection to other tourists, no knowledge of who was who, no faith in their instincts. They seldom sprang into action. There were too many unknowns in an alien environment.

The rod had flown from the downed man's hand. Rolling across the asphalt of the road, it flashed a bluish beam of light. A flashlight; the man had taken a flashlight from his pocket to fight the gloom.

Artie was on his feet and running toward where Walter held the shrieking little man down.

Doughy hands. White. Plump. Dimples for knuckles.

Anna had seen her before, at the first coffee shop meeting. She'd had curly red hair then, but the same hands, the same bag. Whirling, she saw the woman in the pink curler cap drawing on a welding glove, the glove she'd seen peeking from the bag the last time.

One hand gloved, the other dipped into the capacious bag and came out with a can, the flat, squareish, metal kind that holds lighter fluid. She was passing Heath, whose attention was fixed on the tangle of men yelling and wrestling on the green.

"Run, E!" Anna shouted. "Run!" Galvanized by decision, Anna shot across the lawn, legs pumping, lungs filling to bellow again: "Run!"

Heath's head jerked in her direction. "The woman!" Anna screamed.

Ten yards separated her from her goddaughter.

The woman with the lighter fluid dropped her bag. Pinching the can in both hands, she aimed a stream of fluid at Elizabeth's face.

FORTY-FOUR

From out of a swirling mist of blind panic, Elizabeth emerged into focus. Heath felt her blood pressure drop twenty points. Without a glance at her mother, E slid into a chair at a table near Artie. She took her cell phone from her pocket and laid it on the small round tabletop. Heath's fingers closed around her own phone in the pocket of her brightly embroidered tunic. It took all of her self-control not to snatch it out and text E just to feel some small line of connection.

Tearing her eyes from her daughter, Heath forced herself to continue her search of the people straggling from shops or toward the cinema. Anna's WM3 was stopped at the curb. This man had pervert written all over him, from his baggy-butt pajama bottoms to his beetling brow.

Seemingly from nowhere a dark shape, like that of a black bird of prey stooping on an unwary rabbit, crashed into the man so hard his feet left the ground and he flew sideways several yards. Elizabeth squeaked. Heath might have squeaked herself. It was Walter. God bless him, Heath thought. God bless the boy.

Abandoning his laptop, Artie leapt from his table and went to help E's boyfriend. Elizabeth, per Anna's orders, was remaining seated until the all-clear was sounded, but her eyes were as round as a startled child's as she watched her tormentor exposed and laid out by two men.

Heath hadn't recognized the man. He didn't even look familiar. Such was the virulence of the attacks he'd mounted, so imbued with specific hatred, she'd expected Elizabeth's stalker to have a personal agenda. How could a total stranger develop such an oozing rotten loathing of a lovely young woman he'd never even met?

Then again, they might have met. Perhaps a fleeting exchange in a Best Buy or at a Walgreens. Twisting it in his mind, the man had imagined a relationship. Elizabeth failed to play her part, so he imagined betrayal. Then he plotted revenge.

Relief washed through Heath, weakening her, floating her physical fatigue to the surface. Fortunately, they would soon know why and who. Knowing would lay a lot of ghosts to rest. Knowing would keep Heath, and more importantly E, from wondering if black slime underlay the warm smiles and kind words of friends and acquaintances. Heath doubted knowing would promote understanding. Perverts had a perverted way of looking at the world. In their heart of hearts, they believed everyone would behave as badly as they did if they got the chance. Virtue was only a mask. Reality, the pervert believed, was what he lived.

Before Heath could finish drawing in her sigh of relief, she heard a scream.

"Run!"

Anna was pelting across the green, sprinting toward the coffee shop.

Elizabeth looked up from her cell phone.

"Run!" Anna screamed a second time.

Elizabeth half stood, then sat down again, evidently remembering her orders to stay put.

A short woman in a pink curler cap passed Heath, blocking her view of the men struggling on the lawn.

"The woman!" Anna cried.

Confused, Heath turned toward Elizabeth. The stumpy little figure was stopped at Elizabeth's table, standing so close, E couldn't get up without overturning her chair. A large, shiny, purple tote bag slid from the woman's arm, exposing an enormous paw.

It was a hand in a welding glove. In that hand was a can of what looked like lighter fluid.

Heath was easily ten feet from her daughter. Without thought, she dropped her canes and lunged. The legs Leah had crafted from electronics and metal responded to the sudden weight of her upper body moving forward. Dem Bones propelled her at nearly a run. Torso foremost, metal and hinges activated to their utmost, Heath was hurtling toward Elizabeth's attacker, utterly out of control.

The woman raised the can, pointed the nozzle at Elizabeth, and started to squeeze. E shoved her chair back and tried to rise. Heath slammed past the frumpy woman and careened into Elizabeth. Both of them went down in a tangle of arms, legs, and chairs.

"Whore, Jezebel!" a woman's voice drilled into Heath's back. Sizzling and popping like a firecracker booth going up in flames seared the air. The small of Heath's back began to burn.

A loud thud and the crashing of more chairs cut off the shrieked epithets. "Stay down!" she heard Anna yell. "Stay down, God damn you."

"It's on me!" A high-pitched scream. "It's on me."

"Artie!" Anna again. And, "Keep her down."

A gasp came from nearby, and then Heath heard a small voice in her ear. "Mom, you're squishing me."

All of her weight and all of her electronics were pinning Elizabeth to the pavement. Heath tried to lever her upper body off, but her arms were shaking, muscles as weak as overcooked pasta. "I can't move," Heath panted. "Push me."

Small strong hands shoved against her shoulders. Heath was raised far enough that she could see her daughter's face. So beautiful. "Are you all right, E?" Heath's voice quavered with tears. Some good she was in a crisis. Dead wailing weight.

"I think so," Elizabeth said uncertainly.

"Help me! It's on my face!" the obscene woman screamed.

Elizabeth pushed Heath until she could roll off. There she lay on her back, helpless as a stranded beetle, the electronic legs still twisted.

Anna moved into the airspace above. "You okay?" she demanded.

"Yes," Heath managed.

"You?"

Heath heard Elizabeth repeat, "I think so."

"What's that smell? What's making that noise?" Anna asked. Elizabeth was sitting up now; Heath could see her if she craned her neck sideways.

"I don't know," E said.

Heath drew in a breath, tasting the air: singed fabric, burning plastic, a biting acridity. She listened to the sizzling crackling noise coming from beneath her. The small of her back burned like fire. Though there was no flame and no smoke, the woman must have managed to ignite the lighter fluid before Anna tackled her. Some of it must have struck Dem Bones' power pack, where it sat across Heath's hips.

Heath sighed. "I think the smell is me on fire. I'm afraid the racket is the sound of a couple hundred thousand dollars' worth of electronics being destroyed."

Anna had her rolled over and her shirt ripped up the back before Heath could say anything else.

"Artie, call an ambulance," Anna said.

"What's burning? Where is it burning?" Elizabeth was asking.

"No fire," Anna said. "Acid. Battery acid is my guess. E, go into the coffee shop and bring as much clean water as you can and scissors or a sharp knife. Do it now, and do it quickly." Heath felt her hips being jerked sideways and heard what sounded like fabric ripping. Facedown, a view of nothing but table legs and an overturned chair, Heath felt helpless.

Nothing made her angrier than feeling helpless.

"Talk to me!" she said through clenched teeth.

Instead of a reply she felt a cold wet cloth drop onto the small of her back. "Dab gently. As much water as you can without dripping. We don't want to spread the stuff," Anna said.

"Got it," E said.

"Artie, see if you can get Cybercreep to shut the hell up and get some water on her face to dilute the acid," Anna said.

"Talk to me or I'm going to bite you!" Heath said.

"Sorry, Mom." E's voice was shaking as bad as Heath's. "The can had battery acid in it. A little got on your skin above Dem Bones. Anna has cut away the shirt and the straps so we can get anything that has acid on it away from your skin. It ate right through your skirt. It's like horror movie special effects. Dem Bones is practically melting. Most of it got on the power pack."

Heath groaned. "There goes your college education."

A wet sobbing litany of "My face, my face, oh no, my face, she wouldn't be pretty without her face, little baby-faced whore, he wouldn't look at her with no face, not my face, no, no . . ." burbled in a monologue from the other side of the table.

"Are the cuffs on?" Anna asked.

"In front, so she can wash her face," Artie said.

"Help me sit up," Heath told Elizabeth. Before E could start to argue, Heath said, "Please," in a tone that was so pathetic she was almost embarrassed to use it to manipulate her only child.

As they'd done a thousand times before, Elizabeth braced her knees to either side of Heath's and, locking wrists, pulled her to a seated position. Once Heath was stable, E moved behind her and knelt, making herself into a living backrest.

Not more than a couple of yards away the woman in the pink curler cap was sitting on the ground, dribbling words and snot as she dabbed at her face with fat little white hands forced closed with silver handcuffs. Acid had splashed onto one of her cheeks and the side of her mouth. The flesh was red and beginning to blister.

This mewling miserable creature was the person who had filled E's life with threat and filth, then tried to burn her face off with battery acid.

"Who in the hell is this?" Heath asked.

Anna, who was standing slightly behind the woman talking on her cell phone, reached down without interrupting her conversation and pulled off the curler cap and, with it, a red curly wig.

Blond hair tumbled out. Blue-framed glasses fell from her nose. Heath didn't recognize her, although, through the snot, the blistering, and the smeared, mud-colored lipstick, she did seem familiar.

"Mrs. Edleson?" Elizabeth gasped.

FORTY-FIVE

The adrenaline dumped into Anna's system during the excitement of capturing Elizabeth's cybercreep had drained away. Despite the fact that she had slept a good portion of the day, Anna was so tired she could scarcely breathe. Drugged sleep did not refresh the way natural sleep did. Rather than resting, she felt as if she'd spent those hours in a morass of thick oily dreams and mind-numbing traps from which she could not escape into consciousness.

Hunched over the steering wheel of the patrol car used by erstwhile ranger Denise Castle, Anna was aware of her vision tunneling until all she could see was the red taillights in the lane ahead as she followed the second of two ambulances to Mount Desert Hospital.

In the first, with two female officers from the Bar Harbor Police Department, was Mrs. Sam Edleson, the flesh of half her jaw and lower lip eaten away by the acid she'd intended to use to disfigure Elizabeth. Often the why of a crime remained unknown long after the who, what, when, where, and how had been solved. Not so this time. Regardless of the pain talking must have caused with her ruined lip, Terry Edleson wouldn't shut up about why.

According to her, E had lured poor chinless Sam to the dark side with her wanton ways. So bewitched was Sam that he talked of Elizabeth, raved about her firm young flesh, and spied on her through the hedge between the houses.

Abused himself.

First, goodwife Terry had tried to warn E of the dangers of harlotry by destroying her reputation on the Internet, using pornographic images to shock her into good behavior, as well as to make it clear to Sam just what sort of girl he was obsessed with.

Such was the power Elizabeth held over Sam that he actually liked the pornographic images.

Go figure.

Then came the night when Elizabeth was at the Edleson house, when Tiffany had been sent out with her little brother, the night when Elizabeth had all but forced darling Sam to sexually assault her. That was when Terry realized she had to take it to the next level.

She began making threats.

Even then Elizabeth failed to loose her hold on Sam's libido. A couple of off-duty cops roughed Sam up. A rude "uniformed female" visited Terry in her home. That was the handwriting on the wall, Terry told Anna and the Bar Harbor policewomen, and in big black letters it said ELIZABETH WOULD NEVER LEAVE SAM ALONE.

Unless she was made hideous with acid burns to her face.

When her smooth soft flesh was furrowed and scarred, her gentle mouth melted, her brown fawn eyes white with blindness, then and only then would Sam be free.

At that moment, except for the fact that it was illegal to execute an insane individual, Anna could have wrung Terry's fat little neck with as little remorse as a turkey farmer on Thanksgiving eve.

Breathing deeply, Anna banished the wretched Mrs. Edleson from her mental jurisdiction. If the woman died in the ambulance, her face rotted off, if she went to hell, to prison, or back to Boulder—it was all the same to Anna.

Rohypnol hangover and fatigue ruined her powers of concentration. Fantasies of a long sauna to sweat out the toxins, a massage to unknot the muscles, and a husband's shoulder to lay her head on were about all she was willing to hold in her tattered cerebrum for more than a second or two.

That and the taillights.

The second ambulance, the one Anna followed with such dogged determination, carried Heath, E, and Gwen. The area of Heath's back affected by acid burns was small. Most of the acid had struck Dem Bones' power pack, only a small amount hitting bare skin. Cool water, quickly applied, kept the burns superficial, probably second degree at worst. Anna had no way of knowing what Heath's leaping, lunging, falling, and floundering with chairs and girls and electronic exoskeletons had done to the unfeeling half of her friend's body.

The dual red eyes of the taillights wavered as Anna's eyes watered and strained. Blinking, she pushed her face closer to the windshield. The movement set off the scrapes on her butt and heel, scabs cracking, blood oozing. Considering the possibilities, she'd gotten off lightly. Yesterday's contusions, and the shoulder she'd used to take down Terry Edleson, were the worst of it.

After a miserable eternity, the ambulances turned off the winding road out of the town of Bar Harbor and into the front lot of Mount Desert Hospital. As hospitals went, Mount Desert was small. Its age and the warm brick facade robbed it of the sterile futility the sight of most hospitals stirred in Anna's breast.

The ambulances pulled up beneath a bright sign reading EMERGENCY. In a fog, Anna nearly rear-ended the vehicle carrying Heath before she realized the flare of taillights meant it had stopped. Cursing softly, she backed out, drove around the corner into the dimly lit lot, and parked the borrowed Crown Vic.

Levering herself out of the driver's seat, Anna grunted. Gone were the days she could tackle someone and wrestle them to the ground without paying for it. Tomorrow, no doubt, she would discover a medley of bruises where Terry had managed to get in a few licks before she was subdued.

As she walked back to the emergency room entrance, she nearly bumped into Peter Barnes. Staring up at the towering form blocking out the light, she was momentarily disoriented. "Did I call you?" she asked stupidly.

"No," Peter said, taking her arm as if she needed steadying. "Are you okay?"

"Fine," Anna said. "Who called you?"

"Nobody. Anna, let's go in and sit down, maybe get somebody to look at you." He began steering her into the harsh lights of the ER waiting room. "Lily will be here in a sec. Why don't you tell me how it went tonight with your stalker, why you're here."

Peter was talking in the gentle tones used to calm crazy people, or people too sick to stand any kind of shock.

"It went fairly well," Anna said. His assumption of her frailty annoyed her, but since she couldn't think of anything she'd rather do than sit down for a minute, she let him lead her to a chair.

"Who got hurt?" Peter asked.

"Heath, but not badly, I don't think. The perp has facial burns, fairly severe I hope. The stalker was Elizabeth's best friend's mother. A woman who baked the girls cookies. Her husband had a hard-on for Elizabeth, so his wife trashed her on the Internet. A couple of weeks ago, he tried to molest Elizabeth, and the woman went psycho. Blamed E. Tried to squirt acid in Elizabeth's face."

Anna let her head drop back and closed her eyes against the fluorescent lights.

"But you're not hurt?" Peter insisted.

"You mean in addition to being dead?" Anna asked.

"Yes, in addition to that." Peter's chuckle, low and throaty, almost like the purr of a cat, washed reassuringly over her.

"Bumps and bruises," she said. "Other than that, nary a scratch."

"Oh my God! What happened to you!" came an exclamation.

She opened her eyes. Lily Barnes.

It finally occurred to her to wonder why, if she hadn't called him, Peter was here, and why Lily was here at all.

"What happened to you?" Anna countered, wincing as she dragged her butt over the plastic, pulling herself up straight in the chair

"Olivia got real sick," Lily said. "Vomiting, diarrhea, then a seizure. God, it was terrifying. The doctor thinks she may have an allergy or ingested something toxic. We've been wracking our brains. Paint on the bassinet? Dog fur? I'm going to have to go over the whole house with a Q-tip."

"Is she okay?" Anna asked, rubbing her eyes. Fine grit scraped across the sclera as if she'd spent the day at a windy beach.

"Yes. She's sleeping. The doctor thinks she'll be fine. They just want to keep her overnight for observation because of the seizure," Lily said. The young woman's brave smile looked ragged around the edges. Sinking down, she settled on the edge of the chair next to Anna. Lily laid her hand gently on Anna's arm and, with seemingly genuine concern, asked, "What happened to you?"

A nurse pushed through the glass double doors on the far side of the waiting room. One of the doors flashed Anna's reflection at her. The mystery of why people kept asking what happened to her was solved. In the fracas, her braid had come undone; her hair was hanging witchlike around a face drawn and white with fatigue. Unused to wearing makeup, she'd rubbed her eyes until they were ringed with black mascara. What lipstick remained on her lips was only in the crevices, like red stitches.

Anna laughed abruptly. "I'm better than I look." She laughed again. A worried frown formed two lines between Peter's dark eyebrows. "No. I'm good," Anna said to put him out of his misery. "Just tired and, obviously, frighteningly disheveled. No new wounds. I'm sorry about poor little Olivia."

"Why don't you stay at our house?" Lily offered. "It's nearly an hour's drive to Schoodic. We have plenty of room."

Anna accepted gratefully. "I'll be over after I check on Heath," Anna said. "I'll try and be quiet."

"Don't worry," Peter said. "I doubt we'll be getting a whole lot of sleep until we have Olivia home safe and sound." A pained expression crossed his face. "I hate to ask . . ." he began.

"Ask," Anna said.

"Denise forgot a model in her office. She bought it when we went to Hawaii once. I was going to drop it by her apartment as a sort of good-bye peace offering. Given the situation, would you mind?"

Anna would, but she didn't have a baby in seizures, and a checkered past with the model's recipient.

"Not a problem."

"You go ahead and find your friend. I'll stick it in your car." Peter took her keys. "I'll leave these at the front desk."

Anna nodded her thanks and went to find Heath.

FORTY-SIX

Denise watched Peter and Lily leaving the hospital. Hand in hand. Enough to make a person want to puke. When Denise and Peter had been together, Peter wouldn't hold hands in public. Too much like a Hallmark card, he said. Big ranger man was self-conscious showing his softer side, he joked. What a load of crap.

Didn't matter. Tonight he was going to lose that softer side. She wasn't after revenge, Denise told herself. The fact that Peter would suffer was just a perk. Denise was all about justice.

The radio she'd conveniently forgotten to return to the NPS when she retired lay on the passenger seat. She looked from Peter Barnes to the radio. All day she'd had the thing on, waiting for the shit storm about the missing Anna Pigeon to hit the airwaves. Nothing. Either nobody noticed the pigeon's comings and goings or they weren't talking about it. Maybe they booted it upstairs and were quietly waiting for the FBI to come and save their collective ass. Denise didn't believe that. The NPS considered itself the search-and-rescue experts. They would have mounted a search. Everybody would have been on the radio all day to show how important they were.

Never mind, Denise told herself. Not her problem. Silence was golden.

After the adorable Mr. and Mrs. Barnes had driven out of the parking lot, Denise punched a number into her disposable cell phone and waited. Three rings. Four. What was Paulette doing that was so important she couldn't answer the goddam phone?

"Hello," came a whisper in Denise's ear.

"Time to take a smoke break," Denise said. "Bring a face mask, hairnet, and one of those sterile coat thingies." She punched the END CALL button without waiting for her sister's response.

From various trips to Mount Desert Hospital on EMT business, and, once, to have her tonsils out—a thing like mumps or measles, a real bitch when you were an adult—Denise had a fairly good idea of the layout. What she needed from Paulette was specific locations of patients, things that were fluid and couldn't be easily predicted. That, and where there were cameras, if there were any.

Ten minutes later by the dashboard clock in the new SUV, Paulette finally saw fit to emerge from the rear door of the hospital beside the Dumpster. In the wan light of the single security bulb, she looked around furtively, the items Denise had asked for clutched to her breast. Even in pink teddy-bear scrubs she managed to look as guilty as hell.

"Holy shit," Denise breathed. Paulette had to be kept out of any kind of heat that might be generated by this night. She probably lacked the capacity to lie about her age or weight, let alone a felony murder and all the rest.

Denise tried to tell herself that this was good, this was the honest half of herself, this was her innocence lost, but she wasn't buying it. Paulette needed to grow a backbone if they were going to have a good life together. At least for the first couple of years. After that they could let down a little, relax, and enjoy themselves.

Finally deciding the coast was clear, Paulette trotted toward the Volvo.

Denise leaned across the console and pushed the passenger door open. Paulette climbed in. "What are we doing? Oh my gosh! Look at you! In scrubs and the new hair color you could be me." She laughed.

Paulette had a lovely childlike laugh. Denise smiled, feeling better for the moment. They looked more alike. That meant they were more alike. It was the ravages of the world that had driven them apart, even in Denise's mind. This felt better. Them laughing. Or at least, Paulette laughing.

"Did you come to show me the new outfit?" Paulette asked.

Annoyance returned.

Like she'd call her out of the hospital in the middle of the night when the world was about to stop spinning to show off her new hair and matching scrubs. The ignorance wasn't Paulette's fault. Denise's decision not to share tonight's activities with her sister had been a hard but necessary one. She wouldn't change her mind now.

"No," Denise answered, and was proud at how upbeat and normal she sounded. "There's one last thing I have to do before we can—" She started to say, "Leave this shithole," but that, too, was not something Paulette needed to know at this point. "Get on with things," she finished.

This next part was key to her plan working well. Without it, the plan would still work, but it would be a good deal riskier. "Are there any women in the maternity ward who have babies, born babies, I mean, not fetuses?" she asked, trying for nonchalance and managing only monotone.

"There's Mrs. Frazier in 307," Paulette said. Then, "Oh no! You don't mean to take that poor woman's baby! She was in labor for twenty-two hours. The baby is only a day old. Not that it matters how old she is. Honey, I love you for thinking how much I wanted a baby, and I did, but you can't take her baby."

"No, no, nothing like that," Denise lied. "I just wanted to know if you had extra duties or anything that would keep you away from the infant care ward."

"No. Mother and baby are resting comfortably," Paulette said, parroting a phrase she'd heard the real nurses use, Denise assumed.

"There's a camera at the ER doors and one on the nurses' station on the second floor that I know about," Denise said. "Are there any others?"

Paulette thought about that for a moment, then ticked a list off on her fingers. "There is one at the main entrance. One in ICU. One in the infant care observation room. I don't know about the adult rooms on the first or third floor. There aren't any in the patient rooms—patients don't like that. None in the operating rooms or halls—the doctors don't like that. I think that's all. Maybe one in the pharmacy, but I don't know for sure. I've never seen it. Why? Denise, what are you going to do?"

"Where is the infant care observation room?" Denise asked.

"Second floor, between the nurses' station and the stairs. Why? Denise, tell me what you're going to do." Paulette was demanding. That was new. Though she'd wanted her sister to show a little spunk, Denise didn't like it.

"Nothing scary," Denise said. "Tying off a few loose ends."

"Do I have to do anything?" Paulette asked. "I wouldn't like to do anything that would be against doctors' orders or hospital policy."

Denise stifled a sigh of exasperation. This part would soon be over. From then on it would be smooth sailing. "Not a thing," she assured her sister. "All you have to do is stay near the nurses' station where you will be on camera for an hour or so."

"I can't just hang around. People will wonder. I have work to do," Paulette whined.

Whined.

Denise couldn't believe it. They were on the cusp of their new life, with all the things they'd always wanted, and her twin—her twin, for Christ's sake—was whining about what people might think.

"Just stay there, or go to the ER, or find an excuse to go to the main entrance foyer. All that matters is that you stay on camera so you can prove where you were."

"What are you going to do?" Paulette asked again. Tears welled up in her eyes, green and glowing in the light of the dashboard, lending them the sinister effect of eyeballs floating in a poison soup.

"I'm going to save a life," Denise said. "Don't forget to wedge open the door." She handed Paulette an old flip-flop she'd purloined from Paulette's closet. Planning was everything. Rushing was an invitation to disaster. Too bad one seldom got a choice.

She waited until Paulette was back inside the building, then waited five more minutes to give her time to reach the nurses' station. Having squirmed into the sterile yellow paper jacket, Denise used the lighted mirror on the back of the sun visor to tuck all of her hair beneath the hairnet—a white paper cap—then put the face mask on, securing the straps firmly behind her ears and pulling the cap down until not so much as a lobe showed.

She'd overthought this portion of the plan. Cameras wouldn't matter. The fact that she was identical to Candy Striper Paulette Duffy wouldn't matter. The sterile gear hid her identity far better than the Lone Ranger's mask hid his. Surgical gloves finished her preparations. She let herself out of the Volvo, beeped it locked, and walked toward the back door of the hospital.

Denise retrieved the flip-flop Paulette had used to keep the door from closing, tossed it into the Dumpster, and slipped inside. The fire escape stairs were as expected: metal treads, pipe hand-railing, concrete floor and walls and ceiling, no windows, dim lighting, and devoid of human life. Like most people, nurses avoided physical effort in even its most modest guises. Moving quietly, she climbed to the second floor. Opening the heavy metal door an inch, Denise peeked out.

Nothing but a long hallway with doors to either side. Some were open, the light from televisions and reading lamps spilling out along with the desultory murmur of TV shows. A nurse carrying a tray with half a dozen miniature paper cups, the kind hospitals put meds in, walked past the semicircular desk where two other nurses sat, eyes on computer monitors. As far as Denise could see, Paulette had been telling the truth. There were no cameras at either end of the hallway, just a single round black eye pointing at the space in front of the desk. Halfway between the fire stairs and the nurses' station, just as Paulette had said, was a large window beside a glass door.

The observation room.

For no apparent reason, Denise's foot shot out, smacking into the door with a hollow thud. The nurse with the tray of pills stopped. She looked back over her shoulder as if she'd heard. Holding her breath, Denise waited, afraid to move the door even the half inch it would take to close it. Finally the woman shrugged and went about her business.

No worry, no worry, Denise chanted silently. Hospitals had to be full of things that went bump in the night. Bedpans falling, patients banging on their bed rails, doctors dropping wads of cash on the polished floors, interns fornicating in broom closets. Maybe that was only on television; still, hospitals had to have noises.

No worry.

Denise stood stock-still until her breathing slowed, then silently closed the door and began to ascend the steps. Between the second and the third floors was a smell of cigarette smoke. Midstride, she halted. A nurse or doctor too lazy to walk down to the parking lot might have stepped into the fire stairs for a quick puff. Denise waited for the sound of an inhalation, a butt hitting the floor, a door opening or closing. Nothing.

The smoke smelled stale. Maybe it was from earlier, even a day or more earlier. Cat piss had nothing on cigarette smoke when it came to the staying power of the odor. That was a habit Paulette was going to have to break.

Denise did a quick peek around the bend in the stair. No smoking gun. She crept up to the third floor and opened the door a crack for surveillance.

The door closest to the fire escape, from where Denise watched, had a square metal plate with the number 311 on it in black numerals. If the numbers followed the rule of even on one side and odd on the other, 307 would be four doors down and to the right.

The hallway was empty. Denise's fingers scampered over her face and head, reassuring her that the mask and hairnet were in place. They were. Forcing herself not to walk too fast or too slow, Denise went down the hall, noting the numbers on the doors. Room 307 was where it was supposed to be. No light showed from the little rectangular window in the door. Peeking in, Denise could see it was a private room. This was good. Retirement was making her stupid; she hadn't thought what she'd do if it was a double. It wasn't. This was a sign this was meant to happen.

In the single bed was a woman-sized lump limned by the pink of a nightlight. Between the woman and the door was a low crib bed. In it was an infant lying on its belly, a hand no bigger than a quarter spread like a starfish on its cheek. Denise took a deep breath, stepped briskly in, gathered up the infant, turned, and stepped briskly out.

"Point of no return," she whispered as she carried the baby toward the stairs.

The new mom hadn't woken. The child didn't scream.

All good. All signs this was meant to happen.

FORTY-SEVEN

Heath's burns had been dressed, and, as Anna had surmised, they weren't severe. There was bruising of her lower limbs, and a hairline fracture of her left shin. Both her palms were skinned and one finger broken. Given the night's events, all of them had gotten off lightly.

Anna should have taken her leave after the reassuring results of Heath's exam were delivered, but she'd stayed on, feeling a sense of comfort in the company of Heath, Elizabeth, and Gwen. When she'd been younger—like last week—she'd craved solitude and silence, the peace of wide open spaces and infinite sky. Now the small room, crowded with people she cared about, all alive, all warm, fed, and sheltered, wrapped comfortingly around her like a soft blanket.

A loud click announcing the opening of the door startled Anna's eyes open. She had dozed off in the chair beside Heath's bed. A nurse in pale green scrubs stuck her head in. Maybe a hospital shift change; Anna hadn't seen this woman before. She was in her fifties with small, brown, very bright eyes in a narrow lined face. Frowning, she glanced around the room.

"What is it?" Gwen asked.

"Nothing, not a thing," the nurse said. "Sorry to bother you." She pulled her head back and closed the door softly.

"Odd," Gwen said.

"She probably can't remember where she left her last patient," Elizabeth said. "That or visiting hours are over."

"Visiting hours have been over for a while," Heath said.

"Then why—" E began. Heath raised her eyebrows and tilted her head toward Gwen. "Right," E said. "It's who you know.

"I've been thinking, it's going to be weird seeing Tiff," E said after a moment. "After us getting her mom arrested and what not, I don't think we can really be friends anymore. I mean, how would that work?"

"It probably wouldn't," Anna said. "Too much blood under the bridge."

"Too bad," Heath said. "Tiffany is a nice girl. None of this is her fault or," she said, looking pointedly at her daughter, "yours."

"I know," E said. "Even though I know it, it feels like I could have done *something*."

No one argued with her. Anna felt as if there must have been something she could have done or seen or sensed that would have kept things from going as far as they had. Only the fact that Elizabeth wasn't in ICU, blinded with severe acid burns to her face, kept her from dwelling on what might have been.

"What will happen to Mrs. Edleson?" Elizabeth asked Anna.

"She'll be charged with assault—not just attempted; the acid got on Heath. That's a charge she'll have to face here in Maine, I expect. It was Maine law she broke. As for the cyberbullying, I'm not sure if there are statutes in place for that in Colorado or Maine state law. It's my guess she'll get a slap on the wrist. Community service. I doubt she'll do any jail time. If she does, I expect it will only be sixty days or so. If she gets a half-way decent lawyer, he will plead her out with time served and probation. Maybe an order not to go within *X* number of feet of you or your home."

"Not fair!" E cried.

"Life is not fair," Heath said. "Who knew?"

Gwen laughed.

Again the door to the room was opened. In hospitals no one knocks. This time it was a security guard, easily over sixty and overweight. Anna hadn't seen any security around the building or the ER when she'd arrived. Maybe he came on for the night shift.

"'Scuse me, ladies," he said, smiling an apology for the interruption. "I hate busting in on you like this. I just need to take a look in your bathroom."

"Sure," Heath said. In silence they watched him waddle to the bathroom, open the door, and look in. He did the same with the tiny closet.

"What's going on?" Gwen asked.

"Nothing for you to worry about," he said. "Good night." And he was gone.

Gwen got up and smoothed down the front of her blouse. "I'm going to find out what the fuss is about. Anybody want me to bring them back anything? Coffee? Coke?"

Nobody wanted any more caffeine.

"It is getting late," Heath said to Anna. "I think you've saved the world enough times today. Why don't you go home? You look worse than I feel."

"I'm good," Anna said automatically.

"I'm staying," Elizabeth said.

Anna managed a smile. Elizabeth had been attacked by the neighbor lady, shamed before her entire high school, and probably lost her best friend in the bargain, but she was happy. Her joy showed through the layers of concern she had for her mother and for Anna. By E's lights, Walter was the handsome prince on the white horse who had slain her personal dragon. Never mind that Walter had mowed down an innocent man, and managed to lure Artie away from his post, or that her mother had taken a splash of acid meant for Elizabeth, or that Anna had smashed her shoulder and elbow all to hell taking down Terry Edleson.

The cybercreep was out of Elizabeth's life, and a beautiful boy was in it. God was in his heaven and all was right with her world.

Anna wouldn't have had it any other way.

Gwen popped back into the room. "Nothing to be alarmed about," she said. "A baby has been misplaced. It will turn up. They always do." Stifling a yawn, the older woman sank down on the foot of Heath's bed.

"None of you need to stay any longer," Heath said firmly. "We're all worn out. You were snoring, Anna."

"I don't snore," Anna said.

"Hah!" E snorted.

Heath rolled her eyes. "You have taught my child to snort," she accused Anna.

"I taught myself to snort! Anyway, I don't snort," E insisted.

"I'm staying," Gwen said. "Hospitals aren't much about caring for patients anymore. They are about following doctors' orders and medical protocols. Without an advocate, a patient gets about as much TLC as you might expect if we abandoned you under an overpass."

"I'm staying, too," E said.

Anna rubbed her eyes with her fists, smearing more mascara around. Nothing remained for her to do but sleep. "Okay, I'm for bed. If you need me, I'll be at Peter and Lily's."

As she tried to shove herself up from the plastic chair, the shoulder of the arm that had taken a bullet during the Fox River misadventure, the one she'd used to slam Terry Edleson to the ground, locked up. Squeaking, she held herself halfway out of the chair, unable to get up, unable to lower herself back down. "Damn," she said as Elizabeth and Gwen leapt up to help her.

Standing, she shook out her arms. "Good as new," she said, balling her hand into a fist to prove everything was working.

"Get that shoulder X-rayed," Gwen said.

"It's not broken," Anna insisted. "Just banged up."

She had no intention of spending the rest of the night being alternately pestered and ignored by a bunch of people in scrubs. Straightening her back, she walked to the door without limping, wincing, or whimpering. Success beyond her wildest expectations. Fortunately they were on the first floor and not far from the main doors. Anna picked up her keys at the registration desk, then made it to the parking lot without scaring any children with her likeness to a zombie, or attracting unwanted attention from medical personnel.

Having unlocked the Crown Vic, she crawled into the darkness of the rear seat and closed the door. In the privacy of the cramped chamber she managed to escape from the long-tailed shirt. The Velcro straps of her borrowed Kevlar vest—E had worn hers—released with a satisfying ripping sound. Sighing, she let the thing fall to the seat beside her. Beneath the vest, her tank top was soaked with sweat.

For several minutes she sat reveling in freedom from the Kevlar and the grating fluorescent lights of the hospital. Fluorescent lights made Anna feel brittle and tired. Someday scientists would undoubtedly discover the light penetrated flesh and corroded bone matter. Rubbing the ache in her shoulder, she tried to remember whether or not she'd seen a bathtub at Peter and Lily's. A long hot bath would be a passable stand-in for the sauna, the massage, and the husband.

Once she felt sufficiently recovered to drive the six miles to the Barneses' house, she gathered her courage.

For decency's sake, she put on the shirt and fastened a few buttons. Traversing from the rear seat to the front to climb behind the wheel wasn't as easy as she'd pictured it. Finally in place, she closed her eyes and leaned her head back against the headrest for a moment.

"I'm getting too old for this shit," she whispered. Opening her eyes, she saw the item she was to deliver before she could go to bed. A two-foot-long model of a Hawaiian outrigger canoe was sitting on the passenger seat. "And miles to go before I sleep." She groaned and turned on the ignition.

The way to the Barneses' home led back through Bar Harbor, then to the east a quarter of a mile before the road forked, the western fork crossing the narrow land bridge connecting Mount Desert Island to the mainland. Denise's apartment complex was on the way. Anna slowed as she drove by. A light showed in the upstairs apartment where she'd changed into Denise's clothes for the first fruitless attempt at the cybercreep.

Denise's little green Miata wasn't in evidence in the parking spaces beneath the complex. A white Volvo had taken its place. Anna snugged the Crown Vic neatly, and illegally, behind the Volvo. Her errand would only take a second. Even if the car didn't belong to Denise, she should be back to move the Crown Vic before anyone needed to leave the complex.

On her first two visits the stairs had made no impression on Anna: short, one level, a romp in the park. This trip she felt all thirteen. Good deeds were never a good idea. Leaning against the doorframe of Denise's apartment, she knocked, then rang the doorbell. A long silence followed. Relief crept in. Anna wasn't up for even the short exchange of "This is yours" and "You're welcome."

"Who is it?" Denise's voice came from behind the door.

"It's me," Anna said.

There was no peephole.

Feeling foolish, Anna opened her mouth to announce herself properly, but "me" must have been sufficient. Anna heard the slide of bolts and the rattle of a door chain. The knob turned, and the door swung open.

Paulette Duffy stood in the spill of light, her blond hair falling around her face, her pink scrubs rumpled, the front stained, a silver laptop computer held at her side. Anna stared stupidly. Paulette gaped at Anna in absolute shock, mouth open, lips pulled back showing nice, neat front teeth.

Pieces fell like bricks through Anna's mind and into place: the photo by the bed of a younger Denise before she'd gotten the overlapping front teeth fixed, Mrs. Duffy's blond hair, identical twins, Huntington's disease, the uncontrolled movements of chorea, short-term memory loss. Mood swings.

This was Denise. Denise was the other twin.

In the instant it took for this to flash through Anna's mind, she realized that Denise might have murdered Kurt Duffy while Paulette was establishing her alibi in the Acadian Lounge, and here Anna had come gimping up the stairs in the middle of the night with no weapon, no backup, no vest, and no radio.

"Hey, Denise," Anna said. "Love the hair. Peter said you'd left this in your office." She held up the canoe in both hands.

"Thank you," Denise said. She didn't reach out for the canoe.

Anna took a step back.

From within the apartment came the high gasping wail of a baby crying.

Denise swung the laptop at Anna's head. Reflexively, Anna threw up her arms, using the canoe to deflect the blow. Her shoulder locked. The laptop smashed through the thin balsa wood, shattering the model, to strike her above her eye where the knot from her last head trauma had yet to begin to heal.

"You're dead" was the last thing Anna heard.

When she regained consciousness, or what she assumed might be consciousness, she was blind. She tried to open her mouth to scream, but it was sealed shut. Struggling, she tried to figure out where one arm started and the other left off. A soft smelly pillow was hot against her chest. Her legs had been welded into a single unit, like the tail of a mermaid.

"Stay still or you'll kill her."

The whisper was close. Without eyes, Anna couldn't tell if the whisperer was in front of her or behind her. "Denise?" she said. What came to her ears was a muffled "Hunhh?" Duct tape, or something very like, had been put over her mouth. Probably her eyes as well. She could feel the pull on her eyelids when she tried to open them.

"In your arms is a baby. If you fall down, or fight, or do anything except exactly what I tell you to, you might crush her. You might asphyxiate her. You might snap her little neck." As directionless as fog, as sibilant as wind in the eaves, the whisper rasped around Anna. "You might jam your chin through the soft spot in her skull and get baby brains in your mouth."

Words hissing in her ears, Anna became aware of the life she held in her arms. The smell was a dirty diaper, the heat a tiny body, the softness the rounded contours of an infant. Lowering her head, she felt downy hair tickle the underside of her chin. This had to be the baby Gwen had so airily assured them would turn up. Denise had taken it.

Ransom? Anna wondered. Was the child the child of a rich person? Auction the little creature off to a barren couple, or sex traffickers? It seemed a bit ambitious for a retired park ranger. Kidnapping was America's least favorite sport. Hard to pull off, severe penalties, and a live product: Anna doubted law enforcement officers would risk it. At least not sane law enforcement officers.

Denise Castle might not be entirely sane. Huntington's could cause mental disorders; Gwen had said that. If Huntington's mixed with regular craziness, the results might be bizarre.

Peter Barnes had spoken of how Denise looked at Lily, how she looked at Olivia, how she reacted to the mention of her previous home. Was the baby some kind of compensation for losing her relationship?

Did it matter?

Not much, Anna thought. What mattered was the life duct-taped in her arms. If there was life.

There was no movement. If the baby breathed, she couldn't hear it.

Had she crushed it already? Squeezed the little rib cage until the baby couldn't draw breath? While unconscious, had she folded over and smothered the child? Darkness greater than blindness gripped Anna. Her heart grew cold and still. Her hands, each taped tightly to the opposite elbow to provide a cradle for the infant, were useless but for the little finger on her left hand. She could bend that one. Denise had missed it in her wrapping. Gingerly, Anna poked the baby. It didn't move or cry. She poked it again harder.

Feeble squirming, then tiny baby feet kicked into her damaged joint, making it throb. "Thankyoubabyjesus," she meant to say. "Mmmghhh" was what reached the air. Anna allowed her heart to recommence beating.

Craning her neck until her shoulder knifed her in the back in self-defense, Anna managed to nuzzle the infant's face. The baby's mouth was not duct-taped shut. Anna allowed herself a meager trickle of relief. At least the child would be able to breathe as long as Anna could keep her exhausted muscles from collapsing and squashing the poor thing.

"I'm going to cut the tape on your ankles," the whisper said. "You're going to get up and walk quietly where I tell you to." The tip of a sharp object poked into Anna's cheek under her right eye. "If you are not absolutely compliant, I will poke out this eye, then the other, and so on. Nothing I do can be bad because you are a dead pigeon, and dead pigeons have no rights. If you understand, nod your head."

The prick of flesh beneath her eye receded. Anna nodded. Strands of hair were plucked from her head. Her hair had been taped down along with her eyelids and arms, effectively pinioning her head in one place. An image of Gulliver, surrounded by mallet-wielding Lilliputians, his head staked to the ground by his hair, flashed through her mind. The benefits of a reading life, she thought absurdly.

Again she nodded, more firmly this time. Maybe there was some slippage. Maybe she could trade hanks of hair for greater movement. Something to keep in mind.

A hand insinuated itself beneath her left elbow, where it was taped tightly to her ribs. "Up," the voice breathed. The hand pulled. Anna floundered to her knees, mindful of not crushing the baby, of not losing her balance and falling on it, while the voice—Denise Castle's, she assumed—continued popping, "Up, up, you. Get up. Up."

Without sight, the Rohypnol remaining in her system, combined with fatigue and shock, compromised Anna's balance, making her unsteady on her feet, unsure where this "up" was. Her inner ear insisted she was listing to starboard, but when she tried to compensate, she was jerked the other direction by the hand beneath her elbow.

"You hurt that baby and you're dead meat," Denise said, full voice this time.

Anna shuffled her feet further apart, centering her weight carefully around her spine. The sense of toppling to one side diminished. Palpable mist slid over her skin. Anna staggered back.

"It's just a shawl, you stupid bitch. Stand still," Denise ordered. The shawl was arranged around Anna's face. A few more hairs were plucked from her head as Denise tucked the fabric around her arms and the child held in them.

"You are going to be a good little pigeon. Don't even think of trying to fly the coop or make any kind of noise. If you do, you could fall down the stairs and kill the baby," Denise said.

Hands landed hard on Anna's shoulders, sending a crippling wave of agony down her side. The hands propelled her forward. The baby began a thin wail.

"Then your eyes would be gouged out and there'd be no more of your peeking and pecking," Denise said as she turned Anna to the left. They stopped. There was the sound of a door shutting. "Keep that baby quiet."

Again Denise was muttering. They must be out of the apartment, in the hall.

"Stairs," Denise said.

With Denise muttering, "Step, step, step," Anna felt her way down, relying on the hand under her elbow for balance.

Thirteen, Anna counted in her head. They were down in the parking area.

"You can't make anything easy, can you?" Denise growled.

Hands fumbled at Anna's crotch, and she wondered if she was being sexually assaulted, but Denise was only digging the keys to the Crown Vic out of her pocket.

A beep, then Denise poked, prodded, and cursed Anna and her burden into the seat of a car. By the height of it, Anna guessed it was the white SUV parked where the Miata had been on her first visit.

"Stay," Denise ordered. "Or you're dead."

You're dead.

Denise had said that the instant before Anna lost consciousness from the blow to her head with the laptop. It hadn't been a threat; it had been a statement. When Denise first opened the door, her face had gone slack with shock at the sight of Anna.

That was when the scene with the ghost of Hamlet's father should have played out. Anna's one shot at acting in a Shakespeare play and she'd blown it.

No one but Heath's family and Peter knew Anna had been "killed." Denise had gone pale because she believed Anna was dead. Ergo Denise had been the one to dump her body into the sea. Denise and Paulette. Walter had seen two people in the boat.

Anna felt the shoulder strap slide across her arms, pushing the baby more tightly against her chest. A click let her know her seat belt was fastened. Since Denise had killed her once, thrown her into the ocean, then knocked her unconscious and taped her up like a mummy, this nod to safety had to be about the baby. Denise wanted the baby safe, her talk of Anna killing it notwithstanding. The baby was what was important.

Anna was just being moved from point A to point B. Never a good thing for a victim. Point B was always nastier than point A. Once they were there, Anna could be disposed of without interference. That was the reason point B held such an attraction for kidnappers, rapists, and murderers.

The baby continued to whine.

Anna wished she'd called Paul before she'd left the island, wished she had taken the first plane home, never stopped to do her good deed for the day, wished the child would stop crying, while at the same time taking comfort in the fact that it had sufficient air with which to cry.

"Hmm, hmm," she crooned, and brushed the infant's head with her duct-taped lips. The baby wailed louder, its fragile skin abraded by the rough tape.

The driver's door opened. "All set?" Denise asked as if she and Anna were going on a routine campground patrol.

Not knowing what else to do, Anna nodded as much as her netting of hair would allow, then a bit more, hoping to loosen the tape.

"Good," Denise said. Denise had been gone less than two minutes; she had to have put the NPS patrol car in another of the parking spaces beneath the rental units. If the apartment the slot was assigned to was occupied, it would be found as soon as the renter came home and wanted to park. If the apartment was vacant, it could be days. Still, Peter and Lily were expecting Anna. Peter knew where she'd been going. When she didn't show in an hour or two, he'd come looking. He'd find the car.

That was something.

Being on the move seemed to soothe Denise. Gone were the hissing and the hurrying. Anna heard mirrors being adjusted, a seat belt fastened, the engine coming to life. The SUV backed out of the narrow space. Off to point B.

Had Anna decided to set a trap to catch herself, she couldn't have done it more thoroughly. She was alone, unarmed, injured, fog-brained, and had delivered herself into the hands of a deranged kidnapper. The proverbial handwriting had not merely been on the wall, it had been all but tattooed across Anna's forehead. Denise liked to dive at night. Denise had a boat at her disposal. Denise had refused to be seen near Paulette the morning after the murder, was paranoid about Anna being in her apartment, reacted bizarrely when Anna had asked about the photograph where her teeth were identical to Paulette's, showed the same chorea as Paulette Duffy.

Shaking her head, Anna groaned.

"Okay?" Denise asked.

Anna nodded.

The distraction of the cybercreep had kept her from paying attention to what was going on in the park, the park she'd been brought in to help protect and preserve. Instead, she'd played hooky, worked on personal issues, and one of the rangers nominally under her supervision had gotten away with the attempted murder of Anna and, probably, the actual murder of Paulette's husband.

Almost, Anna felt she deserved what she was getting, what she was going to get when Denise reached point B.

Almost.

FORTY-EIGHT

W e're here," Denise announced.

Here, Anna knew, was between fifteen and thirty minutes by car from Denise's apartment. First, Anna guessed, they were headed to Paulette's house, but they didn't go into a house. They went into the woods. Pine needles slithered underfoot as they walked the last hundred yards or so, and the smell of sap was strong in the night air. They were in a shed or garage; Anna surmised. She'd heard the unmistakable sound of a padlock being unlocked.

"Sit," Denise ordered.

Blind, a baby bound to her chest, the best Anna could do was get to her knees and sit back on her heels. Duct tape made for secure bondage. Little of Anna remained mobile.

"God," Denise fumed. "You're such a pain in the ass."

A hand pushed hard on Anna's shoulder, toppling her onto her side. To keep the child from harm, Anna took the full weight of the fall on the point of her left shoulder. Her face was ground into rough carpet as her legs were pulled out of their bend. The baby began to cry, a few decibels higher and angrier than its ongoing pitiful mewling.

Ripping sounds filled Anna's ears; then she felt her legs being taped together again, once at the ankles and once at the knees. Clearly, Denise had a higher opinion of Anna's threat level than Anna did. She doubted she could best a fly even if she had a swatter and a head start.

"There," Denise declared, when Anna was trussed up again. "Sit up."

Struggling like a landed fish, Anna tried to bring her torso up to right angles with her legs. She failed.

An exaggerated sigh heralded the coming assistance. Hands slid under her shoulders and pushed her up.

"This will hurt," Denise said.

Since a significant portion of Anna hurt, she hardly winced as Denise carefully pulled the tape off of her eyes.

"Won't have to get those brows waxed for a couple years," Denise said.

Her face was so close it was all Anna could see, and it was out of focus.

"No reason you can't talk," Denise said. "You can even scream if you want. Nobody will hear you." Crouching in front of Anna, Denise gently worked the duct tape free of Anna's mouth.

Drool ran from her newly freed lips and dripped on the baby's head. Air, constrained by fear and pinched nostrils, rushed in through Anna's mouth. She felt her chest expand against the tight wrapping of tape and the soft bundle of life she held in her arms.

"Better?" Denise asked, her head cocked to one side like that of an alert Chihuahua.

"Yes," Anna said. "Thanks." Absurd as it was, Anna was genuinely grateful for these small kindnesses. Beggars couldn't be choosers, but they could show gratitude for the scraps given them.

As Anna's eyes cleared of tears from the stinging removal of the tape, the room that coalesced around her was not what she had expected from her garage or shed theory. Lit only by the light of a single kerosene lantern was a room built of rough wood. The curtains on the windows were open, showing a warm sunny forest outside. They weren't windows, she realized dazedly, but mullions and frames over a painting of a summer forest scene. A crib with a stuffed bear in it sat in the corner. Beside it were a child's tiny chair and a potty-training toilet

Denise had brought her—and the baby—to a nursery.

"Nice, isn't it?" Denise sat down in a rocking chair with low arms and looked around the small space with obvious pride. "It's a shame we won't get to use it. We'll have to build another just like it at our new place. It could be like a playhouse."

Despite the kindly light of the kerosene lamp, Anna's captor's face looked drawn and pale. The youthful glow the blond hair lent her had faded.

"Tired," Denise said, as if affirming Anna's thought. Dragging her hand down over her face, fingers pressing gently on her eyelids, she mimicked a gesture that Anna equated with the living closing the eyes of the dead.

A thousand questions boiled in Anna's mind with such fury that she couldn't get any to separate themselves from the maelstrom to form words. Her palms, each fastened tightly to the opposite forearm to make a basket for the infant, were growing numb. She could no longer feel the child breathing, but, with her eyes uncovered, she could see the tiny baby she held. Snot bubbled out of a nose as small and soft as a peony petal. The crying had stopped. Now the child looked up into Anna's face with vaguely trusting gray-blue eyes.

"You took the baby from the woman in the hospital," Anna said to Denise. Her voice cracked from a throat so dry Anna could barely swallow. Without being asked, Denise got up, crossed to a shelf, and took out a bottle of water from half a dozen stored there. There were also several army surplus MREs, the kind Anna hadn't seen for years, and two pairs of handcuffs. Anna looked longingly at the cuffs. After her time in duct tape, they looked positively humane.

"Sort of took the woman's baby, but not exactly," Denise said, unscrewing the cap on the water bottle. She held it while Anna drank. Water was a fluid of many magical properties. Anna's throat opened; her mind perked up; hope flickered where the water left its trail of strength.

"What do you mean sort of?" Anna asked. "How do you sort of take a baby?"

Denise smirked as she regained her seat in the rocker. "That isn't the baby you think it is. Guess who you're holding?"

Anna stared down into the baby's face. To her, all babies looked pretty much alike. This one was pink and round with a blank little face and wide open eyes. Why would she be expected to know this baby?

Disparate facts, stored in unrelated places in her cerebrum, began to flock together like blackbirds into a pine tree: Paulette Duffy, an infant care LPN, Peter and Denise together, Peter and Denise apart, Lily and Olivia, Denise's sudden retirement, Olivia mysteriously ill and transported to the hospital where Duffy worked.

"Peter Barnes's baby," Anna said.

"My baby," Denise flared. "Olivia. What a stupid name. We'll give her a better one."

"Olivia wasn't the baby that went missing," Anna said.

"Hah!" Denise leaned forward, her elbows on her knees so her face was on a level with Anna's. "The camera over the door in the infant care observation room is pointed at the crib. I walked in, back to the camera, carrying one baby, backed out, still not facing the camera, with another baby. Peter doesn't even know his child has gone missing. That's how much he cares about her. Do you think the baby should have water?" Denise asked, her face suddenly worried.

"Probably, but done up like she is, I'm afraid she would choke. Don't you want to hold her?" That was a question new mothers and grandmothers asked Anna. For some reason, women were supposed to want to hold infants. If Denise was among them, maybe Anna would be given an opportunity to do . . . well, some damn thing.

For a long moment, Denise sat, chin in hands, elbows on knees, studying Anna and the baby. "I don't want to hold it," she admitted at last. Anna didn't think Denise was talking to her so much as thinking out loud. "I thought I would. I really thought it would be like when my sister and I realized we were two parts of a whole. But when I carried the baby out of the hospital and didn't feel much, I figured it was because things were so, you know, tense. Then back at my apartment all she did was cry. I tried holding her, doing the rocking thing. She kept on crying. She didn't feel like a part of me, not like Paulette, more like a fish trying to flop its way out of a soggy newspaper."

"Babies aren't for everybody," Anna said sympathetically. "No big deal. I never went much for babies. Tell you what, nobody knows she's gone. We could take her back and nobody would be the wiser."

Denise straightened up. She actually appeared to be considering the suggestion, and Anna felt a tiny spark of hope.

Then Denise shook her head. "No," she said firmly. "The closeness will come. It will just take a while."

"Why don't you cut the tape so we can let her out of my arms? Then at least she can have water," Anna said.

"Soon," Denise promised. "If Paulette comes back from work and everything is hunky-dory, we won't need you for a hostage. Then we'll leave, and in a few hours, I'll send an anonymous message saying where you are and that will be that. No muss, no fuss."

Anna doubted she would be left alive. In their previous encounter, Denise had proved to be an individual who chose not to strain the quality of mercy in any meaningful way. A bullet to the back of the head or a one-way night dive was more likely.

Again Denise wiped her face, fingertips pressing on her eyelids. Anna took the opportunity to see if she could bite the duct tape closest to her chin. She couldn't, not without crushing the baby.

"I know Paulette is your sister," Anna said.

Denise laughed. "My identical twin sister." Shaking her head, she smiled to herself. "I'm still having trouble believing it's true. Too good to be true usually isn't."

"Oh, it's true," Anna said. "I know a lot about your family."

Denise had lifted the water bottle she'd used to give Anna a drink partway to her mouth. Her arm froze, suspending it midway between the chair's arm and her face. Her eyes narrowed. It didn't take a psychic to see the aura of paranoia and suspicion that darkened her visage. Paranoia: That was one of the symptoms Gwen had mentioned for Huntington's. Committing murder could make a person a tad jumpy as well. Kidnapping, Anna suspected, was hell on the nerves. Denise would have to be crazy not to be paranoid.

Since Anna had nothing to lose, she chose to feed it.

"I know she's your identical twin," Anna said, shooting for the tone of someone starting on a long list of sins. "I know the woman who delivered you as babies. I know the legacy that your biological mother wanted to share with you."

The water bottle flew from Denise's hand. Rolling, it left a dark wet trail across the rag rug where Anna sat. Denise hadn't thrown the water intentionally. Her hand had spasmed.

"Now look what you've done," Denise cried. Rising from the chair, she retrieved the bottle and set it on a small table beneath the pretend window. Hair whipping wildly, Denise looked around the room. "There's nothing to wipe it up with."

"It's only water. It will dry," Anna said calmly. "I know about your dropping things, too. You didn't used to be clumsy; now you drop things. Same with Paulette." Anna wasn't quite sure where she was going with this, just hoping that things would shake loose in a way that was more conducive to her surviving the night.

Denise growled, or grunted—a sound associated with animals, not humans. Reaching behind her back, she drew something from her waistband.

No surprise, a SIG Sauer 9 mm. Most likely the one Anna lost that night on Schoodic. The gun had never looked as big in Anna's hand as it did in Denise's. Viewed from the wrong end, the gun barrel seemed to take up half the room.

"Stop playing games with me," Denise said coldly. "If you know something, tell me. Otherwise, I'll blow your head off. I might do it anyway. You are supposed to be dead already, so what difference would it make?"

The thin yellow flame from the lantern reflected in Denise's eyes. There wasn't much else there that Anna could see. Not the panic at the spilled water, the confusion at not wanting to hold "her" child, the warmth when she spoke of her sister: Her face reminded Anna of a patient her sister, a psychiatrist, treated. Molly had taken Anna along on a visit to the mental health facility to see a woman who suffered from severe autism. A screaming fight between three other patients had overloaded the woman's senses and she'd shut down.

Denise had that same look, as if the soul had moved a very long way from the windows, so far it almost couldn't be seen. Denise didn't look insane. In fact, she looked saner than anyone Anna had ever seen, if sanity could be measured by control. She exuded the vibe of an individual totally detached and completely dedicated to the task at hand.

A few times in her life Anna had thought she might be going to die. She thought that now. No one knew anything about death. No one came back to report on how it went down, what followed. Dead people gave no interviews, wrote no books.

Perhaps that was the reason that, though afraid, Anna wasn't nearly as afraid as she would have been if she'd been asked to speak in front of a crowd, or crawl down a skinny cave passage. Those things were real and scary. Death wasn't real. It was the last page, the fade to black. It was hard to be truly terrified of an event that wasn't quantifiable, that wasn't quite real.

"No games," Anna said evenly. The baby quieted. Glancing down, she checked to see if it had expired. Olivia's eyelashes were unbelievably long. They quivered on her round cheeks as her eyes moved beneath the closed lids. Still alive.

"No games," Anna repeated. "A woman I know, Dr. Gwen Littleton, delivered twin girls forty-some years ago. The babies were given up for adoption. Gwen and the mother became friends. The mother's health was failing, and she decided to try and find her daughters."

"Makes sense," Denise said. "She's about to kick the bucket. Don't want to die with abandoning two little girls on your conscience. Might go to hell. Tidy up with a quick 'so sorry I fucked up your lives,' and off to heaven goes Mommy."

Denise's voice, hands, and trigger finger were rock steady. If she'd gone over the edge in the past few minutes, she hadn't landed on Anna's side. "Is there anything you want to get off your chest?" Denise asked in a flat voice. "I'm the closest thing you're going to get to final absolution."

"You'll lose your hostage," Anna said. She'd wanted to sound reasonable, but her voice cracked, and she had to swallow to clear her throat.

"We can work around it," Denise said, and her finger tightened on the trigger.

"If you shoot me, you could hit your baby daughter," Anna said.

"I'm a crack shot," Denise said.

"No. You used to be a crack shot. The legacy is you have Huntington's disease; you can't control your hands," Anna said. "You put three bullets in Kurt Duffy from no more than ten feet away and none of them were anywhere near fatal."

"Bullshit." Denise pressed the muzzle of the gun hard against Anna's forehead. "Now I can't miss."

"Wait," Anna begged desperately. "You pull the trigger, this close, and the report will deafen Olivia. Rupture her eardrums. She'll be deaf as a post her whole life, and it will be all your fault."

"Put your fingers in her ears," Denise snarled.

"I can't," Anna said.

Denise glared at her. Turning suddenly, she yanked open the door and stormed out of the room. Through the open doorway all was in darkness until, about forty yards away, the overhead light in the SUV came on. Denise dove into the vehicle, only her legs sticking out.

Anna took the time to look around the room. The place was child-proofed. Nothing that could be used as a weapon, even if she had use of her arms and hands, came to her attention.

A squawk made Anna's heart lurch; then a voice called her number, then Artie's. An NPS radio lay on the low table under the fake windows.

The caller was the superintendent. They'd discovered Olivia was miss-ing. Panic vibrated in his voice. Anna had to stop herself from shouting that Olivia was okay, that she had her. Not only would Peter not hear, but Denise would be interrupted in whatever she was doing in the Volvo and hurry back to the shed.

Without fingers or even toes, pushing the TALK button on the side of the radio to reply would be an interesting exercise in ingenuity. Since that was Anna's only option, she wriggled around until her back was to the ra-dio and, shoving with her heels, began pushing herself along the rag rug an inch at a time toward the low table. "Sorry, Olivia," Anna said as she managed to lever herself to her knees by bracing one elbow on the tiny chair by the crib. If she'd already killed Peter's child, it wouldn't matter. If she hadn't, this wouldn't be the fatal move.

Anna nosed the unit over to the wall, then pressed her chin as hard as she could into the TALK button. Maybe she depressed it a hair, maybe not; still she said, "Anna Pigeon, maybe near the Duffy house. Help!"

Denise banged back into the shed, slamming the door behind her. "Stupid bitch," she hissed. In two strides she'd crossed the room. The radio was slapped onto the floor. "Sit." Denise shoved Anna until she fell back against the wall and her rump slid down to the floor.

A pair of Bose earphones was in Denise's free hand. She squatted beside Anna, then carefully settled the phones over the baby's ears.

"There!" she said, standing. Snatching the gun out of the waistband of her pants, she pressed the muzzle to Anna's temple. "This time, promise me you'll die."

Anna closed her eyes and wondered what a person was supposed to think at a time like this.

"Denise? Honey?" The door was pushed open. Paulette stood in the faint spill of lamplight, her pink scrubs as rumpled as pajamas in the morning. "My God!" She stepped in and closed the door behind her. "Denise, what are you doing? Put that gun down." Her eyes on the baby, she stepped onto the rug in front of Anna. Dropping to her knees, she wailed, "No! You promised you wouldn't take the baby." She reached out as if she'd scoop it out of Anna's tape-and-bone bassinet, then froze. "This isn't the Frazier baby. Denise! What have you done?"

"She's kidnapped Peter Barnes's daughter, Olivia," Anna said. "The baby is sick. It was in the hospital for observation."

"Shut up!" Denise snarled.

"You're dead!" Paulette exclaimed, noticing Anna for the first time.

"Yes I am," Anna replied, wondering if it was true. "I've come back to save this child. If we don't get her back to the hospital, she'll die."

"Olivia Barnes? The three-month-old admitted for a seizure? Denise, you said you were going to save a life!" She looked up at her twin accusingly.

"I did, Paulette," Denise said, the gun lowered to her side. "I did. It was the only way. Lily, her mom, has Munchausen-by-proxy syndrome. She poisoned Olivia with ergotamine so she could go to the hospital and be the big hero. If we don't get the baby away, eventually Lily will kill her."

Paulette rocked back on her heels. "How could any mother . . . Oh, Denise! This is so awful. What can we do?"

"We have to get the baby and ourselves away from here, leave no hint to where we've gone, or that it was us who saved the baby," Denise said.

Mood swings was an understatement; she sounded so rational, so believable, that for a second Anna wondered if it could be true. "Ergotamine," Anna said suddenly. "How do you know the baby was poisoned with ergotamine?"

Paulette looked from her sister to Anna, then back to her sister. "The doctors didn't know what made the baby sick," Paulette said. Tears flooded her eyes. "Oh, Denise! You did it! You poisoned one of my babies. You . . .

"Help!" she screamed, scrambling to her feet. "Help! Somebody help me!" She reached the door and pulled it open.

The gun rose from Denise's side, leveled on Paulette's back.

"Gun!" Anna yelled because that's what she'd been trained to do.

A flash of muzzle fire and a blast, so loud in the small room that it numbed Anna's eardrums, shook the shed. Denise was turning, gun in hand. Before she could aim a second shot, Anna fell to her side, the baby affixed to her chest toppling with her, and whipped her legs out, knocking Denise's feet from under her. The gun hit the floor and skittered to the center of the round rug.

Cursing, Denise crawled for it. Whiplashing her feet, Anna managed to kick the SIG Sauer. The pistol slid over and stopped against Paulette's thigh. Paulette Duffy lay facedown, halfway in and halfway out of the nursery, a stain of blood blooming across the pink teddy bears on the back of her scrubs. There might have been life left in the woman, but Anna doubted it. The bullet had entered the left side of Paulette Duffy's back below the shoulder blade near the spine. The heart had probably been next on its trajectory.

Denise followed the gun. Trying to beat her to it, though the gun was out of her reach now and, she expected, forever, Anna flipped open and shut like a broken jackknife, getting nowhere. No crying from the baby. She hoped she hadn't smashed it.

Denise didn't grab up the SIG Sauer. Coming to her knees beside her sister's bleeding body, she covered her mouth with both hands. Moving in slow motion, she turned her head toward Anna. The hands floated down.

"What have I done?" she asked in a bewildered tone.

"You've killed your identical twin sister," Anna said. "Shot her in the back."

With a keening wail, Denise dragged Paulette up from the floor, cradling her in her lap. Denise's newly blond hair fell over Paulette's face, mingling with Paulette's bleached mess until no difference could be seen between them. Identical noses close, one face in repose, the other in a rictus of grief, Denise's tears dripped onto Paulette's cheeks.

From somewhere in the room the radio crackled. "Anna . . . Duffy house . . . Roadblocks . . ." Anna's message had gotten through.

Arms wrapped her around her sister, Denise began to rock. As if an invisible hand arrested her movement, she stopped suddenly. Misery blinked out, cheeks still awash with tears, Denise looked almost happy. Anna watched as her hand dipped into the pocket of Paulette's smock. Pulling out an empty unused syringe, she held it up to the lantern light and smiled.

Using her teeth, Denise uncapped the needle. Thumb on the plunger, she jammed the needle into her carotid artery and ripped downward. Blood sprayed out in a crimson wave, then pulsed ever smaller fountains of red. The sisters' blood mixed until both were dyed red with it and Anna couldn't tell where Denise began and Paulette left off.

Sirens sounded in the distance. "Your daddy is coming," Anna whispered to Olivia.

Expelling a sigh, Anna looked away from the tragedy clogging the door, her eyes moving to the painted sunlight through the fake windows.

There had been an instant, a moment in time, when Anna might have been able to say or do something that would have stopped Denise, saved her life.

But it would not have been a kindness.

We hope that you've enjoyed reading
Nevada Barr's nineteenth Anna Pigeon mystery.

Don't miss the previous Anna Pigeon book in the series . . .

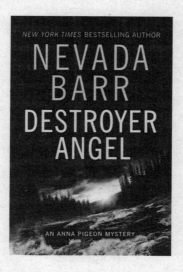

After a summer fighting wildfire, US Park Ranger Anna
Pigeon sets off on a camping trip to the Iron Range in
upstate Minnesota. With her are four women: Heath,
Leah and their two teenage daughters. For Heath, who
is paraplegic, it is the chance to test out a new, cutting edge
line of outdoor equipment, designed by Leah to make the
wilderness more accessible to disabled campers.

On their second night, Anna takes a canoe out on the Fox River
but when she returns, she finds that a band of kidnappers,
armed with rifles, pistols and knives, has taken the group
hostage. With limited resources and no access to the outside
world, it is up to Anna to track them across the treacherous
landscape and rescue her friends before it is too late . . .

HEADLINE